Microsurgical Reconstruction of the Extremities

Microsurgical Reconstruction of the Extremities

Indications, Technique, and Postoperative Care

Leonard Gordon, M.B.B.Ch.

Associate Clinical Professor of Orthopaedic Surgery
Lecturer, Department of Anatomy
University of California, San Francisco

Illustrations by James Brodale and Susan Taft

With 135 Figures in 538 Parts, 156 in Color

Springer-Verlag
New York Berlin Heidelberg
London Paris Tokyo

Leonard Gordon, M.B.B.Ch.
Director, Hand and Microsurgery Service, Department of Orthopaedic Surgery, University of California, San Francisco and Mt. Zion Hospital Medical Center
Microsurgery Consultant, Oak Knoll Naval Base and Letterman Army Medical Center

Library of Congress Cataloging-in-Publication Data
Gordon, Leonard
Microsurgical reconstruction of the extremities.
Includes bibliographies and index.
1. Extremities (Anatomy) – Surgery. 2. Microsurgery.
3. Extremities (Anatomy) – Transplantation.
4. Postoperative care. I. Title. [DNLM: 1. Extremities – transplantation. 2. Microsurgery – methods.
3. Postoperative Care. 4. Replantation. WE 800 G663 m]
RD551.G65 1988 617'.58059 87-32362

Softcover reprint of the hardcover 1st edition 1988

9 8 7 6 5 4 3 2 1

ISBN-13: 978-1-4612-8358-4 e-ISBN-13: 978-1-4612-3802-7
DOI: 10.1007/978-1-4612-3802-7

To my wife Chandra
and "the boys" –
Danny, Josh, and Coby,

and

in memory of
my friend and teacher,
Richard J. Smith, M.D.

Foreword

On April 23, 1906, Alexis Carrel presented his manuscript entitled "The Surgery of Blood Vessels" to the Johns Hopkins Medical Society. His work on the technique of small vessel anastomosis and the transplantation of visceral organs earned him the Nobel Prize in 1912. The use of magnification in operative surgery began in 1921 with the work of Nylén, who first employed the microscope for reconstructive procedures in the middle ear. Jacobson and Suarez published their initial observations on the use of microsurgery for the anastomosis of small vessels in 1960, and two years later, Malt reported the historic replantation of an upper extremity.

To surgeons involved in reconstruction of the extremities, the evolution of microsurgery has provided the most significant advances of the past three decades. The dramatic clinical successes of replantation surgery and free tissue transfer have substantially improved functional and cosmetic results in addition to decreasing morbidity in patients who present with complex reconstructive problems. *Microsurgical Reconstruction of the Extremities* crosses the traditional surgical disciplines and will be invaluable to orthopaedic surgeons, plastic surgeons, hand surgeons, and general surgeons, as well as to residents and fellows.

Much of our knowledge in the field of reconstructive microsurgery has been published in a variety of journals, and, up to now, this information has not been readily available to the reconstructive surgeon. The dispersion of information is especially apparent when attempting to locate descriptions of surgical techniques for performing the various free tissue transfers. Dr. Gordon has carefully collated the existing literature pertinent to microsurgical reconstruction of the extremities, and presented an organized text describing the indications, techniques, and postoperative care that are based on his unique experience with complex reconstruction problems. For the first time, here is a text that presents a detailed description of the anatomy and dissection techniques required for performing free tissue transplantation relevant to extremity reconstruction. The excellent bibliography at the end of each chapter cites and summarizes publications that directly relate to the specific free tissue transfer procedures.

This volume is clearly the result of an extraordinary effort, and Dr. Gordon deserves our gratitude for providing us with a comprehensive approach to deal with reconstruction of complex injuries of the extremities.

Andrew J. Weiland, M.D.
Professor of Orthopaedic and Plastic Surgery
The Johns Hopkins University School of Medicine
Baltimore, Maryland

Foreword

Preface

The purpose of this book is to provide the extremity surgeon with practical information on microvascular repair and reconstruction. To be successful, the surgeon performing a microvascular procedure must have an intimate knowledge of vascular anatomy and be able to apply this knowledge in performing a meticulous surgical dissection. Unfortunately, the anatomy required for microvascular procedures is not found in standard anatomy texts or atlases because many of the vessels used in microvascular procedures have not previously been regarded as having great anatomic importance. This book evolved from the repeated requests of residents and fellows for clarification on points of anatomy and surgical dissection as they prepared for microvascular procedures.

A thorough knowledge of the various procedures that can be used to treat a particular clinical problem is equally important. Options must necessarily include well-established nonmicrosurgical techniques as well as an analysis and comparison of the various microsurgical alternatives. Each surgeon must establish his or her own philosophy for the use of these procedures. One such approach is given here.

A microsurgical armamentarium is presented which will allow the care of almost any clinical problem where microsurgical technique may be appropriate. With this in mind, transplants of various tissues and sizes are described. There are many microvascular procedures that have not been included, and I have done my best to provide a rationale behind procedure selection. Each surgeon will necessarily prefer certain procedures over others, and no surgeon will use all of the transplants available. This practice is to be encouraged to foster proficiency. Reconstructive possibilities are limited only by the imagination and skills of the surgeon, and my hope is that this text will be used as a foundation on which each practitioner can build.

The bibliographies consist of only those journal articles that deal with indications and surgical technique. Many outstanding contributions have not been included to avoid duplication of information and to make the text as simple to use as possible. Toward this end, each entry includes a brief description to help the reader determine whether a detailed study of the article will be valuable.

Tissue survival rates of over 95% should be attained. This can only be accomplished by first mastering the techniques of microsurgical anastomosis in the laboratory. There are many practical courses and texts that offer detailed instruction, but there is no substitute for the many hours of laboratory practice required to perfect these techniques. Combining meticulous microsurgical technique with appropriate cadaver dissections to prepare for these procedures, and having a clear understanding of the indications and postoperative program will ensure a successful outcome.

LEONARD GORDON

Acknowledgements

In our specialized world, most endeavors require a team approach. Both the successful outcomes of the microsurgical procedures documented herein and the presentation of this text are evidence of this. Neither would have been possible without the immense contributions of many in the Department of Orthopaedic Surgery at the University of California, San Francisco.

The bibliography of microsurgery was electronically compiled by Elaine Chiu, who made possible the review and selection of articles. I thank her for obtaining and helping to summarize each of these papers, as well as for assisting in the anatomic cadaver dissections. The enormous editing project was ably done by Judith Simon. Microsurgeons performing these procedures would do well to adopt her meticulous attention to detail. Jackie Benson deserves my special thanks and appreciation for her prodigious effort in typing, retyping, and printing out the many drafts of the manuscript. I also wish to compliment Chong Lee and Ellen Caruthers for producing the hundreds of excellent black-and-white prints.

All of the patients presented in this book are from my personal practice except the two provided by Hill Hastings II, M.D. I greatly appreciate his contributing these outstanding cases which illustrate the wrap-around procedure and the radial forearm flap. I am indebted to Enrique Monsanto, M.D. who was an able cosurgeon for most of the cases presented in the surgical technique sections, and I extend praise and thanks to Pam Silverman, O.T.R./A.S.H.T., both for her contribution to the text and the excellent therapy she has provided to almost all of the patients presented. The University of California, San Francisco operating room team and recovery room and ward nurses are also to be commended for their fastidious care of these patients.

I am grateful to Dr. William Murray and the orthopaedic faculty for their support of the Hand and Microsurgery Service, and to the many residents who helped in these procedures. Finally, I thank my many teachers and colleagues who have shared their knowledge and inventiveness. In so doing, they have established our current fund of knowledge and ensured the continued prolific growth of microsurgery.

Contents

Foreword by Andrew J. Weiland vii
Preface ix
Acknowledgements xi

Chapter 1 Muscle Transplantation 1

1.1 Overview 1
1.2 Indications 1
1.3 Choice of Transplant 24
1.4 Gracilis Muscle Transplantation 26
1.5 Serratus Anterior and Latissimus Dorsi Muscle Transplantation . . . 30
1.6 Tensor Fasciae Latae Musculocutaneous Transplant 42
1.7 Postoperative Care 46
1.8 Selected Bibliography 46

Chapter 2 Cutaneous Transplantation 49

2.1 Overview 49
2.2 Indications 49
2.3 Choice of Transplant 51
2.4 Lateral Arm Flap 58
2.5 Scapular Flap 60
2.6 Dorsalis Pedis Flap 63
2.7 Radial Forearm Flap 65
2.8 Postoperative Care 66
2.9 Selected Bibliography 66

Chapter 3 Vascularized Bone Transplantation 69

3.1 Overview 69
3.2 Indications 69
3.3 Choice of Transplant 79
3.4 Vascularized Fibula Transplantation 82
3.5 Vascularized Iliac Crest Transplantation 88
3.6 Postoperative Care 92
3.7 Selected Bibliography 92

Chapter 4 Toe Transplantation for Hand Reconstruction 95

4.1 Overview 95
4.2 Indications 96

4.3 Choice of Transplant 97
4.4 Preoperative Planning 101
4.5 Anatomy 117
4.6 Surgical Technique 120
4.6.1 Whole Great Toe Transplantation 120
4.6.2 Toe Wrap-Around Procedure 124
4.6.3 Second-Toe Transplantation 126
4.6.4 Partial Toe Transplantation 129
4.6.5 Toe Joint Transplantation 131
4.7 Postoperative Care 134
4.8 Selected Bibliography 134

Chapter 5 Replantation 139

5.1 Indications 139
5.2 Contraindications 149
5.3 Emergency Department Care 150
5.4 Surgical Technique – General Considerations 151
5.5 Postoperative Care 158
5.6 Surgical Technique 163
5.6.1 Thumb Replantation 163
5.6.2 Digital Replantation 164
5.6.3 Ring Avulsion Injury 167
5.6.4 Vein Graft Harvesting 168
5.7 Selected Bibliography 169

Chapter 6 Regional Indications 173

6.1 Soft Tissue 173
6.2 Bone 174
6.3 Composite Loss 174
6.4 Selected Bibliography 175

Chapter 7 Recipient Site Preparation 177

Chapter 8 Monitoring 179

Index 183

1 Muscle Transplantation

1.1 Overview

Muscle tissue is composed of closely packed bundles of fibers which are separated by connective tissue. Blood vessels run through these connective tissue septa and branch out to form a generous capillary network among the individual muscle fibers. This superior vascularity of muscle tissue combined with its density and ability to contour and fill "dead space" appear to make it better than skin with subcutaneous fat for treating the various clinical problems described in this chapter.

Initially, muscle pedicle flaps were the only method of transferring muscle tissue, but with this technique, a muscle cannot be moved beyond its arc of rotation without compromising its vascular and nerve supply. The advent of microsurgical muscle transplantation has expanded the versatility of muscle tissue transfer, and muscles of various sizes can now be placed in almost any anatomic location.

Four muscle transplants are described in this chapter – the *latissimus dorsi*, the *gracilis*, the lowest digitations of the *serratus anterior*, and the *tensor fasciae latae*. These four muscles can effectively treat almost any wound requiring muscle tissue because they can provide the full range of sizes and shapes that may be required.

The *latissimus dorsi* and underlying *serratus anterior* have a common proximal vascular pedicle, which makes the approach to harvesting these two muscles similar. Either the latissimus dorsi, the lowest digitations of the serratus anterior, or both can be harvested (Harii et al. 1982). They may also be used where there is a large dead space. This dead space can be filled by the serratus anterior with the overlying latissimus used for soft-tissue cover. The serratus anterior is small and flat, whereas the latissimus dorsi is large and flat and can cover extremely extensive soft-tissue wounds. The *gracilis* is intermediate in size, longer, and somewhat cylindrical for long and narrow wounds. The *tensor fasciae latae* is a large bulky muscle used as a musculocutaneous transplant (Fig. 1-1). It can fill large defects, but its principal advantage lies in the cutaneous sensation it can provide with the lateral femoral cutaneous nerve.

1.2 Indications

1.2.1 Wound Coverage (May et al. 1984, Swartz and Mears 1985)

Muscle tissue is effective in covering wounds complicated by infection. The mechanism involved remains unclear, but as mentioned above, it may relate to the excellent vascularity of muscle, its density, and its ability to contour and fill the wound's dead space. These characteristics make it ideal for covering wounds of the following kind.

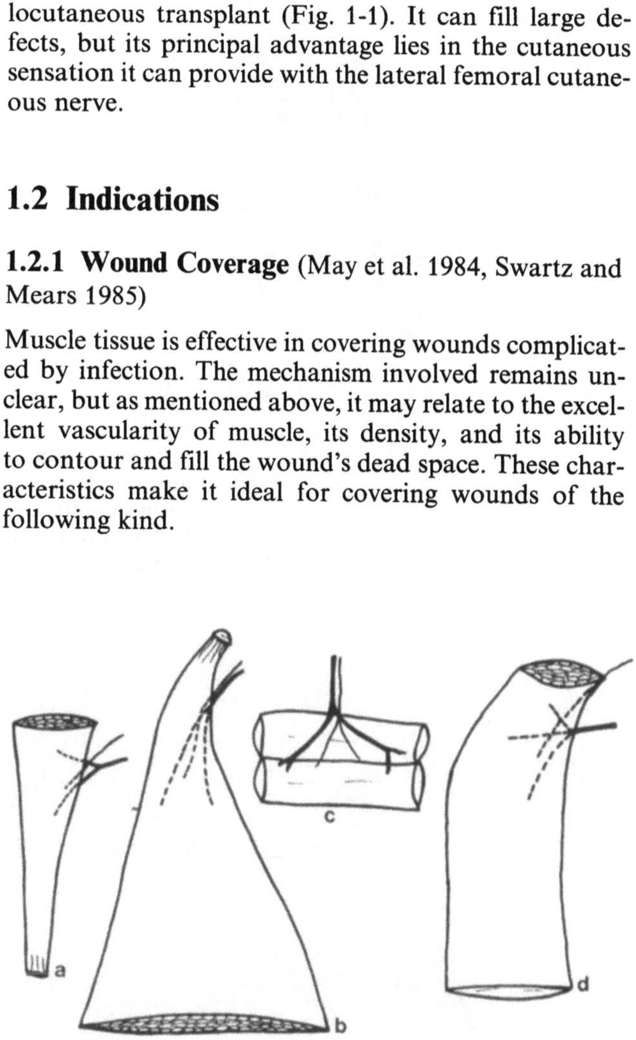

Fig. 1-1 a–d. The relative sizes and shapes of various muscle transplants are shown. **a.** Gracilis: 5 × 20 cm. **b.** Latissimus dorsi: 15 × 25–30 cm. **c.** Serratus anterior: 2 × 8 cm (each digitation). **d.** Tensor fasciae latae: 8 × 25 cm.

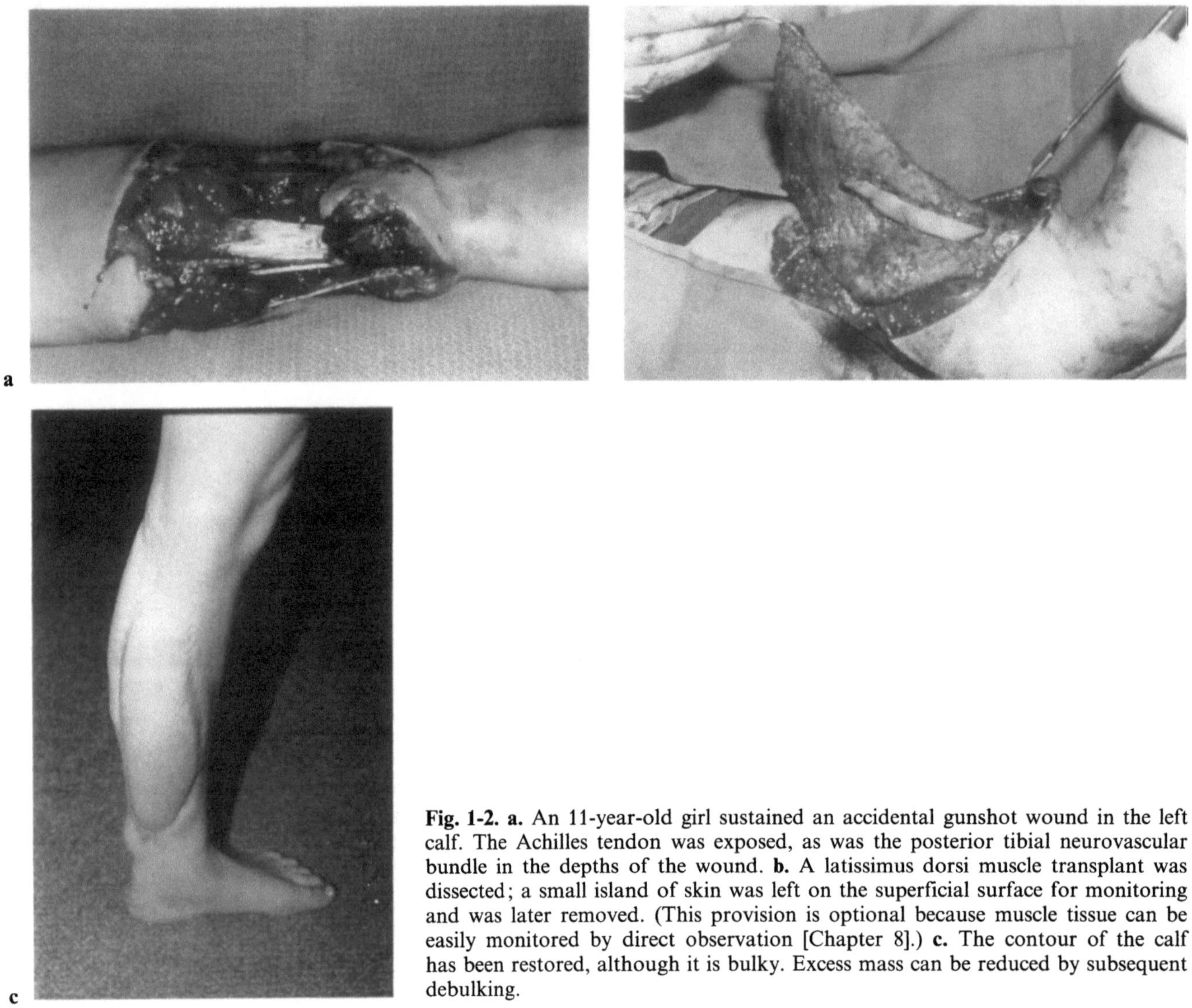

Fig. 1-2. a. An 11-year-old girl sustained an accidental gunshot wound in the left calf. The Achilles tendon was exposed, as was the posterior tibial neurovascular bundle in the depths of the wound. b. A latissimus dorsi muscle transplant was dissected; a small island of skin was left on the superficial surface for monitoring and was later removed. (This provision is optional because muscle tissue can be easily monitored by direct observation [Chapter 8].) c. The contour of the calf has been restored, although it is bulky. Excess mass can be reduced by subsequent debulking.

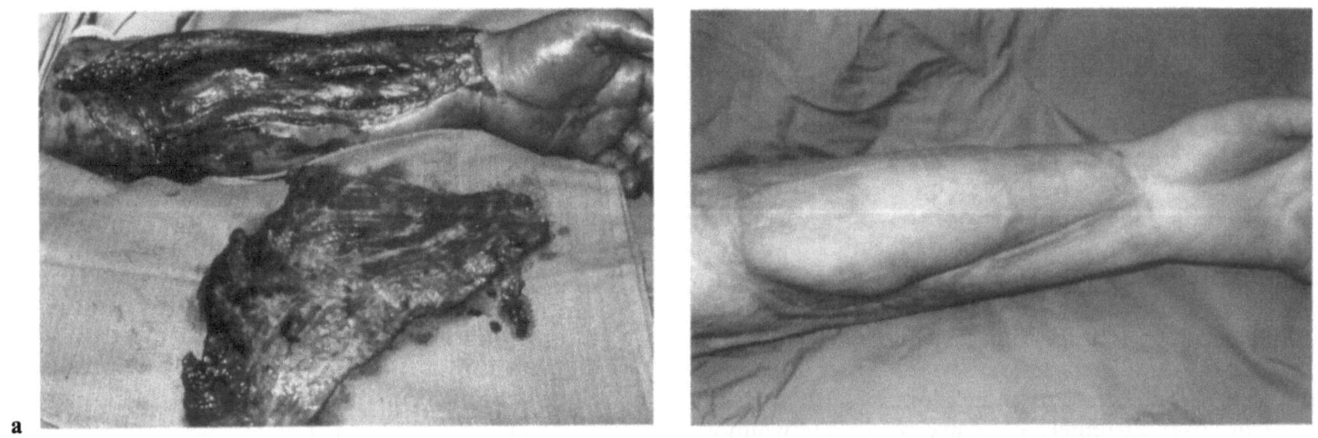

Fig. 1-3. a. This 32-year-old man caught his left arm between two rollers of a press and was trapped in this position for 8 hours. He was referred at 6 weeks with unstable fractures, delayed soft-tissue healing, and infection. The wound was debrided and the forearm bones were plated. Because of continued infection and the size of the wound, a latissimus dorsi muscle transplant was chosen. The latissimus muscle can be seen ready to cover the wound. **b.** Six months later, excellent cover had been achieved with a split-thickness skin graft used over the latissimus dorsi, and good pinch had been restored in his hand.

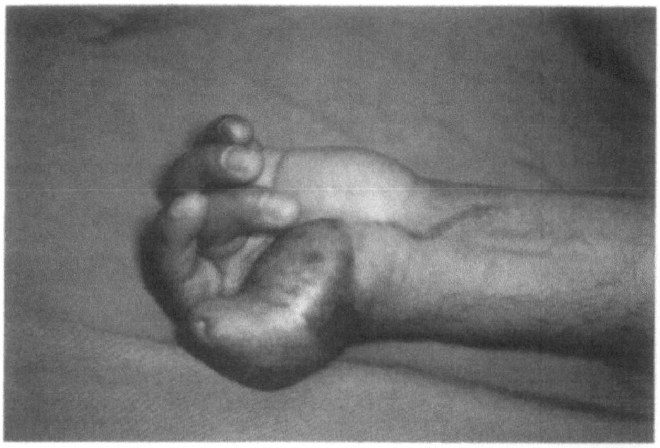
a

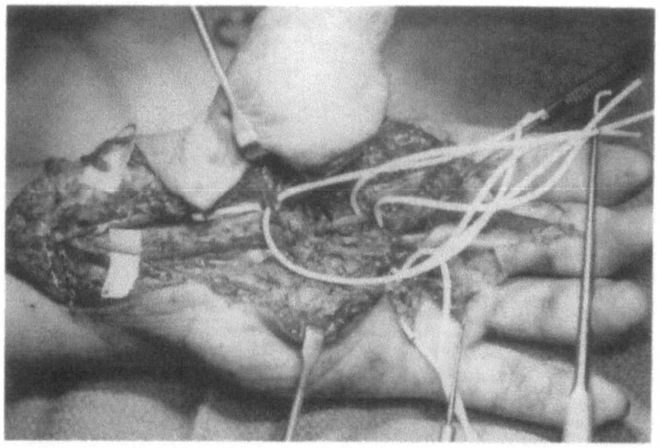
b

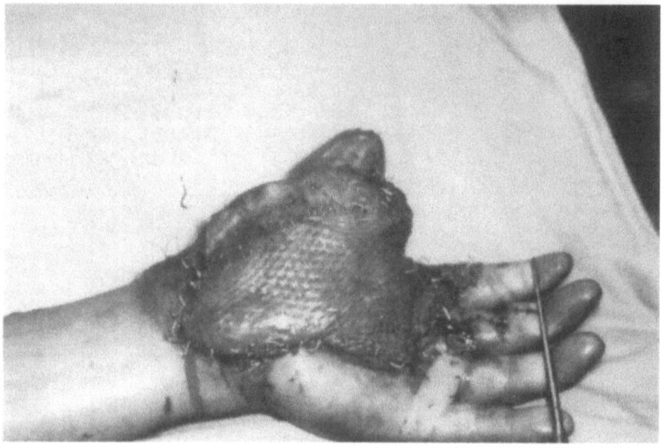
c

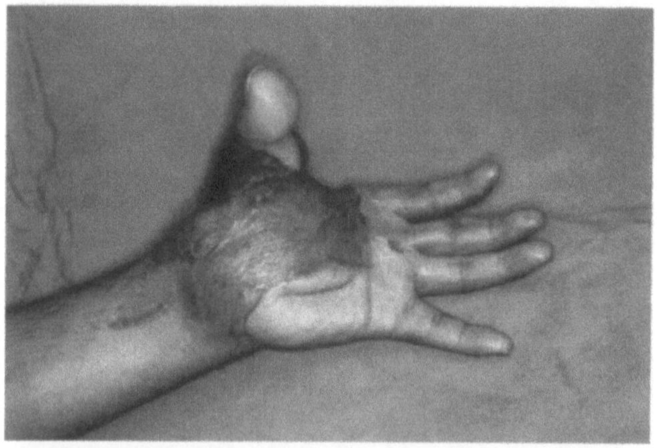
d

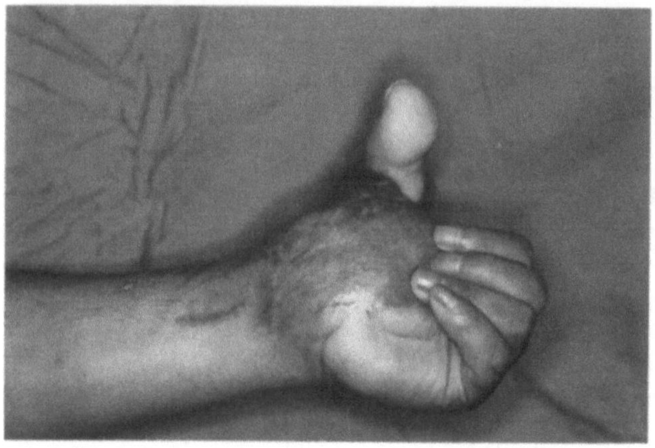
e

Fig. 1-4. a. This laborer sustained a saw injury across his palm along with amputation of his thumb. A pedicle groin flap had been applied around the thumb. This photograph shows his poor finger extension due to severe scarring in the palm. He also had a fixed adduction contracture of the thumb amputation stump. The hand was functionless. **b.** After releasing the contracture and all of the soft tissues of the palm, fingers, and thumb, an extensive defect remained. **c.** The serratus anterior muscle was placed in the palm and covered with a split-thickness skin graft. **d** and **e.** Six months later, a toe transplant was performed. The patient maintained excellent extension of all his fingers as well as good flexion of all but the long finger, which he learned to trap with the ring finger (he usually wore a buddy tape between the long and ring fingers). The serratus anterior provided a good palmar surface.

1.2.1.1 Traumatic Wounds – Acute Stage (Within the First Week of Injury) (Byrd et al. 1985, Godina 1986, Swartz and Mears 1985).

Extensive acute wounds in the *lower extremity* (Sec. 6.1.4-6), if covered with transplanted muscle after thorough debridement, will usually heal within a few weeks. The infection rate is extremely low, and the advantage the procedure offers through prompt healing and enabling early bone grafting is substantial (Figs. 1-2 and 3-4). In the *upper extremity* (Sec. 6.1.1-3), *smaller wounds* in which local flaps are inadequate are often amenable to standard groin or abdominal pedicle flaps. However, after severe trauma or in other situations where hand stiffness and edema are major problems, microvascular transplantation is needed to allow early elevation of the extremity and mobilization of the joints. Cutaneous microvascular flaps such as the lateral arm and scapular flaps are indicated in such situations (Sec. 2.1, 2.3). More *extensive wounds* or those with marked potential for infection should be treated by muscle transplantation (Fig. 1-3). A serratus anterior muscle transplant covered with skin grafts is effective in covering the *palm* (Sec. 6.1.1, 1.5.2.1) because it results in less shearing of the transplant on the deeper tissues compared with cutaneous flaps (Fig. 1-4). These

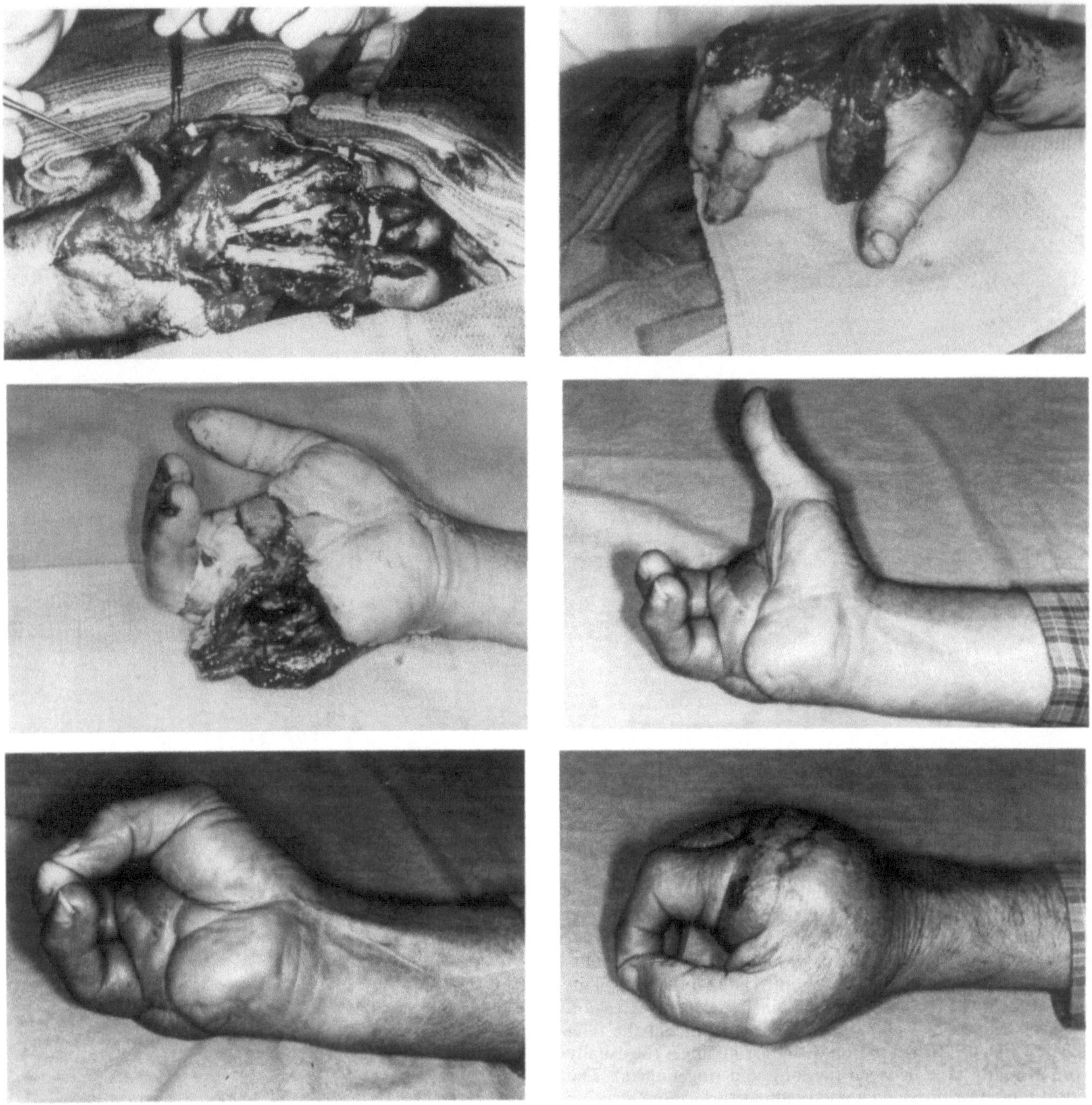

a b c d e f

Fig. 1-5. a. This laborer suffered a severe crush injury that resulted in a hand wound requiring extensive soft-tissue reconstruction of both the palmar and dorsal surfaces. **b.** Two slips of the serratus anterior were separated to provide the dorsal cover; the third slip (the largest slip) was routed across the first web space to provide cover in the palm. **c.** The patient ultimately lost his ring and small fingers because of vascular problems, but the muscle provided excellent soft-tissue cover on both sides of the hand. **d–f.** Ultimate function was good for both large and small object grasp.

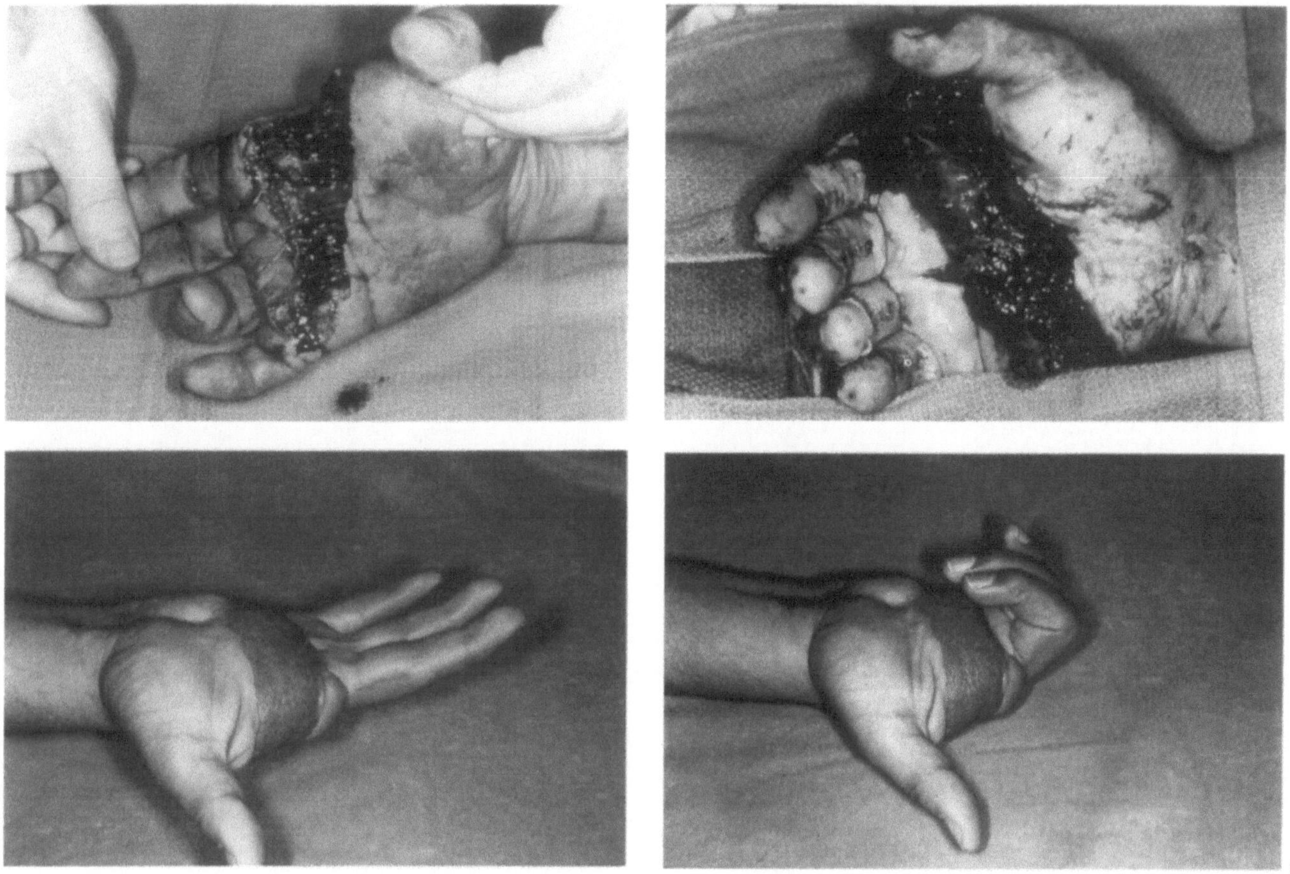

a b c d

Fig. 1-6. a. A 24-year-old laborer sustained a crush injury to his palm with devascularization of the index, long, and ring fingers. Vein grafting was required. **b.** There was substantial necrosis of palmar skin, exposing the vein grafts, tendons, and nerves. One week after the injury, a single slip of the serratus anterior was used across the palm to provide good vascularized cover; this in turn was covered with a split-thickness skin graft. A ray amputation of the index finger had to be performed because vascularity could not be maintained. **c** and **d.** Subsequently, tendon and nerve grafting were required; this restored good flexion of the fingers. The palmar skin has proved to be a durable surface, and the patient continues to work as a laborer 3 years later.

muscle slips are particularly useful if the cover must be "tailored" to the contour of the defect. This need occurs in multiple digit wounds (Figs. 1-5 and 1-6) or those involving both the palm and dorsum of the hand (Fig. 1-7). Tendon reconstruction beneath a serratus transplant to the hand generally requires silicone tendon rods. Placement of these rods, which can sometimes be performed at the time of the muscle transplant, is done as the first of a two-stage reconstruction. On the *dorsum of the hand* (Sec. 6.1.1), cutaneous transplants are preferable because they more closely simulate the pliable skin of this region, especially if subsequent tendon reconstruction is anticipated. For extensive defects of the palm and dorsum, where attempts at hand salvage are appropriate, a combination latissimus dorsi and serratus anterior transplant can be used (Fig. 1-8).

The *timing* of debridement and flap coverage is of the utmost importance. If treated within a week of injury, wounds have the lowest rate of infection and flaps have the highest rate of success. Meticulously thorough debridement of the entire wound is essential. The margins and base of the wound should be sharply debrided back to healthy tissue. After this stage, the tissues, including the recipient vessels, become increasingly edematous and inflamed. There are two situations in which performing a flap in the acute stage is unwise: when a patient's general condition makes major surgery risky, and when the extent of tissue necrosis cannot be assessed.

If a flap cannot be done early, some surgeons advocate placing temporary skin grafts to allow as much healing as possible until the inflammation and swelling have subsided. This generally takes 6–8 weeks, at which time the microvascular flap can be safely done. Of course, the decision to perform such a flap involves many clinical factors, and if bone, nerve, or tendons are exposed, a transplant may be necessary even in the presence of swelling. If so, particular care must be taken to use recipient vessels well outside the zone of injury. (Godina et al. [1986] described "banking" an amputated hand for several months by connecting the vessels of the hand to the thoracodorsal vessels in the axilla while burns in the more proximal part of the extremity could be evaluated and treated.)

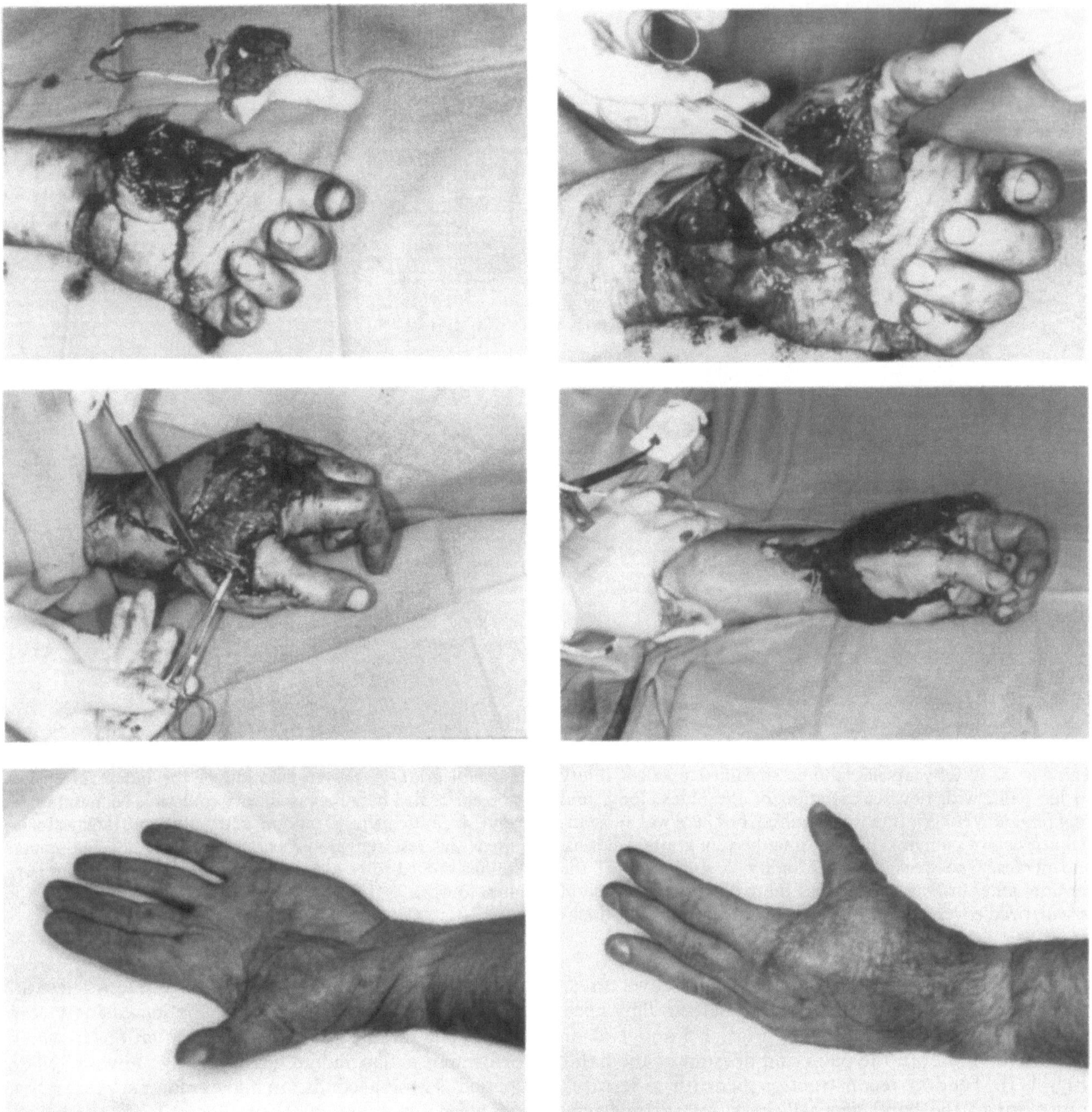

a b c d e f

Fig. 1-7. a. This patient sustained an avulsion of his thumb and thenar eminence in a motor racing accident. **b.** The thumb was revascularized with vein grafts to replace the damaged artery, and the flexor tendon and nerves were repaired. **c.** Vein grafts were also used to reconstruct venous outflow, and the extensor tendons were repaired on the dorsum of the thumb. Soft-tissue cover was required on both sides. **d.** The serratus anterior pedicle was hooked into the radial artery with slips brought around the thumb on the palmar and dorsal surfaces. **e** and **f.** Excellent cover was achieved along with good function. The muscle, which was covered with split-thickness skin graft, has flattened out.

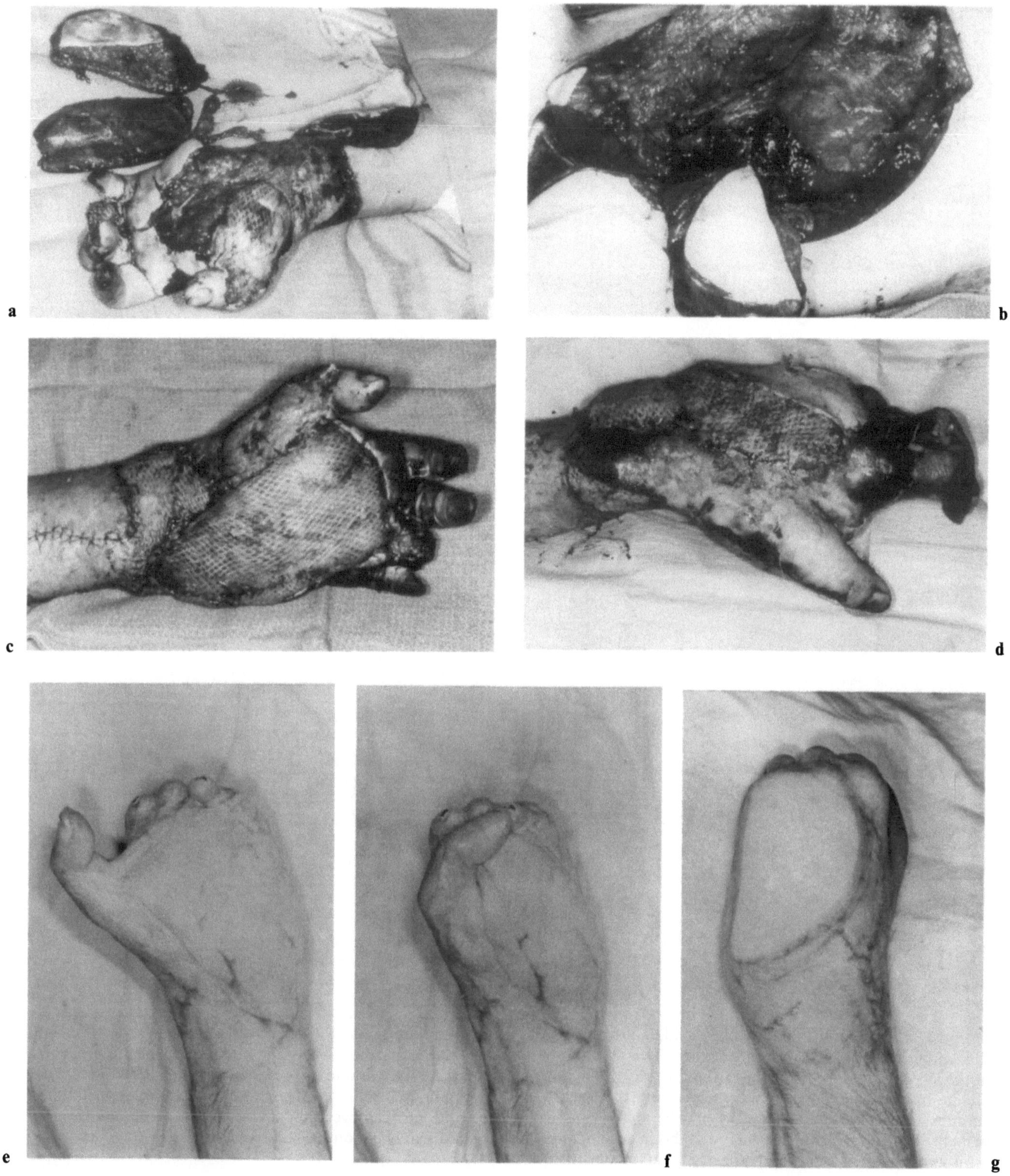

Fig. 1-8. **a.** A 31-year-old man crushed his hand in an industrial machine, devascularizing all of the fingers and the palm. The thumb was revascularized. Cover of the dorsum and palm was needed to salvage the hand. A combined latissimus dorsi-serratus anterior muscle transplant based on the thoracodorsal vessels was dissected from the right thorax. **b.** The combined transplant can be seen prior to its removal from the chest. **c** and **d.** The transplant was anastomosed into the ulnar vessels end-to-side, using the serratus anterior for cover on the palm and the latissimus dorsi musculocutaneous portion for the dorsum. All of the fingers became necrotic and were amputated. **e–g.** The patient regained thumb function and good cover on both the dorsum and palm. Subsequent toe transplantation was done to provide an opposable digit (Fig. 4–14).

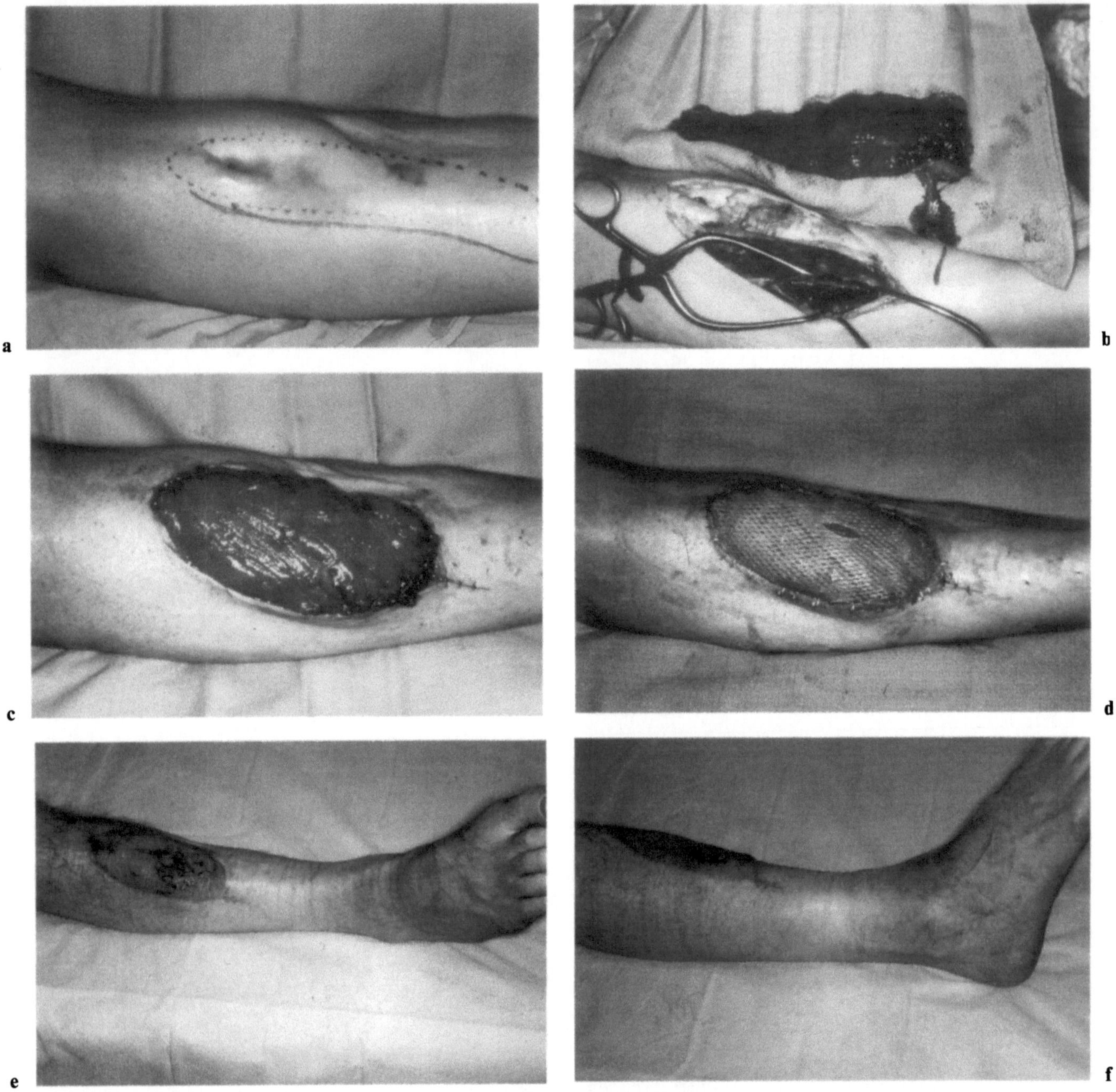

Fig. 1-9. a. A 46-year-old engineer had had osteomyelitis with repeated drainage and intermittent swelling subsequent to a tibial fracture sustained 17 years earlier. The anterior part of the leg was unsightly and the skin continually broke down. **b.** The scarred soft tissues were removed and the bone was curetted to prepare the defect. The gracilis muscle was harvested. The anterior tibial artery and both accompanying veins were dissected in the leg, preparing them for anastomosis to the gracilis muscle pedicle. **c.** The gracilis muscle was sutured into the edges of the wound. **d.** A meshed, split-thickness skin graft was stapled over the muscle. The entire procedure took 2.5 hours. **e** and **f.** In the final result, good soft-tissue cover has been achieved. The muscle has completely flattened out and profiles evenly with the surrounding tissues after approximately 6 months.

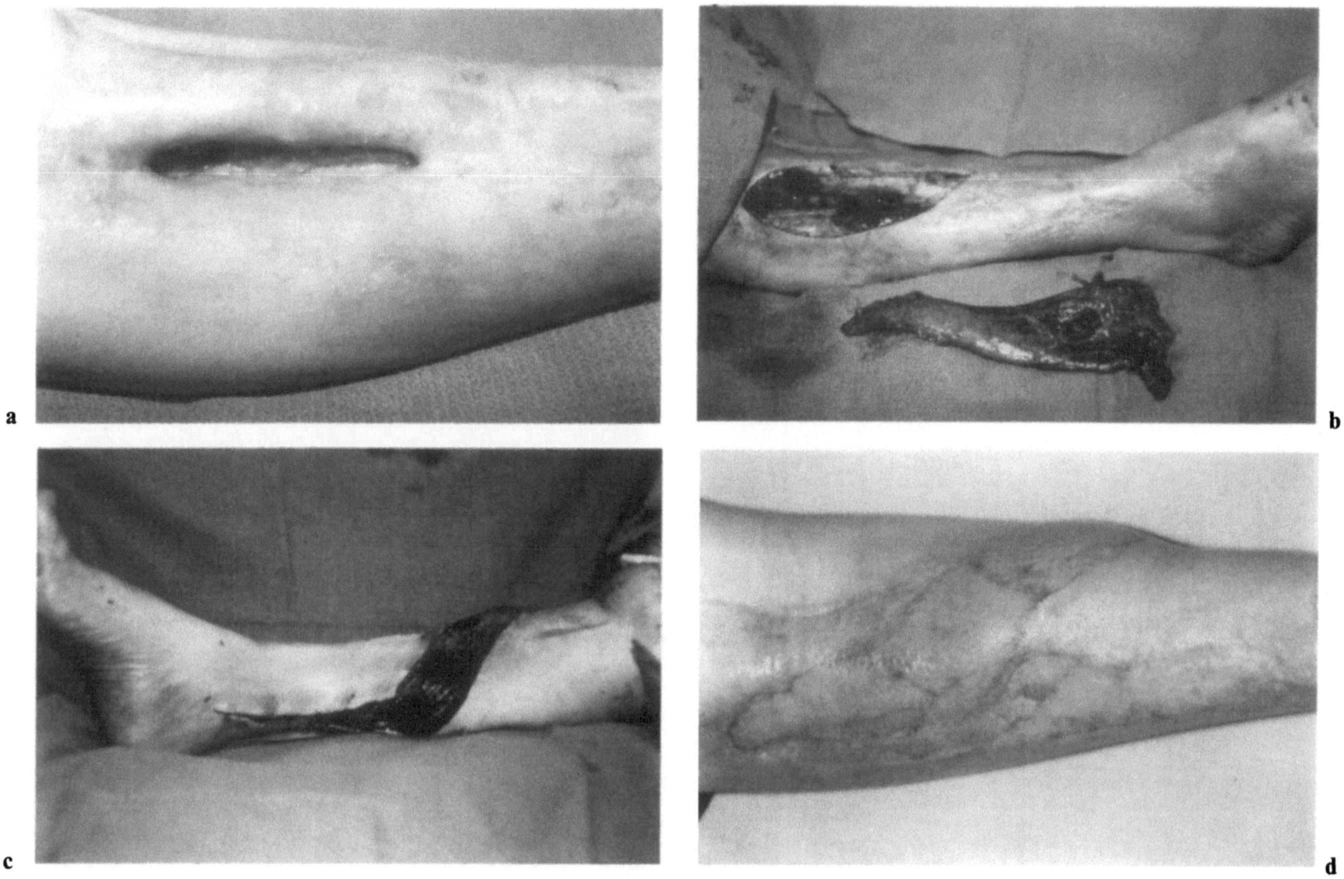

Fig. 1-10. **a.** A 46-year-old woman had had chronic osteomyelitis since being injured in a car accident 20 years earlier. The affected area, a wound located on the proximal lateral aspect of the leg, had been debrided many times but continued to drain, was inflamed, and had poor soft-tissue cover. The choice of recipient vessels was either the anterior tibial artery distal to the lesion, used in retrograde fashion, or the posterior tibial artery, which would require that the muscle course over the crest of the tibia. This latter option was chosen because of scarring around the anterior tibial vessel. (One of the most common causes of vascular problems following transplantation is the use of a vessel in the zone of injury.) **b.** Thorough debridement of the wound involved removing both soft tissue and bone. A local muscle pedicle flap was considered, but following appropriate debridement, it would probably not contour and fill all the dead space as completely as would a microvascular transplant. The gracilis muscle is shown ready to be placed in the defect. **c.** The microvascular transplant was connected end-to-side to the posterior tibial artery, and both gracilis veins were anastomosed to the venae comitantes. **d.** The transplant was covered with a split-thickness skin graft. Six months later excellent contour and adequate, well-vascularized soft-tissue cover was the result.

1.2.1.2 Traumatic Wounds – Chronic Stage, Wounds Surrounded by Irradiated Tissue, Osteomyelitis, and Infected Nonunions (Gordon and Chiu 1988, Mathes et al. 1982, May et al. 1984, Weiland et al. 1984).

In patients with *chronic osteomyelitis*, muscle tissue cover after debridement can usually control infection and reduce or eliminate drainage and other symptoms (Figs. 1-9 and 1-10). Muscle tissue holds up well when used to cover a variety of infected bone and soft-tissue wounds (Figs. 1-11 and 1-12). In wounds that have been previously infected, appropriate debridement is the cornerstone of treatment. Thorough debridement can be done with confidence, knowing that the resultant defect can be effectively covered with a muscle transplant (Figs. 3-3 and 3-5). To achieve a clean wound, several visits to the operating room may be required. Quantitative bacterial counts are valuable in establishing when wound cover should be performed. When that time has come, the muscle of appropriate size to cover the defect can then be selected (Fig. 1-13). Whereas *irradiated wounds* will often not heal, muscle transplants can introduce additional blood supply and effectively enable healing. Care must be taken to debride the wound adequately and place the vascular anastomoses beyond the irradiated region (Fig. 1-14).

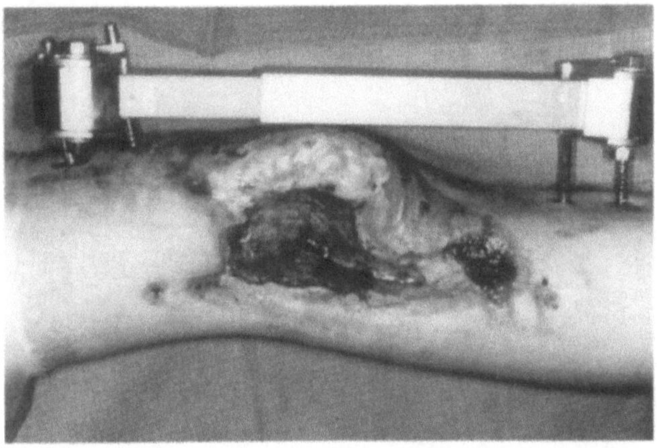
a

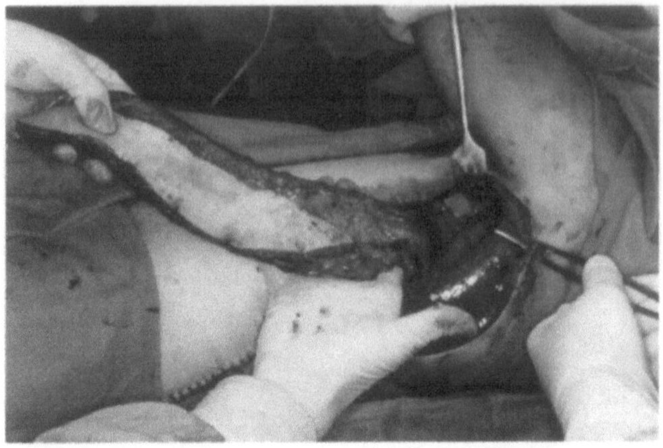
b

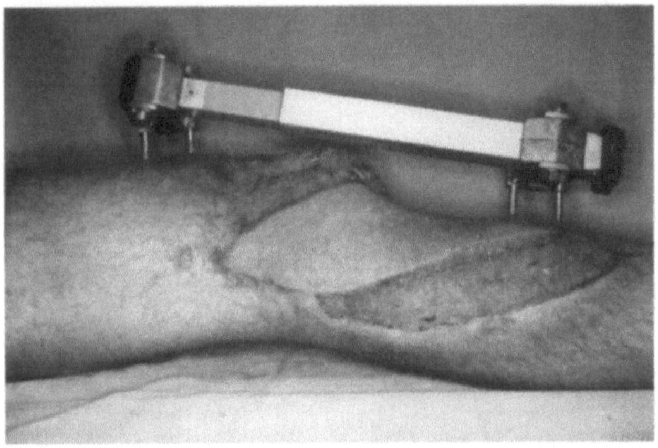
c

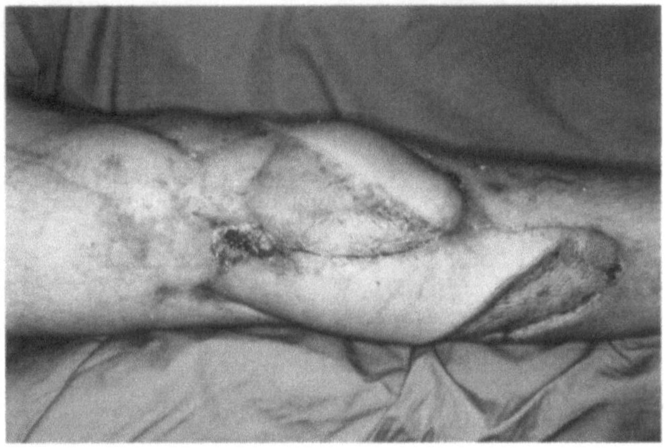
d

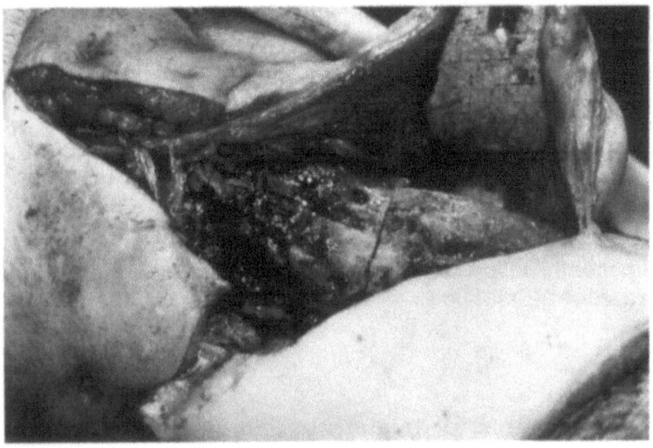
e

Fig. 1-11. a. An 18-year-old boy had an infected wound and osteomyelitis with inadequate soft-tissue cover involving the entire knee region. An external fixator with half-pins placed medially was used to stabilize the bones so that the anterior tibial vessels could be used distally on the lateral side of the leg. **b.** A latissimus dorsi musculocutaneous transplant was harvested from the left chest, and the pedicle was dissected. **c.** The latissimus dorsi flap covered the lateral defect, but anterior cover remained poor for any subsequent reconstruction. **d.** A second latissimus dorsi musculocutaneous transplant was used to provide good cover anteriorly. **e.** The cover was adequate for subsequent knee fusion using an external fixator. After osseous healing, no further drainage occurred despite the fact that the bone appeared infected at surgery. Both bone and soft tissues have remained healed and 2 years later the patient is fully weight bearing.

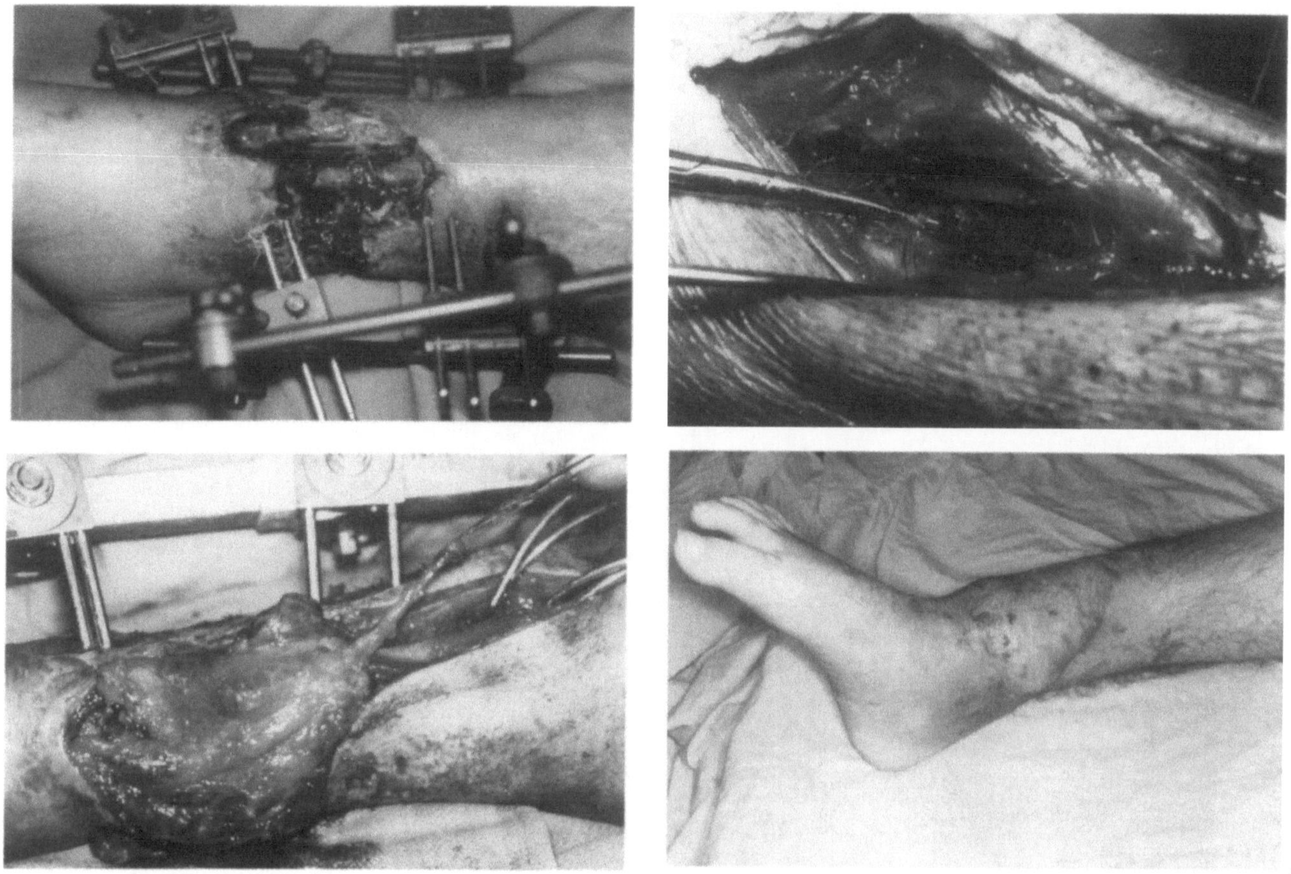

a b c d

Fig. 1-12. a. This 22-year-old man suffered injuries in a motorcycle accident. This 1-month-old infected wound was too small for a latissimus dorsi muscle transplant unless only a small portion of the muscle were to be harvested. The defect was too wide for a gracilis transplant, but the lowest slips of the serratus anterior could be shaped to fit it well. **b.** In dissecting down to the recipient anterior tibial vessels, small vessels could be seen coursing between the tibialis anterior and extensor hallucis longus. These vessels easily led to the anterior tibial neurovascular bundle. **c.** The serratus anterior was harvested and fit the shape of the debrided wound. The muscle was sutured to the wound margins and the vessels were anastomosed. The muscle was covered with a split-thickness skin graft. **d.** The healed wound approximately 3 months later.

1.2.1.3 Exposed Metal (Plates, Prostheses) and Vital Anatomic Structures

A microvascular muscle transplant has the ability to cover foreign material because of its excellent vascularity and ability to closely contour the wound surface. Once again, meticulous debridement is essential (Figs. 1-15 and 1-28).

1.2.1.4 Contour Defects and Dead Space

Muscle tissue is excellent for filling the dead space of large wounds, especially those resulting from the loss of muscle or bone, or from debridement for infection (Fig. 1-16). Large cavities may also result from the removal of infected total joint prostheses where repeated infection has made salvage of the prosthesis impossible, or from tumor extirpation. In these situations, edema, fibrosis, and irradiated tissue frequently make local flaps unwise (Fig. 1-17). In general, excellent contour can be restored. Such defects can be covered with musculocutaneous transplants, or else the muscle tissue can be used alone and then covered with a split-thickness skin graft. The choice depends on the bulk needed to fill the defect and cover the wound.

1.2.1.5 Heel Wounds (Sec. 6.1.4)

Severe heel wounds can be covered with muscle tissue. The ultimate contour will usually be good, but care must be taken to choose a muscle of appropriate size. A musculocutaneous transplant is used for cutaneous cover over the weight-bearing region (Figs. 1-18 and 1-19). Although the latissimus dorsi is used most frequently for this purpose, the gracilis can be used as a musculocutaneous transplant. The cutaneous portion must be kept over the muscle and positioned in its proximal half (Fig. 1-20). For very extensive wounds with a large tissue defect, the tensor fasciae latae should be used. This muscle is particularly useful for heel wounds because the lateral femoral cutaneous nerve can be sutured to a nerve in the recipient area, restoring sensory return in the transplant (Fig. 1-21).

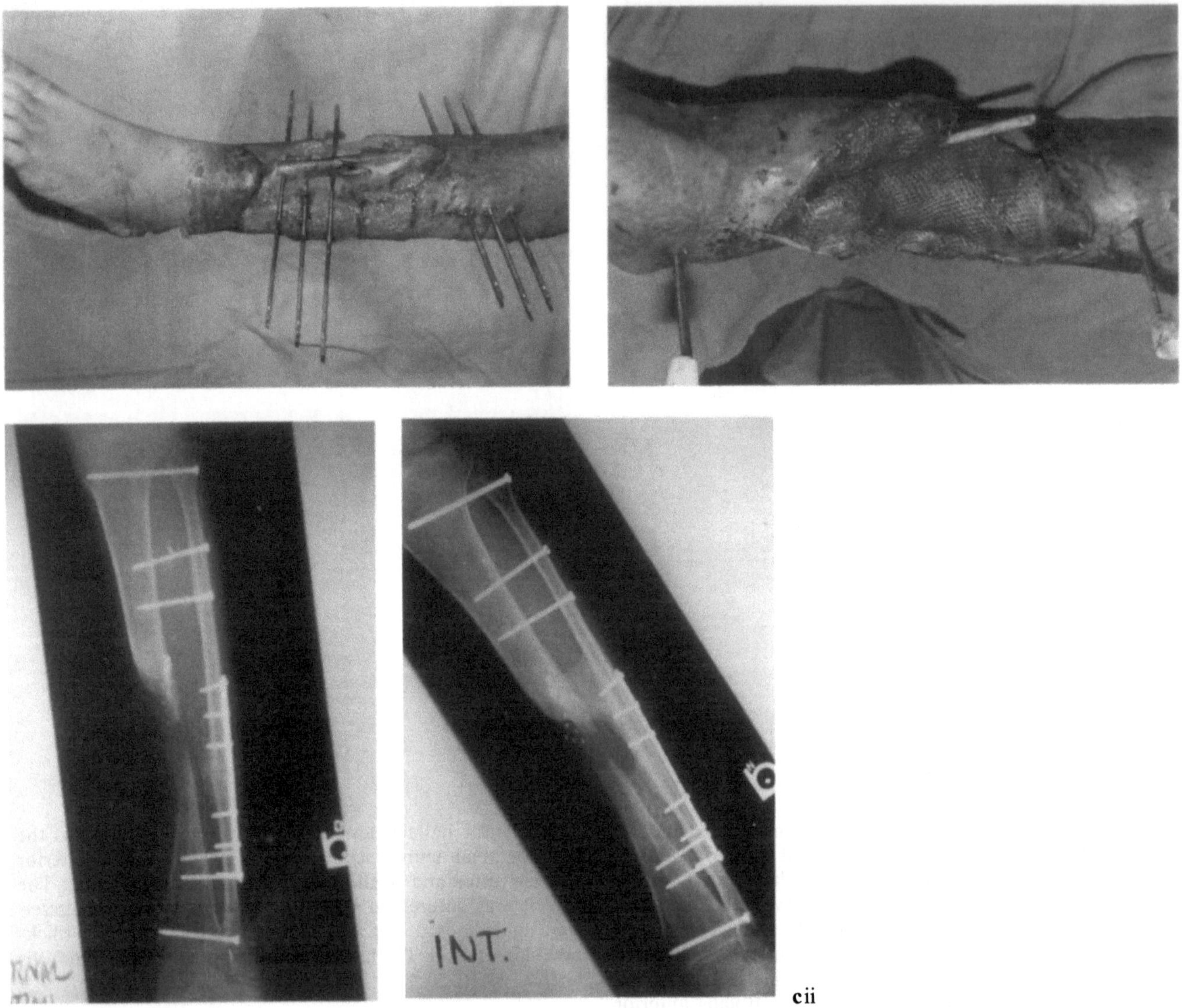

a b ci cii

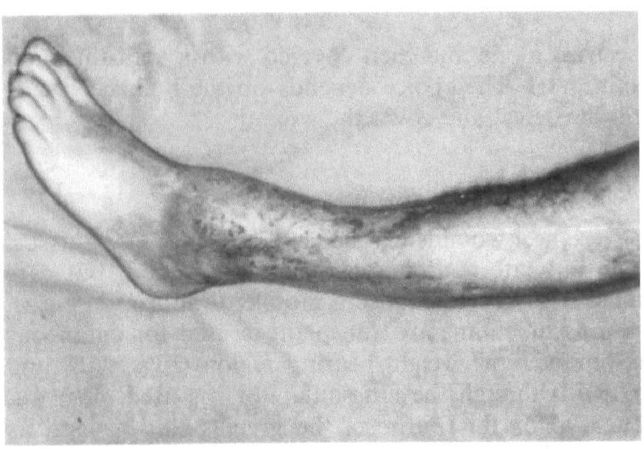

d

Fig. 1-13. a. An 18-year-old boy developed an infected leg wound 3 months after sustaining an open fracture of the tibia and fibula in a motorcycle accident. The necrotic bone and purulent drainage are seen. **b.** The external fixator was replaced so that the half-pins stood away from the wound. The wound was debrided and a latissimus dorsi muscle transplant was used for cover. **c.** Six months later the wound was entirely healed, allowing further osseous reconstruction. Because of the severity of the initial *Pseudomonas* infection, obtaining fibular healing with a plate (i) followed by a proximal and distal tibiofibular synostosis (ii) was decided upon. With this approach, the previously infected region was avoided during the subsequent bone grafting. (Courtesy of Dr. Floyd Jergesen, San Francisco, who performed the tibiofibular synostosis.) **d.** Three years later, the patient was fully weight bearing without difficulty and walked with a slight limp. Radiography showed a solid proximal and distal tibiofibular synostosis.

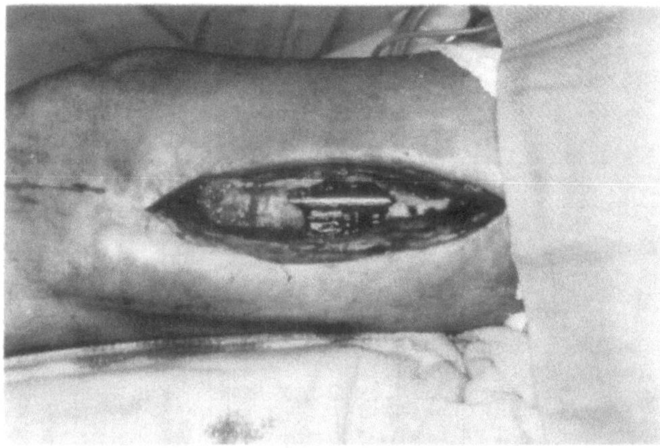
a

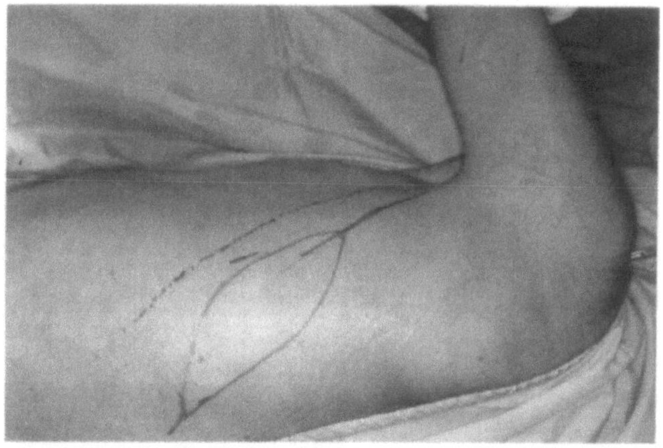
b

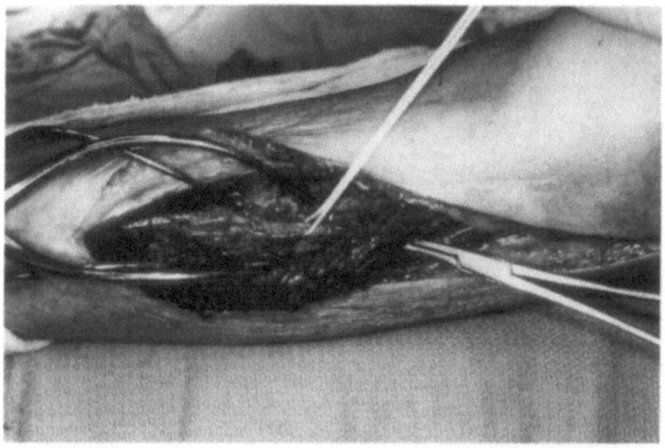
c

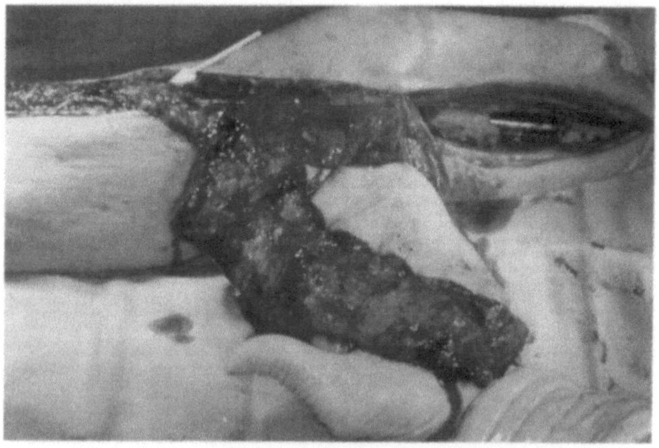
d

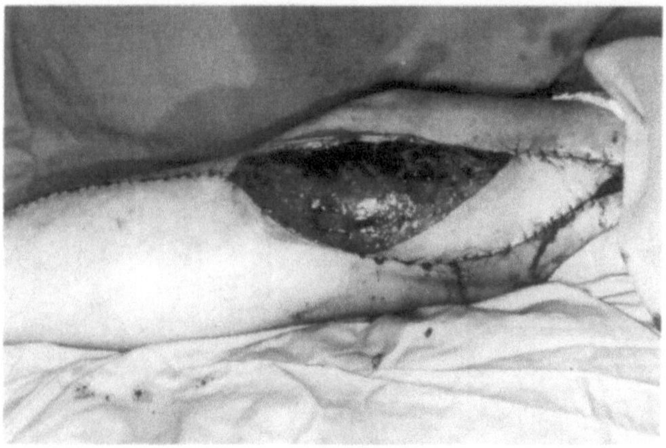
e

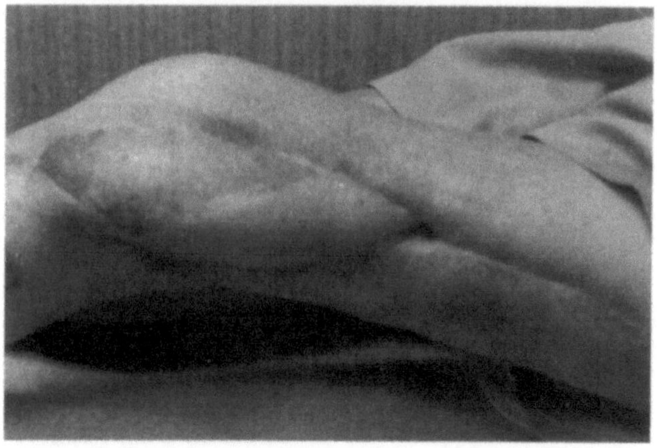
f

Fig. 1-14. a. Following the removal of a low-grade sarcoma, this intramedullary rod was exposed. An irradiated wound on the lateral aspect of the thigh was complicated by chronic infection. After debridement, a transplant was needed that would fill the dead space and introduce well-vascularized tissue. **b.** A latissimus dorsi musculocutaneous transplant was therefore planned to fill the defect and cover the wound. **c.** In the leg, the anterior tibial vessels were dissected (*in the vessel loop*), divided distally, and "swung" back under the tibialis anterior to be used as the donor vessels on the lateral aspect of the knee. **d.** The arrow indicates the location of the vascular anastomoses; the muscle is ready to be set into the defect. **e.** The muscle and skin provided excellent cover. A skin graft was used to cover the part of the muscle still exposed. **f.** The final result. The patient continues to use a cane, although the bone healed spontaneously on the medial aspect.

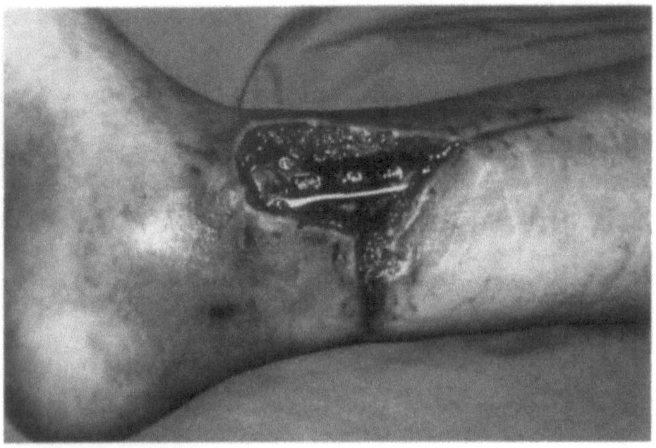
a

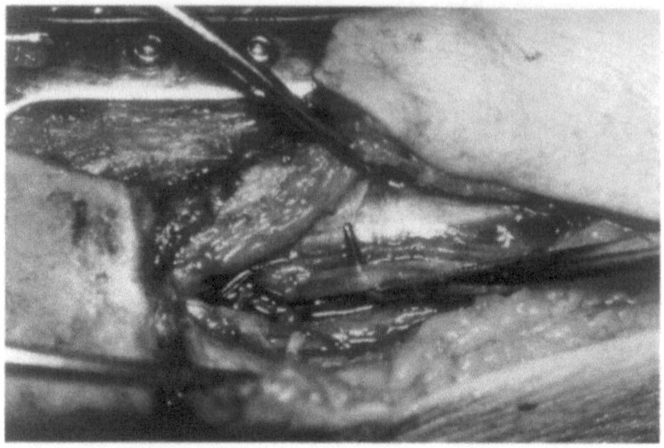
b

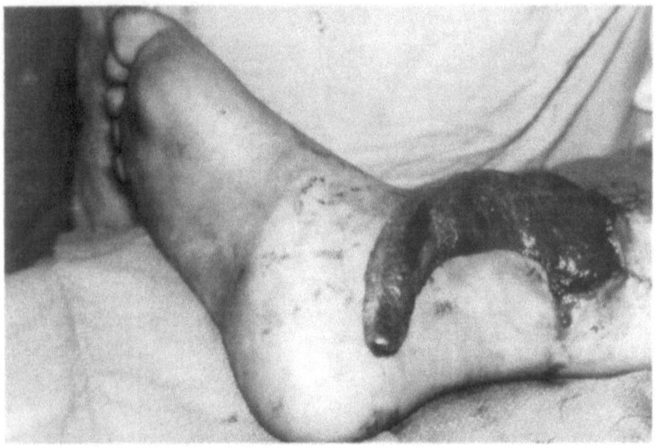
c

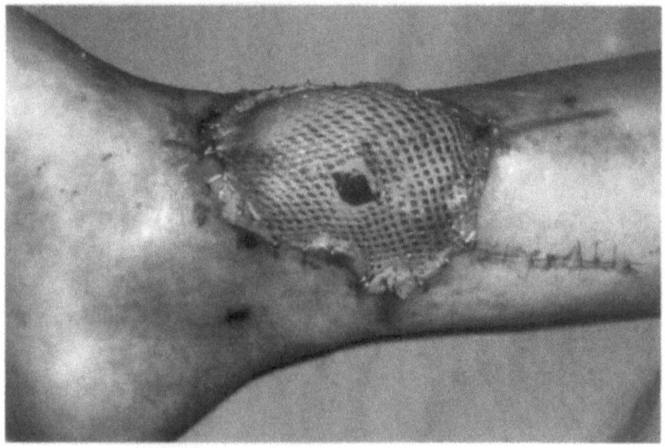
d

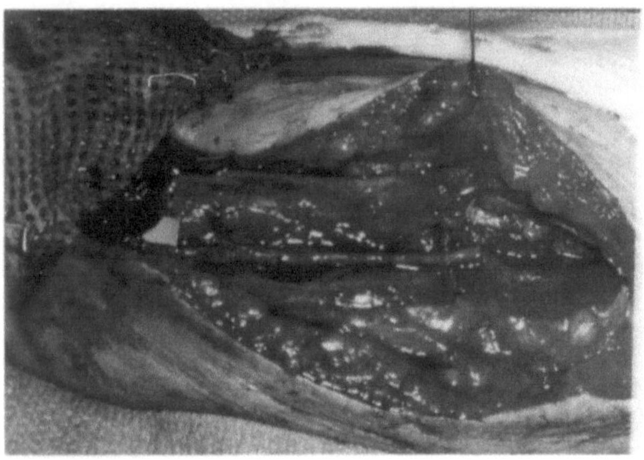
e

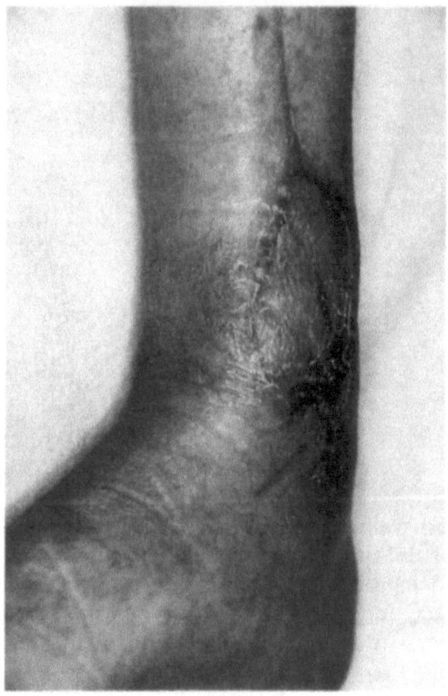
f

Fig. 1-15. a. A 60-year-old man sustained a comminuted fracture of the ankle requiring this plate. The crush injury caused the wound to break down. **b.** The posterior tibial vessels were dissected and the wound was meticulously cleaned and debrided. A close-up of these vessels is seen here. **c.** This wound was thought to be of ideal size and shape for a gracilis transplant, although the serratus anterior would also have fitted well. The gracilis muscle was loosely set into the defect while the vascular anastomoses were performed. **d.** The muscle was trimmed distally, set into the defect, and then covered with a split-thickness skin graft. **e.** Although it was felt that good vascularity was present initially, arterial thrombosis occurred approximately 3 hours later and an 8-cm vein graft was used to anastomose to the posterior tibial vessels more proximally in the leg. The initial repair was probably done with damaged vessels in the zone of injury. **f.** Excellent soft-tissue cover could be seen 4 months later.

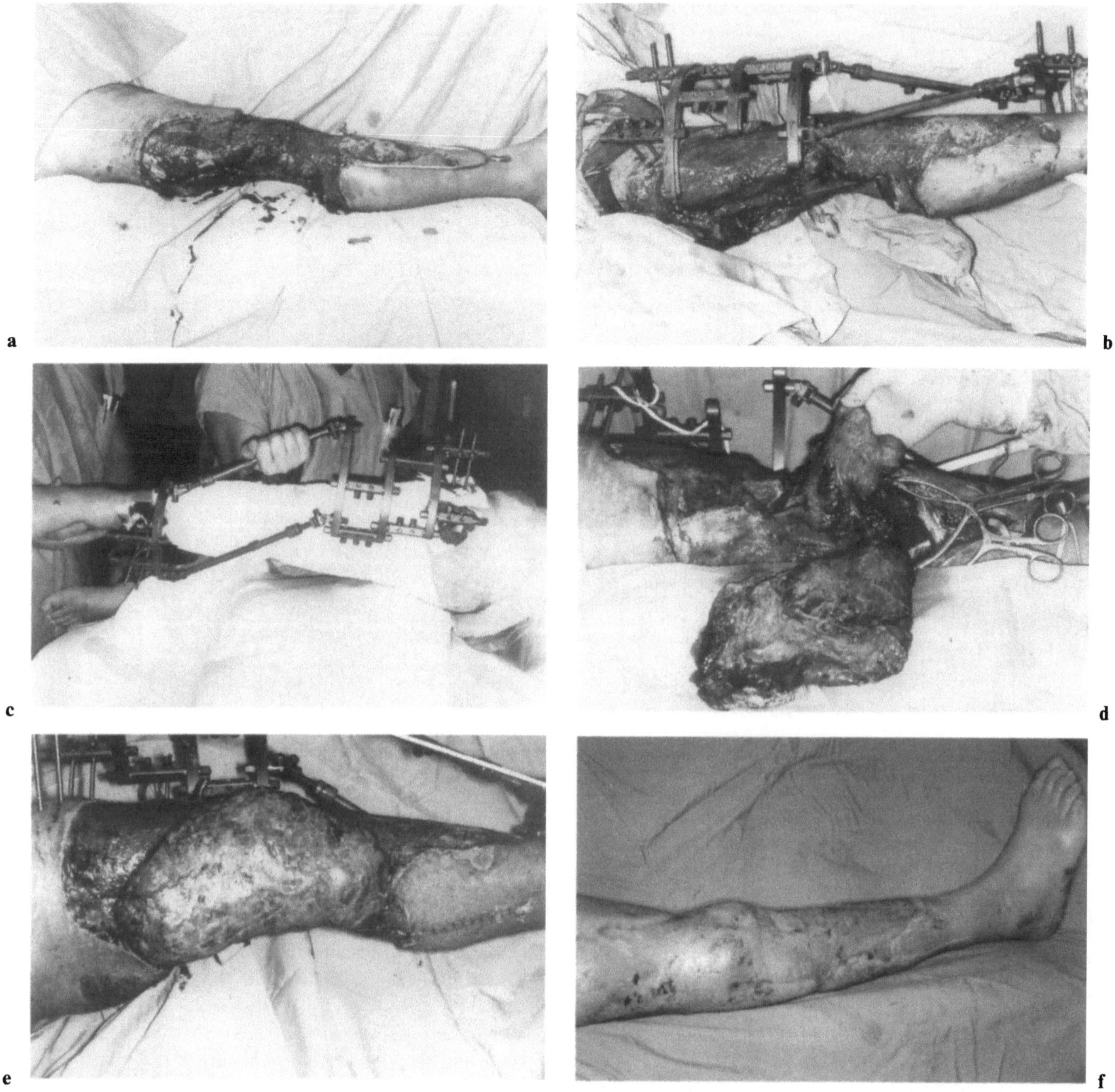

Fig. 1-16. a. This patient was a pedestrian when hit by a car. He sustained a supracondylar fracture with an open knee joint and this extensive amount of dead space and contour defect. The wound was circumferential, extending around the entire extremity. *Pseudomonas* and *Enterobacter* were found when the wound was cultured 10 days after the injury. **b.** An external fixation device with half-pins was placed which allowed access to the anterior tibial and posterior tibial vessels distal to the wound. The pins were placed in the skin so as not to interfere with subsequent muscle placement. (The external fixator must be placed to allow appropriate exposure of the entire wound and vessels. Familiarity with a versatile fixation device is essential.) Two radical debridement procedures were performed to ensure that the wound was as clean as possible and all necrotic material had been removed. **c.** This external fixator provided stability for the bones in all planes and simplified the six hourly dressing changes. **d.** The posterior aspect of the knee is shown. A combined latissimus dorsi-serratus anterior transplant was planned. The serratus anterior was used to fill the dead space and cover the knee joint and fracture, while the latissimus dorsi provided overlying soft-tissue cover. Suction-irrigation tubes were placed in the medial aspect of the knee and remained there until culture results from the tubes were negative, which was about 7 days later. **e.** The latissimus transplant is seen overlying the area of the defect and the serratus muscle. The vessels were anastomosed to the posterior tibial vessels, distal to the injury. **f.** The defect was covered with a split-thickness skin graft, and healing was achieved within 2 weeks. The leg is seen here 3 months later. A knee fusion performed 4 months after injury involved elevating the transplant and placing bone graft. A solid fusion was obtained.

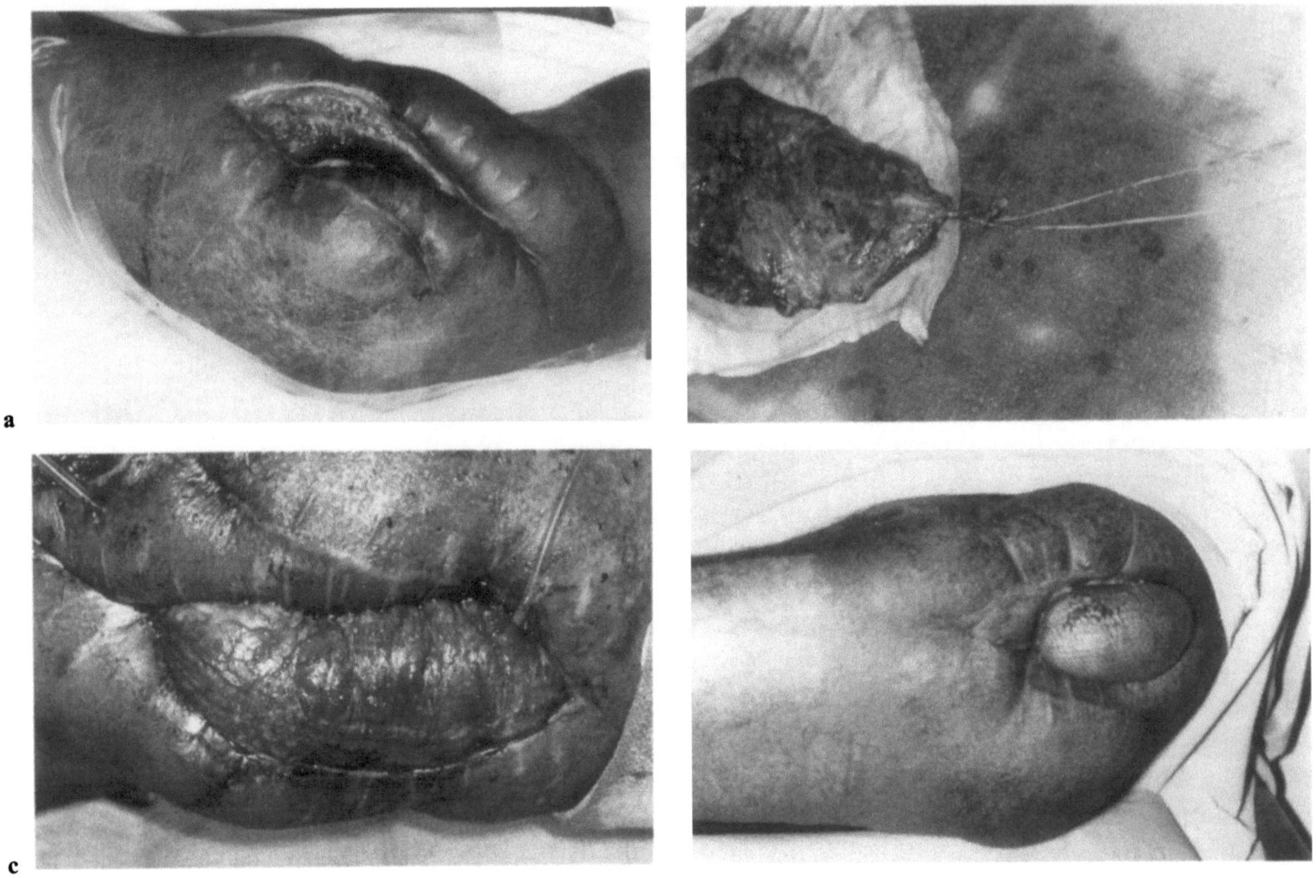

Fig. 1-17. a. A 28-year-old patient with sickle cell disease was left with this large infected wound extending down to the acetabulum and proximal femur following removal of an infected total hip prosthesis. After four attempts at total hip replacement, a Girdlestone procedure was decided upon. Several local flaps had failed, resulting in extensive fibrosis around the hip region. Because of the sickle cell disease, the patient was given an exchange transfusion preoperatively. **b.** A latissimus dorsi muscle transplant was chosen to fill this extensive defect. Because of the extremely poor surrounding tissues, 18-cm vein grafts were harvested; on a separate table in the operating room, these vein grafts were anastomosed to the thoracodorsal artery and vein prior to insertion of the muscle into the defect. The inferior epigastric vessels were used as the recipient vessels. **c.** The latissimus dorsi can be seen filling the defect. Suction and irrigation tubes were placed in the depths of the wound and left there for approximately 5 days. **d.** The transplant was covered with a split-thickness skin graft, and it healed without subsequent problems. At the 4-year follow-up examination, no problems or recurrent infection had been experienced, and the patient was able to fully bear weight with a limp following the Girdlestone procedure.

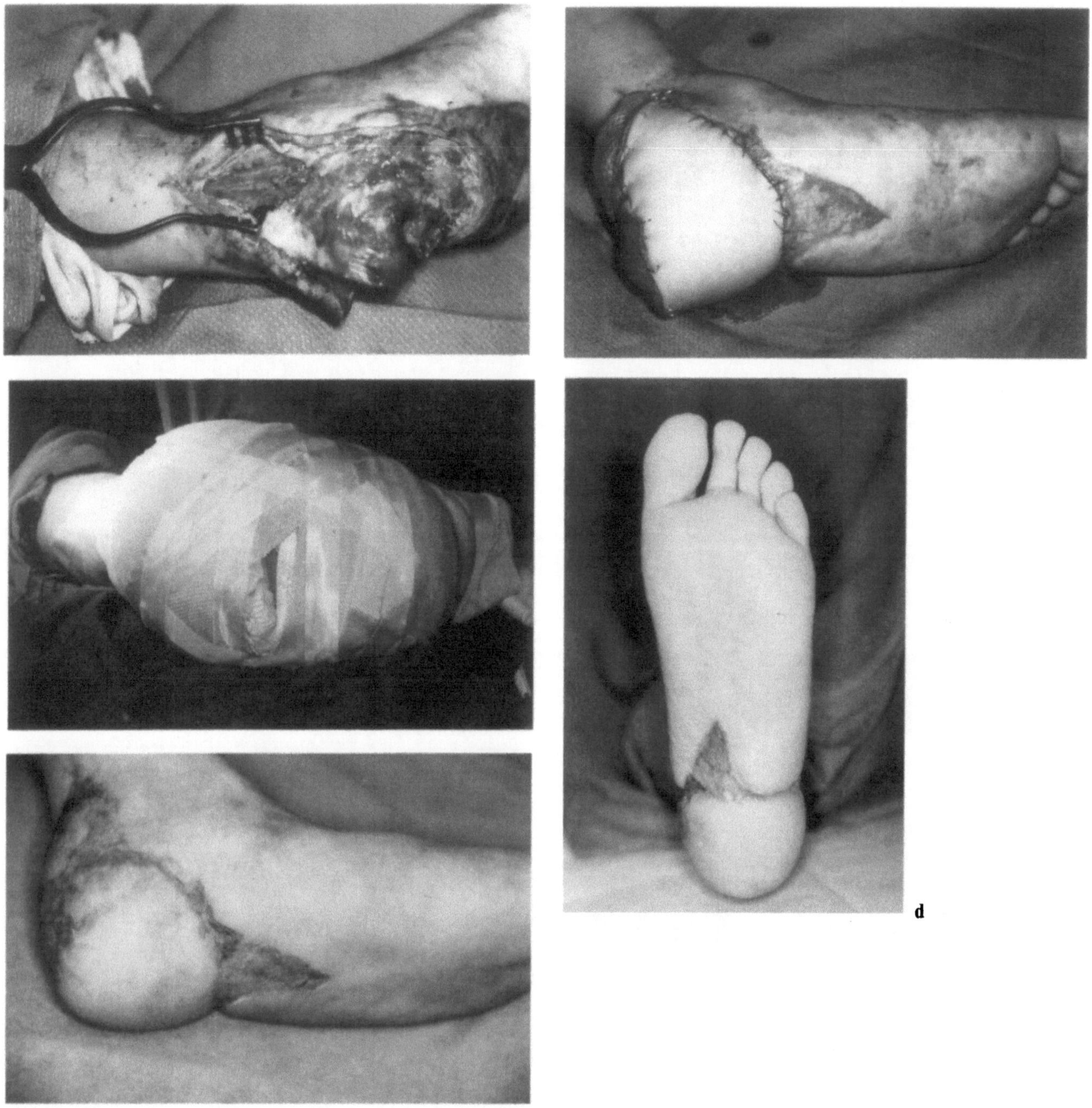

Fig. 1-18. a. A 22-year-old sailor sustained an avulsive injury to the heel which subsequently became infected. The wound was debrided and the posterior tibial artery and accompanying veins were dissected as recipient vessels. **b.** A latissimus dorsi musculocutaneous transplant was used, with the muscle filling the dead space and the cutaneous portion providing cover over the heel. **c.** A window through all levels of the dressing allowed the vascularity of the transplant to be monitored postoperatively. **d** and **e.** One year later the transplant had atrophied considerably, providing good contour. The patient is able to walk normally with special footwear. (I thank Charlotte Alexander, M.D., Oak Knoll Naval Hospital, who was the cosurgeon on this procedure.)

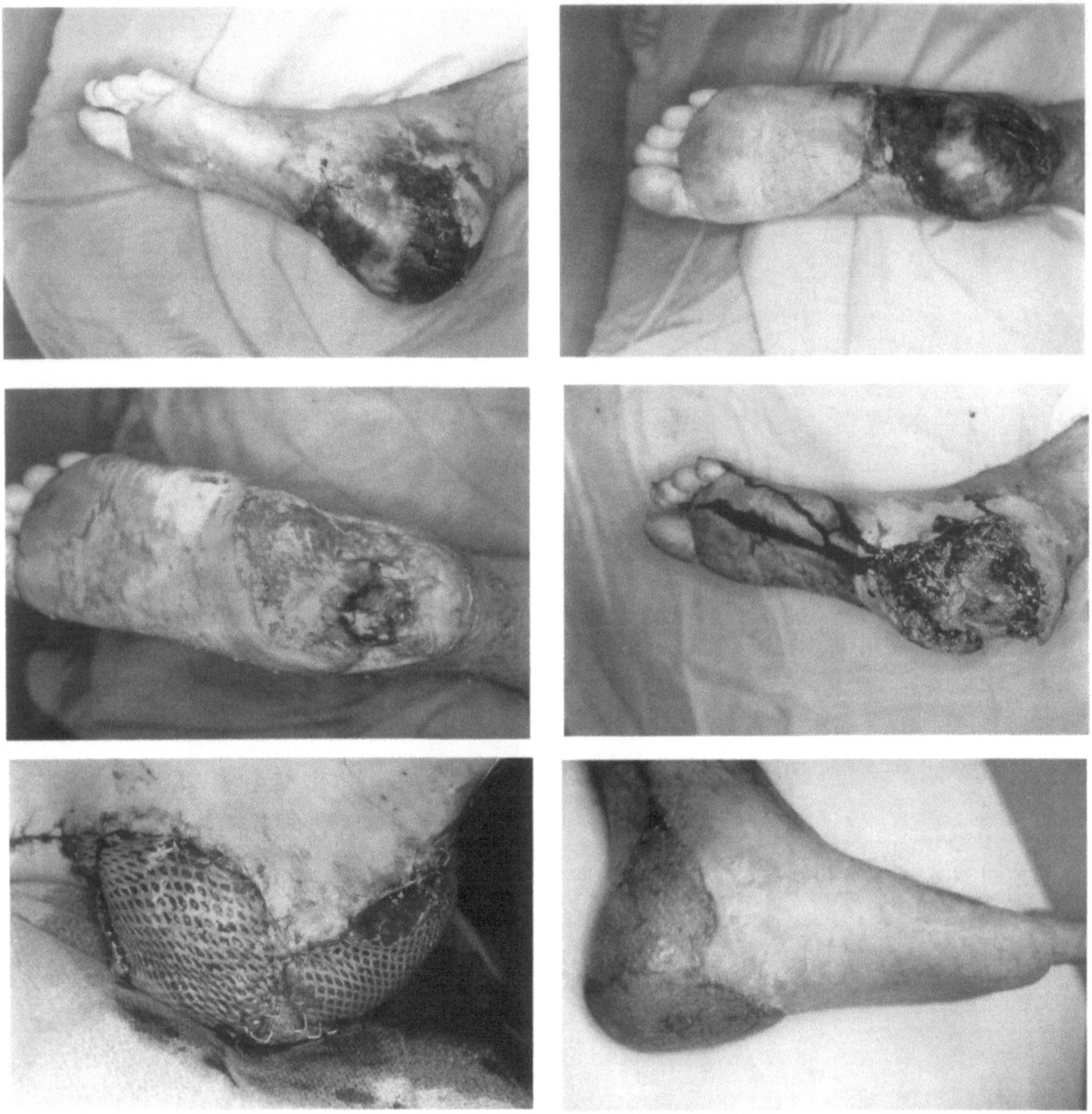

Fig. 1-19. a and **b.** A forklift crushed the heel of this laborer and also caused an underlying fracture of the calcaneus. The heel initially appeared viable but became necrotic 10 days later. (Necrosis of the heel only becomes evident after 7–10 days.) **c** and **d**. Debridement of the necrotic tissue left an extensive defect in the weight-bearing portion of the heel. **e.** The defect was covered with a latissimus dorsi musculocutaneous transplant. The cutaneous part was used over the heel, and the rest of the muscle was covered with a split-thickness skin graft. **f.** The contour is good, and the split-thickness skin graft on the weight-bearing part of the sole can be removed as the muscle atrophies. The patient is able to fully bear weight and walk without a limp, but occasionally has trouble with breakdown that requires him to stay off his heel. He found it necessary to change to a sedentary occupation.

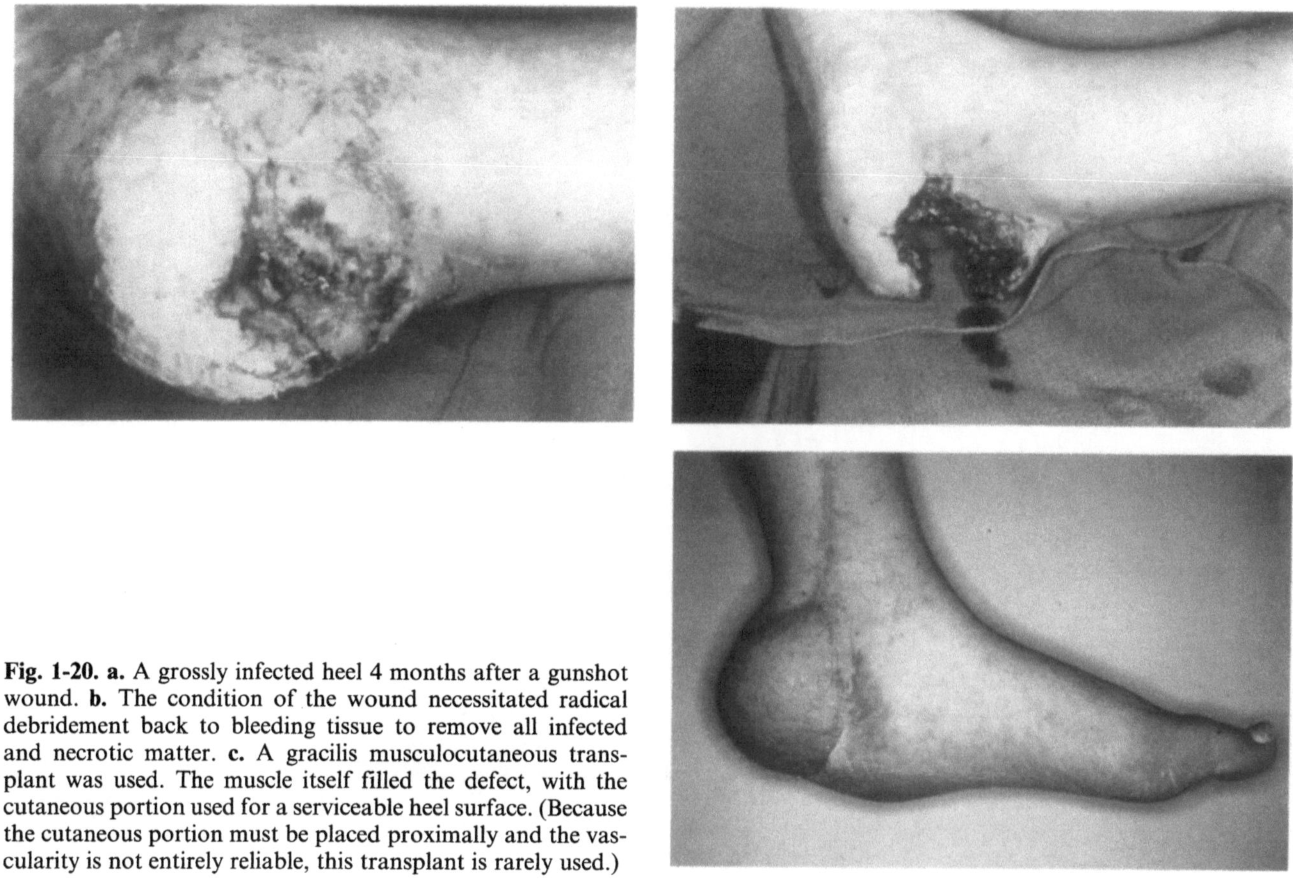

a b c

Fig. 1-20. a. A grossly infected heel 4 months after a gunshot wound. **b.** The condition of the wound necessitated radical debridement back to bleeding tissue to remove all infected and necrotic matter. **c.** A gracilis musculocutaneous transplant was used. The muscle itself filled the defect, with the cutaneous portion used for a serviceable heel surface. (Because the cutaneous portion must be placed proximally and the vascularity is not entirely reliable, this transplant is rarely used.)

1.2.1.6 Amputation Stumps (Sec. 6.1.6)

Short *below-knee or below-elbow amputation stumps* can be covered with a muscle or musculocutaneous transplant. Such cover obviates the need to shorten a stump that is already too short. It is very important to save the knee or elbow joint and make a below-elbow or below-knee prosthesis possible (Fig. 1-22).

1.2.1.7 Complex Wounds

When wounds involve the loss of several different tissues, such as muscle, bone, and nerve, a decision must be made as to whether extremity salvage is wise. This decision partly depends on whether a muscle transplant can achieve vascularized cover without the complication of infection. Extremity salvage may not be appropriate if there is loss of bone and muscle in the presence of infection, especially with gram-negative organisms. For this reason, in such complex wounds, I prefer to treat the problem in stages. First, muscle tissue is used to achieve a healed wound. If no infection is present, vascularized or conventional bone grafting is done 2–3 months later (Chapter 3). Attempting to reconstruct the entire area with simultaneous bone and muscle transplantation is risky and will often fail because of infection and poor healing.

1.2.1.8 Wounds in High-Risk Patients

Whereas conventional solutions are often doomed to failure if not impossible, muscle transplantation can frequently salvage an extremity in "high-risk" clinical situations. To do so, great care in preoperative planning is essential. Some patients who could be considered as high risk are those who are morbidly obese (Fig. 1-23), diabetic, and those who have sickle cell disease (Fig. 1-17). Also in this category are the elderly (Fig. 2-3), the infirm, and those who have a serious illness but need rapid and effective cover to allow them more mobility. None of these factors contraindicate microvascular procedures. Careful judgement is important because major surgery may be too risky. At times, however, microsurgical alternatives are the simplest and best method of mobilizing such patients.

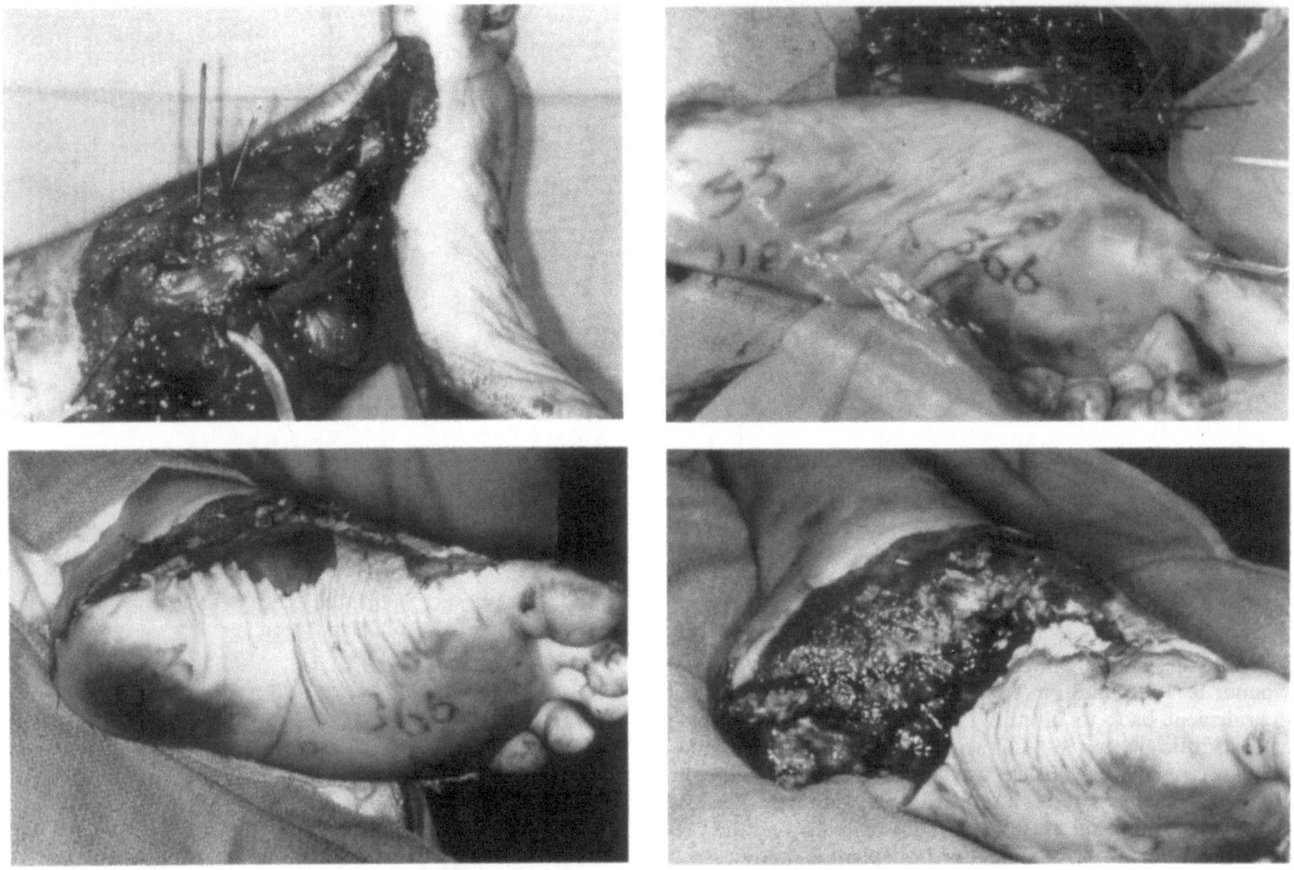

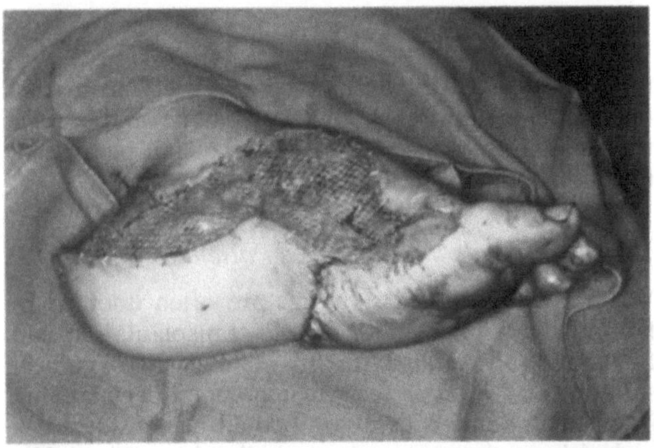

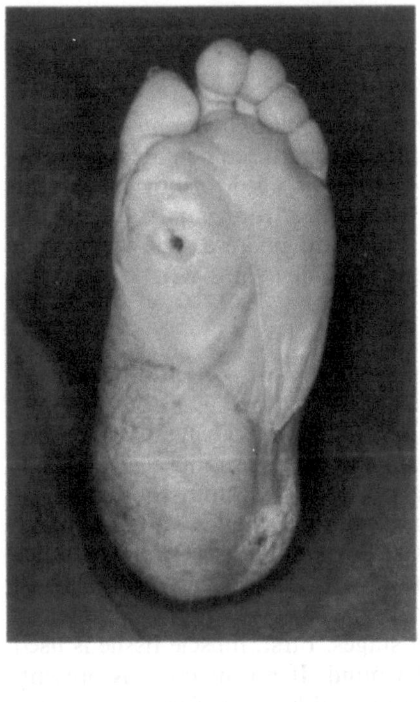

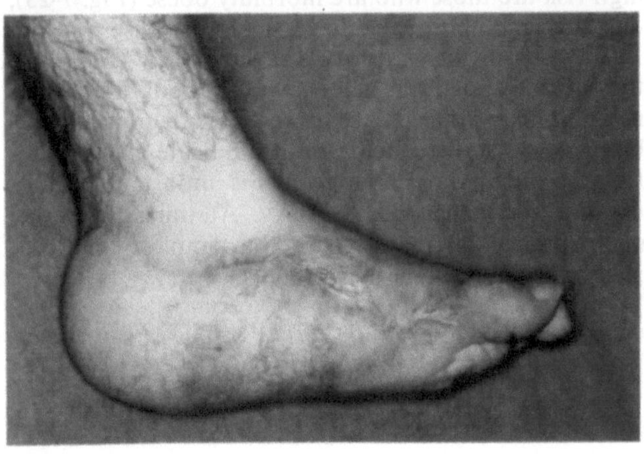

a b c d e f g

Fig. 1-21. a. The entire heel of this 21-year-old man was avulsed in a motorcycle accident. Revascularization was not possible because of damage to the plantar vessels. **b.** The amount of heel that would survive was initially unknown, although the heel appeared to have reasonable vascularity. The dermal fluorimeter was used in an attempt to provide

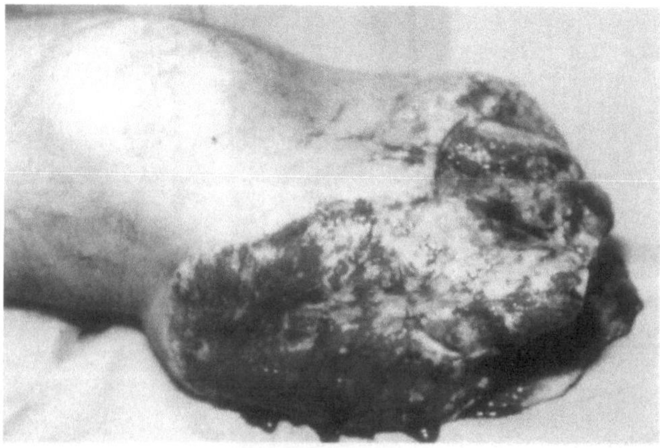
a

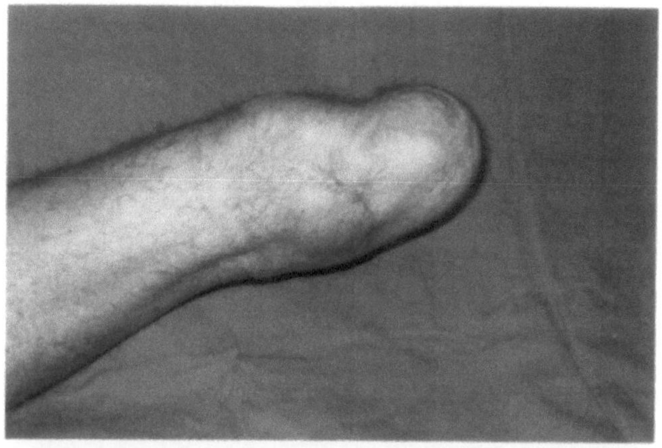
b

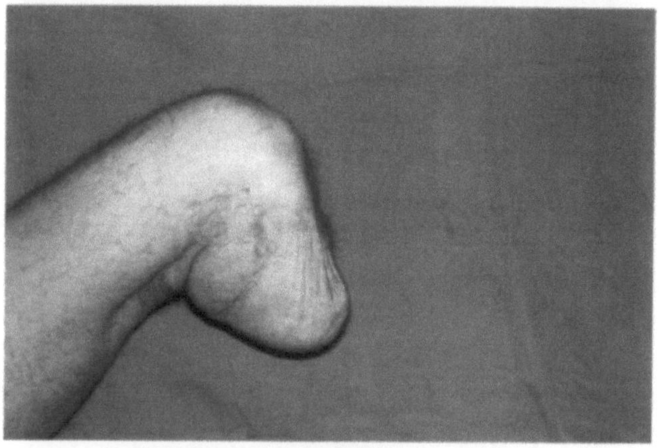
c

Fig. 1-22. a. This 38-year-old man was involved in a logging accident in which his right leg was crushed and amputated below the knee. The short below-knee bone stump had a sagittal fracture without extension into the knee, and the soft tissues were severely crushed. After thorough debridement, a latissimus dorsi musculocutaneous transplant was used to cover the amputation stump. Because the patient had severe injuries to his other leg, salvage of the knee joint was particularly desirable. **b** and **c.** Good cover was achieved but the flap became redundant and there was breakdown over the split-thickness skin-grafted portion. Two debulking procedures were necessary, and a tissue expander was used to bring both the medial and lateral skin over the amputation stump so that it was covered almost entirely with full-thickness skin. The patient regained 90° of knee motion and is able to wear a below-knee prosthesis without difficulty or limp.

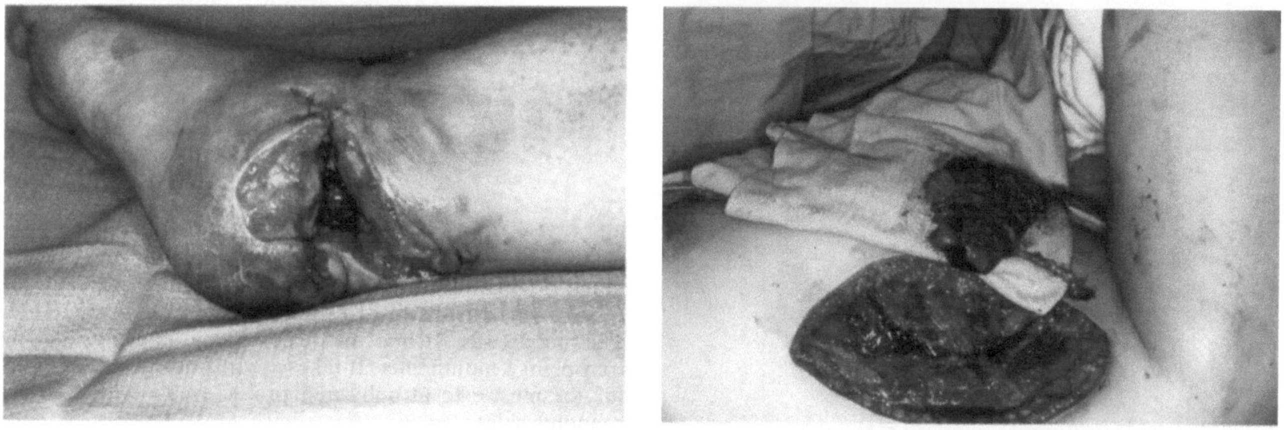
a b

Fig. 1-23. a. A morbidly obese teenager had fractured femurs and other injuries after a car accident. This chronically infected wound of the ankle with calcaneal osteomyelitis needed debridement and filling of the defect with good vascularized tissue. Although it was not large, the wound was deep and would not heal. (The serratus anterior muscle is ideal for this type of problem.) **b.** The serratus anterior was harvested. Only the lowest two digitations were removed. Note the long vascular pedicle (Continued.).

◁

a prognosis. The readings before and after intravenous injection of 1 cc of fluorescein are shown. **c.** The flap was loosely sutured back into position. After approximately 8 days, the amount of necrosis in the heel could be assessed (see also Fig. 1-33). **d.** The necrotic skin was resected, leaving an extensive defect. **e.** A tensor fasciae latae musculocutaneous transplant was used to fill the defect and provide cutaneous cover. (It is important to place this transplant longitudinally if at all possible when used in the heel. If not, it will be bulky and contour will be poor.) Part of the transplant on the medial aspect of the foot was covered with a split-thickness skin graft. **f** and **g.** After debulking, the heel had good contour and cover. This patient was subsequently able to pass the mile run and other tests required to become a fire fighter. In a 4-year period, the patient experienced one episode of temporary breakdown, but the area healed spontaneously.

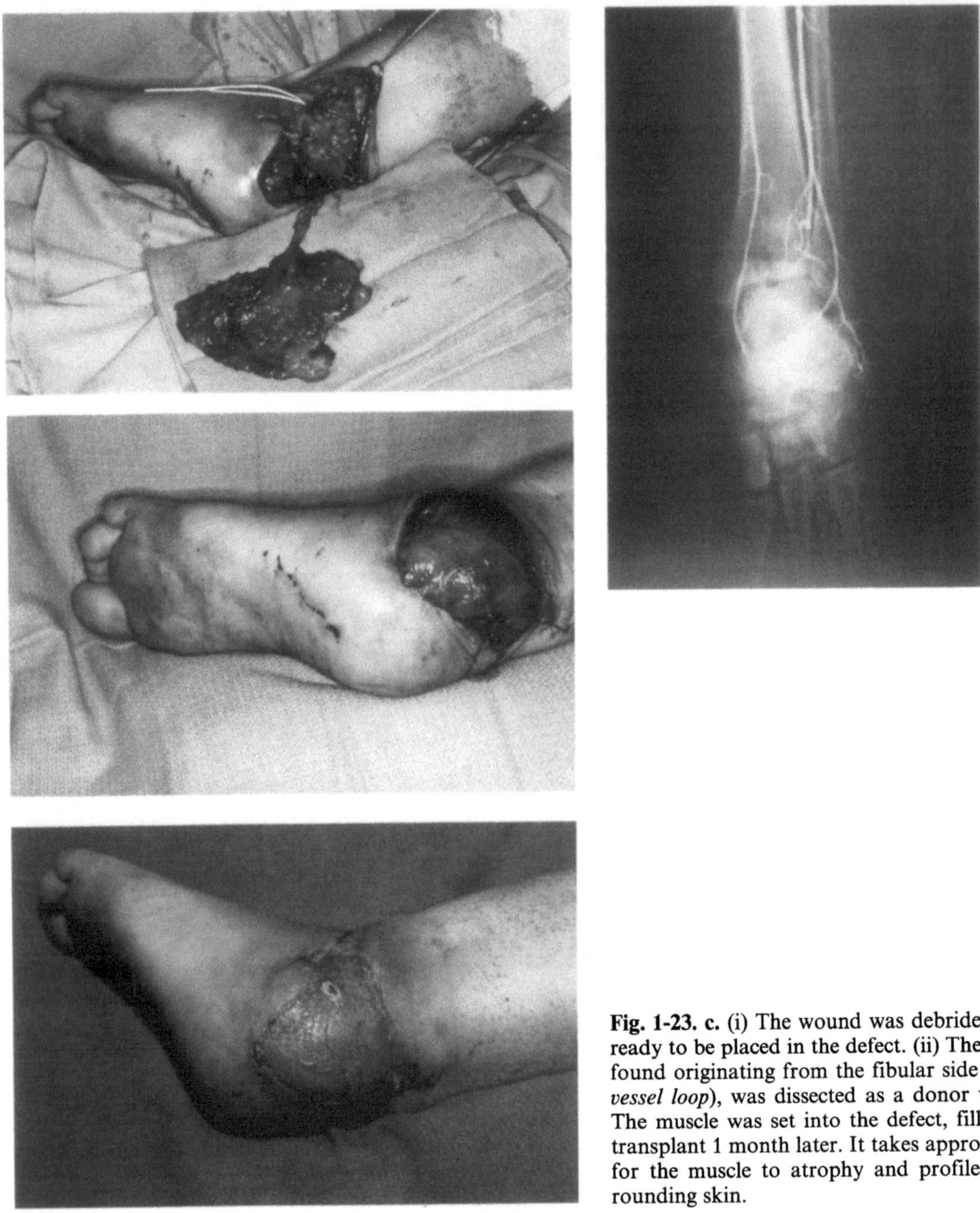

ci cii d e

Fig. 1-23. c. (i) The wound was debrided and the flap is seen ready to be placed in the defect. (ii) The anterior tibial artery, found originating from the fibular side in this patient (*in the vessel loop*), was dissected as a donor vessel (Plate 4-III). **d.** The muscle was set into the defect, filling its depths. **e.** The transplant 1 month later. It takes approximately 6–12 months for the muscle to atrophy and profile evenly with the surrounding skin.

1.2.2 Functional Muscle Transplantation

(Manktelow and McKee 1979, O'Brien et al. 1982)

The need for functional muscle transplantation arises where massive *muscle loss* has occurred, such as after Volkmann's ischemia or a crush, blast, or avulsive injury. This procedure is indicated only if no other tendon transfers are possible. Muscle transplantation cannot be used after severe nerve injuries (such as brachial plexus avulsions), as no recipient nerve will be available. The *finger flexors* are the muscle group most frequently substituted, but reconstruction of the *finger extensors* may occasionally be indicated using a functional muscle transplant. Following this procedure, the muscle can be expected to lose 30–50% of its original strength (Terzis et al. 1978), but enough strength and excursion will remain for functional range of motion of the fingers with useful pinch and grip. *Elbow flexion* is usually restored with the pectoralis major, latissimus dorsi, or forearm flexors. If none of these are available and a recipient nerve is present, a microvascular muscle transplant may then be used. Functional muscle transplanta-

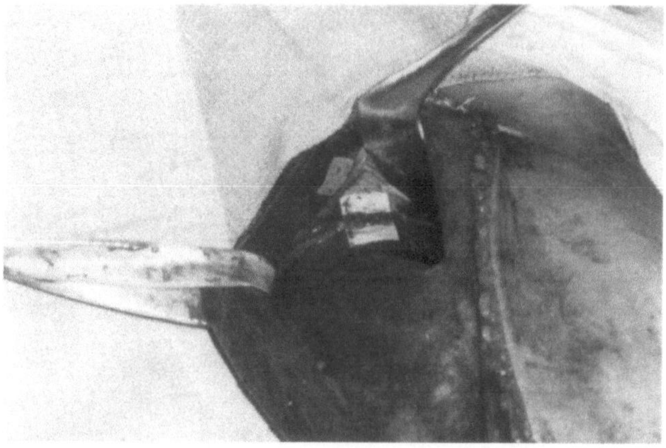

a

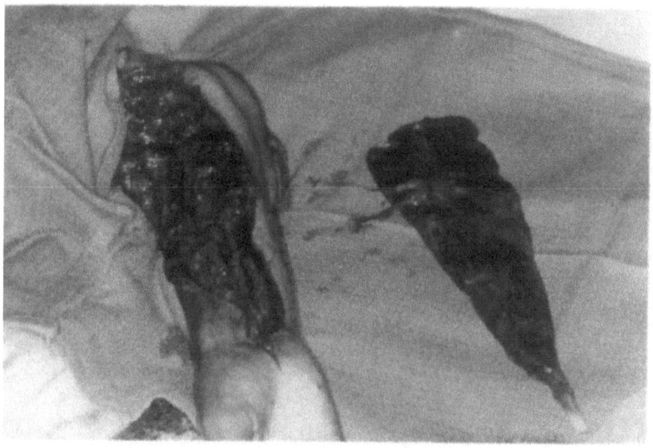

b

Fig. 1-24. a. The gracilis muscle has been dissected (*shown in the Penrose drain*). The adductor longus muscle is being retracted, and the vascular pedicle (*under the blue background*) can be seen coursing under this muscle to supply the gracilis. A pedicle measuring 7 cm has been dissected. The anterior branch of the obturator nerve (*under the yellow background*) superficial to the adductor brevis can be seen joining the vascular pedicle at the neurovascular hilus. **b.** The muscle has been removed and the proximal and distal tendons divided. The vascular and nerve pedicles are seen entering the muscle.

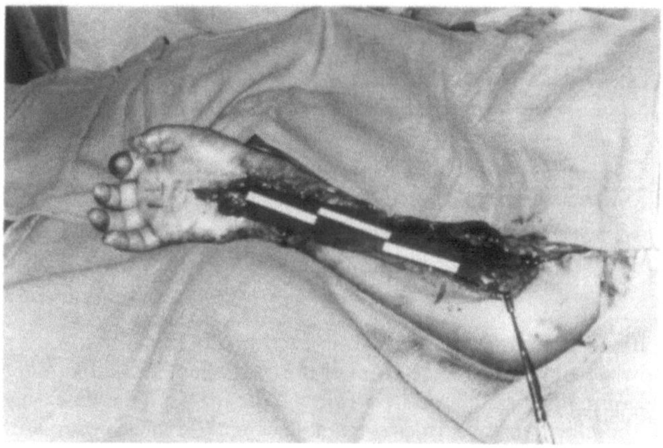

a

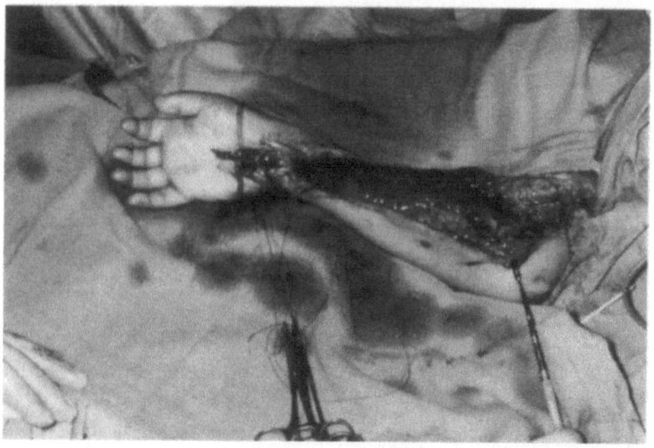

b

Fig. 1-25. a. This 8-year-old boy lost his right forearm flexor muscles after sustaining a supracondylar fracture and Volkmann's ischemia. The gracilis muscle can be seen in position. The proximal tendon (taken from the pubis) was attached to the medial epicondyle, and the distal tendon was attached to the flexor digitorum profundus tendons at the wrist. Next, the vasculature was restored, and the obturator nerve (supplying the gracilis) was sutured to the anterior interosseous nerve. **b.** It is important that the muscle fibers enjoy the same resting length in the transplant site as they did in the donor site. To ensure this, sutures or other markers should be placed every 5 cm along the muscle prior to dividing either of the tendons in the thigh. These markers should remain the same distance apart after the muscle has been sutured proximally and distally in the forearm. If adequate skin is present, the muscle is buried, but it will function just as well if covered with a split-thickness skin graft.

tion for *lower-extremity problems* has not been used with success. The excursion, size, and single nerve supply of the *gracilis* make this muscle useful as a substitute for long finger flexors and other muscles (Fig. 1-24). However, functional muscle transplantation depends on the presence of a recipient motor nerve. In the forearm, the anterior interosseous is the nerve most commonly used for this purpose (Fig. 1-25), but in some circumstances the motor fascicles of the ulnar nerve may be used.

Other muscles such as the latissimus dorsi and pectoralis major have also occasionally been used as functional muscle transplants. These are strong muscles but with less excursion than the gracilis. In rare circumstances, the slips of the serratus anterior can be used for both cover and restoring thumb opposition; in this situation, the recipient motor nerve used is the recurrent branch of the median nerve, which is repaired to the fascicles of the long thoracic nerve supplying the lowest digitations of the muscle (Fig. 4-8) (Gordon et al. 1984).

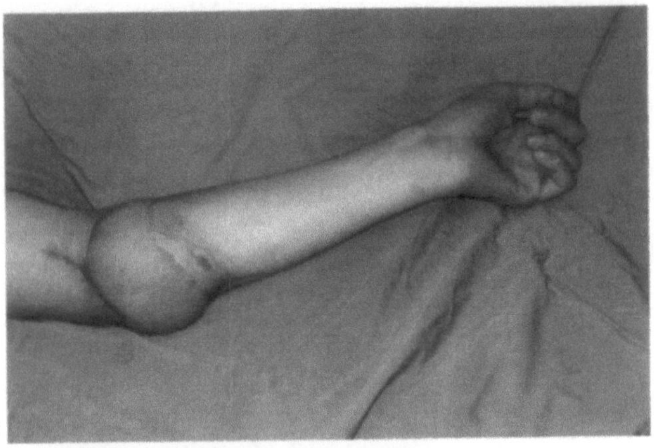

a

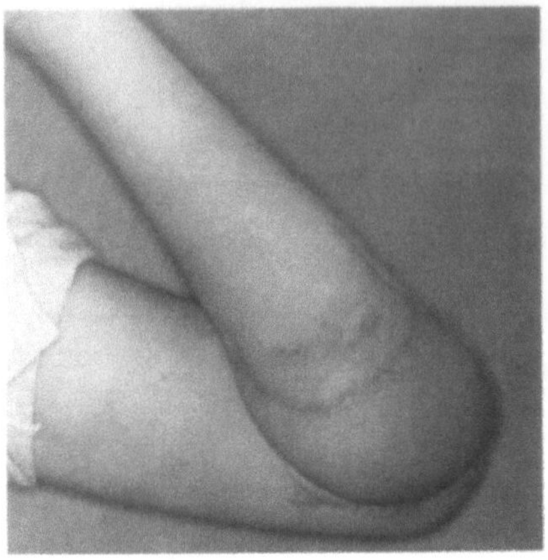

b

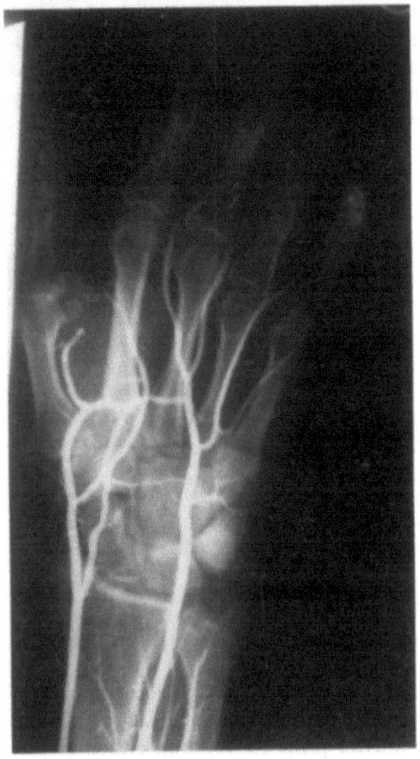

c

Fig. 1-26. a and **b.** A latissimus dorsi transplant was used in this patient to cover an extensive medial elbow wound that involved loss of the medial collateral ligament and part of the elbow joint. The cutaneous portion of the transplant was used to cover the region of the elbow crease to prevent later breakdown. Subsequent nerve grafting was done under this flap. **c.** The arteriogram showed the presence of *separate* radial and ulnar arterial supplies to the hand. For this reason, the radial artery could not be used in retrograde fashion as a recipient artery (see Chapter 7).

1.3 Choice of Muscle Transplant

The *pedicle* of any reliable muscle transplant must have a constant anatomic location and be the dominant vascular supply to the muscle (Mathes and Nahai 1981). Transplantation is considerably easier if the length and diameter of the pedicle is large; preferably, it should average 2 mm in external diameter and be long enough to allow positioning of the anastomosis away from the zone of injury. Each of the four muscle transplants described in this chapter have these features. The dimensions of the vessels supplying these flaps are given in Table 1-1.

The latissimus pedicle consists of the thoracodorsal artery and a single large and patulous vena comitans. The latissimus dorsi is composed of a large amount of muscle tissue, and when the artery is anastomosed to a major vessel in the lower extremity, the inflow and outflow are great. The somewhat sclerotic veins of the lower extremity may not dilate sufficiently to

Table 1-1. Vessel parameters of various muscle transplants.

Transplant	Length (cm)	Artery diameter (mm)	Vein diameter (mm)
Latissimus dorsi	6	2	2.0–2.5 (one only)
Gracilis	5	1.5	1.0–1.5 (two veins)
Serratus anterior	10	2	2.0–2.5 (one only)
Tensor fasciae latae	4	2	1.5–2.0 (two veins)

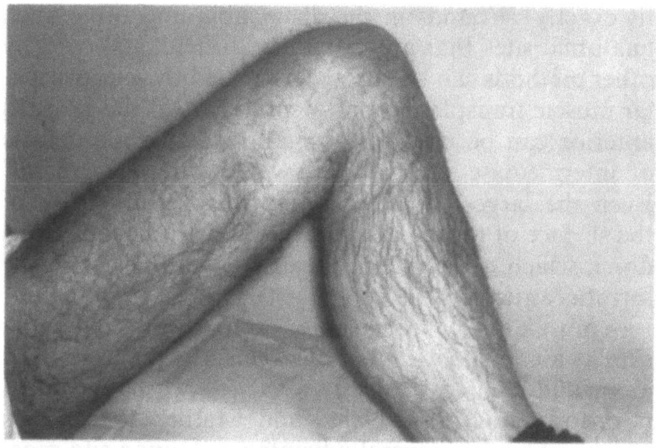
a

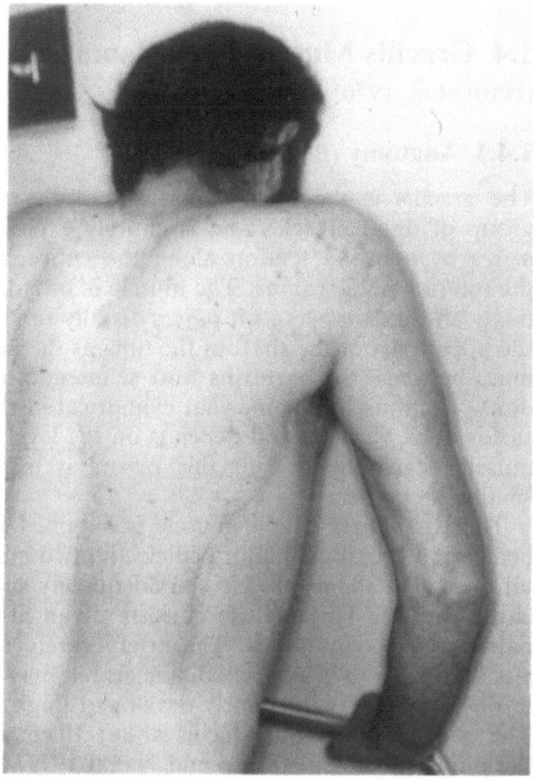
bi

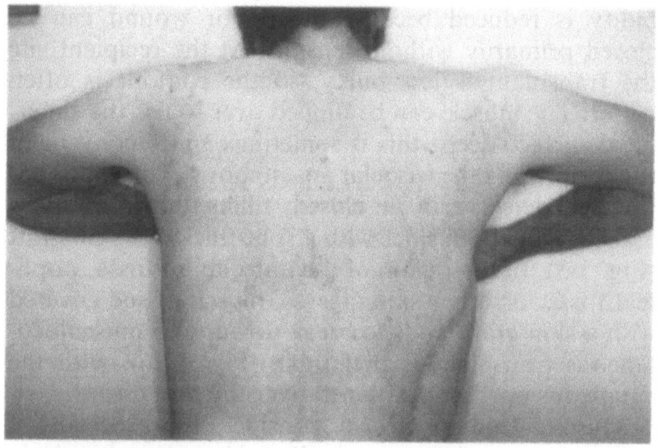
bii

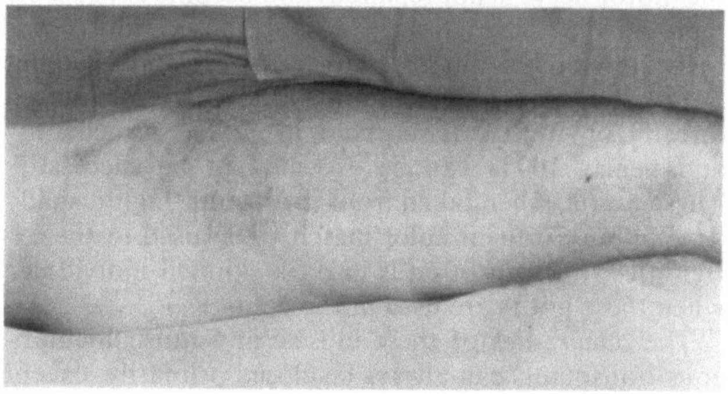
c

Fig. 1-27. a. The donor site following excision of the *gracilis transplant* is inconspicuous and situated on the medial aspect of the thigh. **b.** (i) A contour defect may result at the *latissimus dorsi donor site* in muscular individuals, but it is in a fairly inconspicuous location. (ii) The donor site of the *serratus anterior* is similar to that of the latissimus dorsi, but there is no contour defect. A mild amount of scapular winging can occur but is not functionally significant. **c.** The donor site following excision of the *tensor fasciae latae transplant* can usually be closed primarily with an excellent cosmetic result. If it is too wide, split-thickness skin grafting is required and the appearance is poor because of the contour defect.

allow enough venous drainage, especially if there has been some venous disease; if that is the case, a smaller muscle transplant should be chosen if possible. Also in patients with chronic venous disease, the venae comitantes may have thinner, more dilatable walls, which would make them better recipient veins than those in the saphenous system. The serratus anterior pedicle is usually dissected proximal to the origin of the thoracodorsal vessels to provide a very long pedicle. The pedicle can also be used closer to the muscle where it consists of the serratus branch of the thoracodorsal vessel. The gracilis and tensor fasciae latae pedicles contain one artery and two venae comitantes (Table 1-1).

Variable size and shape are among the greatest virtues of muscle transplantation (Fig. 1-1). The appropriate size muscle can be chosen and then contoured to the form of the defect being treated. Muscle size varies with the stature of the individual. For example, older female patients have small gracilis muscles. In an average individual, the gracilis is approximately 5×20 cm; the latissimus dorsi, 15×25–30 cm; the serratus, 2×8 cm for each digitation (a total of three digitations may be used); and the tensor fasciae latae, 8×25 cm.

When choosing the size of transplant needed, one should take into account (1) that further debridement may be required at the time of surgery; (2) the location of the vascular anastomosis, which must be outside the zone of injury; and (3) the volume of dead space to be filled. One should choose a muscle slightly larger than the defect so that the muscle can be trimmed to fit exactly. Wounds in the distal tibia and other such anatomic sites that are extremely difficult to cover by other methods can be effectively treated by microvascular muscle transplantation. A small part of the serratus anterior can be used for a small defect, while defects of intermediate size can be covered with the gracilis. Even the largest of defects involving the majority of the surface of the leg can be covered with the latissimus dorsi, which, as mentioned, can be combined with the serratus anterior.

A muscle can be transplanted along with its overlying skin as a *musculocutaneous transplant*, or it can be used alone and then covered with a *split-thickness skin graft* (Gordon et al. 1984, Nahai and Mathes 1984). This latter option has several advantages. Donor site morbidity is reduced because the donor wound can be closed primarily without tension. At the recipient site the transplant is less bulky, so the contour is often better. The muscle can be flipped over to use the superficial surface deep; this is sometimes more convenient for performing the vascular anastomosis. Through-and-through defects can be closed, filling the dead space and covering both sides with a split-thickness skin graft (Fig. 3-3). In the region of the antecubital fossa, popliteal fossa, or other skin creases, muscle tissue covered with a skin graft tends to break down, so a musculocutaneous transplant is preferable (Fig. 1-26), with the cutaneous portion positioned over the skin crease.

Muscles tend to *atrophy* considerably (especially if the motor nerve is not repaired) and become extensively replaced by fibrous tissue. Initially the contour tends to be too bulky, but it "settles down" and becomes flat over the next 6 to 12 months. The *skin grafts* placed directly on muscle tissue tend to "take" excellently, and nearly 100% can be expected to be successful. These grafts, when taken from the lateral thigh, usually develop an excellent color match when used in the extremities; one exception is in dark-skinned individuals when these grafts are used in the palm.

The *donor sites* of these muscle and musculocutaneous transplants can always be closed primarily, except for that of the tensor fasciae latae; this transplant should be kept quite narrow to allow primary closure (Fig. 1-27). If that is not possible, skin grafting, which is quite unsightly, will be required. At a later date, a tissue expander can be used so that the skin graft can be removed (Sec. 1.6.2.2).

The *gracilis* is entirely expendable, as the rest of the adductor muscle group takes over its function. The gracilis incision is made on the medial aspect of the thigh and is well concealed.

Removal of the *latissimus dorsi* produces a contour defect in muscular individuals, but one that is not very noticeable. The scar on the lateral chest is inconspicuous. Except in some avid athletes, removal of the latissimus dorsi is unlikely to result in any noticeable weakness, and even patients who swim regularly have not experienced a significant problem.

The *serratus anterior* scar is inconspicuous and similar to that of the latissimus dorsi. The lowest digitations are removed, retaining the integrity of the nerve supply to the upper six digitations and, therefore, muscle function. There is usually a minor amount of scapular winging on very careful scrutiny, but experience has shown that patients have no symptoms following this transplant.

Following *tensor fasciae latae* transplantation, there is no detectable motor functional deficit, but the cosmetic problem can be substantial if skin grafting is needed.

1.4 Gracilis Muscle Transplantation

(Harii et al. 1976)

1.4.1 Anatomy (Plates 1-I and 1-II)

The gracilis is the most superficial of the adductor group of thigh muscles and is entirely expendable. It *arises* by a broad tendon along the entire length of the inferior pubic ramus. The muscle is broader proximally and then tapers as it passes distally to *insert* into the upper part of the shaft of the tibia as the pes anserinus, between the sartorius and semitendinosus tendons. The muscle is somewhat cylindrical in shape. Its size is quite variable and depends on the level of thigh muscle development. For this reason it is generally smaller in women.

The *vascularity* of the muscle is supplied by three pedicles: a proximal, major pedicle and two minor, distal ones. The *major pedicle* can adequately supply the entire muscle. This pedicle consists of an artery and paired venae comitantes. The artery rarely measures less than 1.5 mm in external diameter, but may be small in obese women with poorly developed thigh muscles. The pedicle enters the gracilis about 10 cm distal to the pubic tubercle (Mathes and Nahai 1979). It arises from the medial circumflex artery deep to the adductor longus muscle, and lies on the adductor magnus before entering the deep surface of the gracilis somewhat nearer its anterior than its posterior margin. It often divides into two branches – one ascending and one descending – before entering the gracilis. Pedicle length is 6-8 cm if taken back to the medial circumflex vessels. Along its course, it gives several branches to the adductor longus and other surrounding muscles.

The *obturator nerve* (L2–L4) exits the obturator foramen and divides into an *anterior* and a posterior branch which travel anterior and posterior to the adductor brevis muscle, respectively. The anterior branch then lies on the adductor magnus to join the vascular pedicle near its entry into the gracilis.

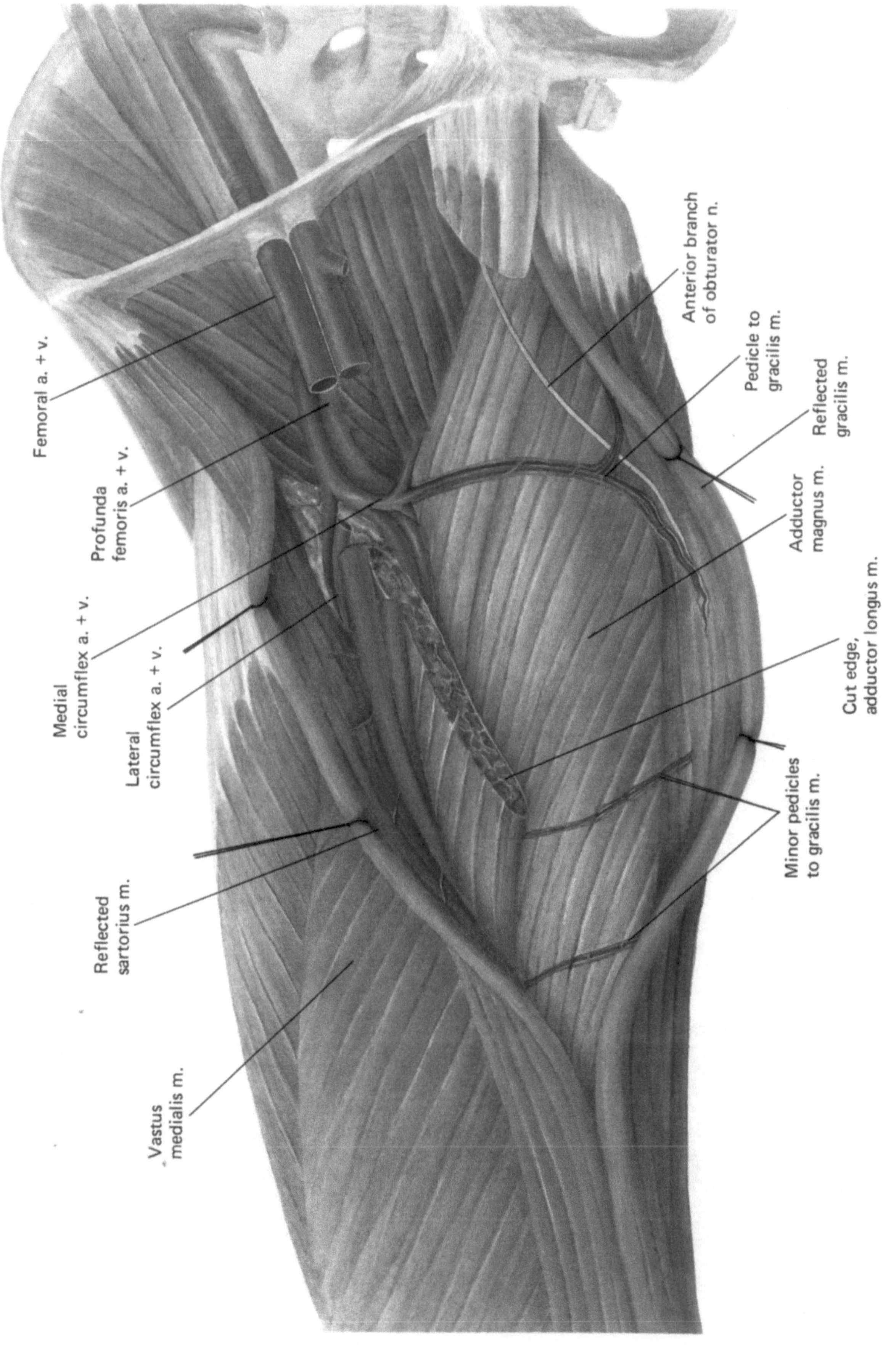

Plate 1-I. Anatomy of the gracilis muscle transplant.

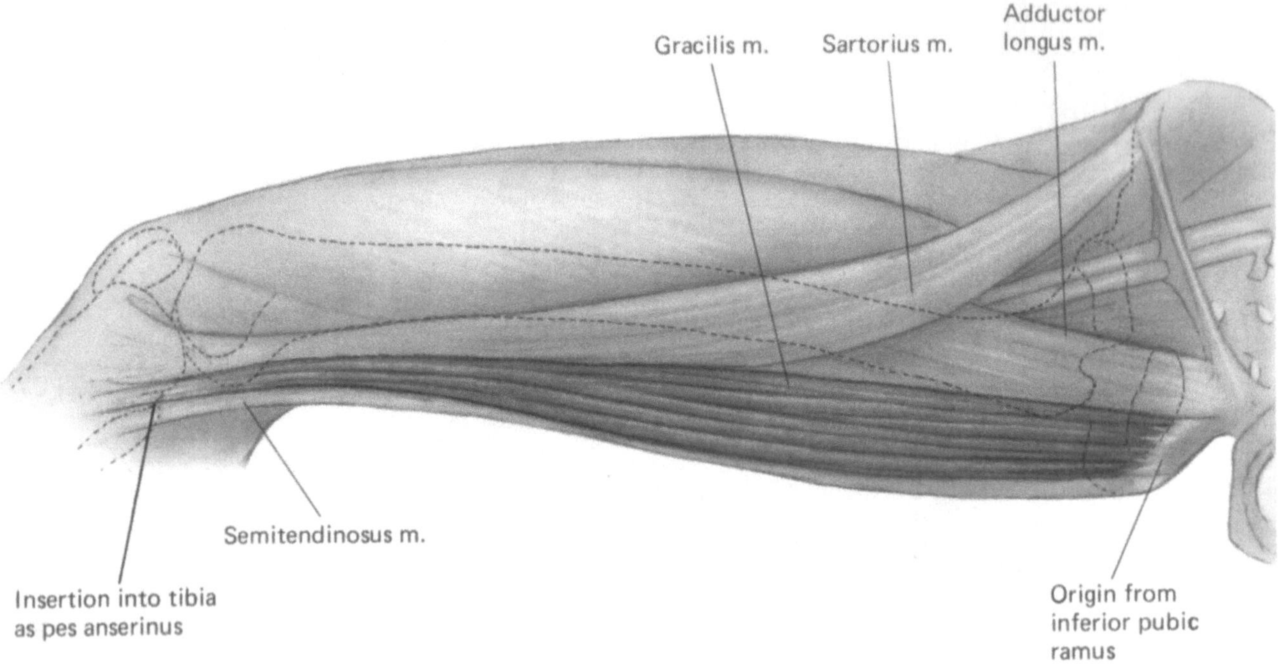

Plate 1-II. Origin, insertion, and relationships of the gracilis.

1.4.2 Surgical Technique

(Fig. 1-28; see also Fig. 1-15)

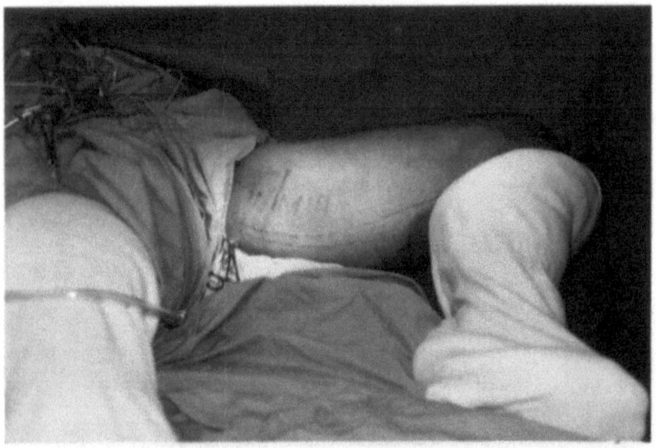

a

a. The position of the patient for dissection of the gracilis muscle is shown. The hip is abducted and externally rotated, and the knee is flexed, putting the gracilis muscle on stretch.

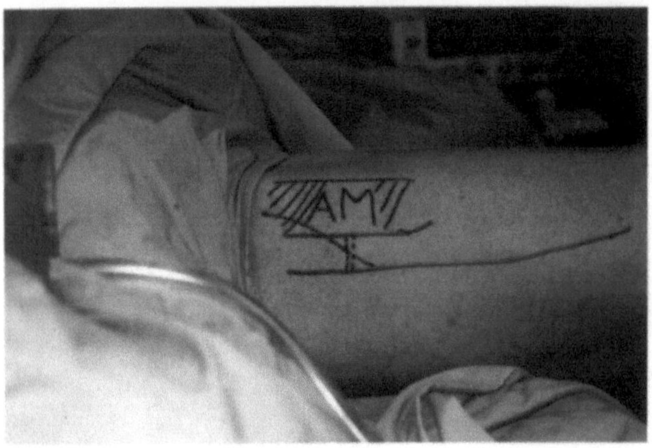

b

b. The proposed incision and relevant structures are outlined. The adductor longus muscle (AM) can be palpated as a firm band on the medial aspect of the thigh. The axis of the gracilis is parallel and 1–2 in. posterior to this band. (There is a tendency to make the incision too anterior.) The anticipated position of the vascular pedicle is marked approximately 10 cm from the pubic tubercle. The position of the anterior branch of the obturator nerve is also outlined.

c. The position of the gracilis muscle is identified, noting the direction of its fibers. The sartorius is more anterior, with fibers traveling proximally and laterally toward the anterior superior iliac spine. A Penrose drain is placed around the muscle distally. One of the two or three minor pedicles of the gracilis is shown here.

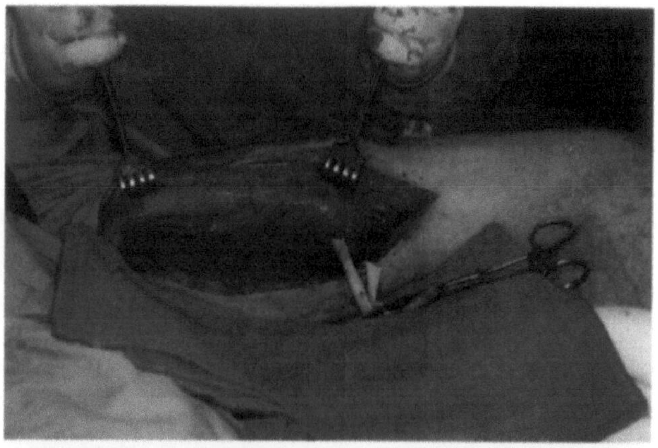

c

d. By lifting on the Penrose drain, the muscle is easily separated from the surrounding tissues by finger dissection, and the minor pedicles are divided.

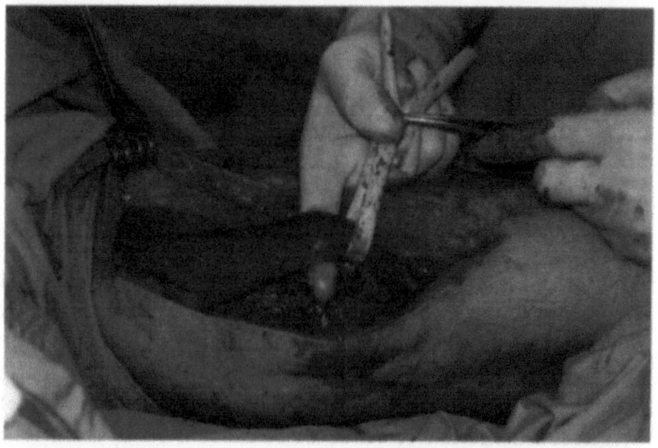

d

e. As dissection proceeds to the proximal third of the muscle, the vascular pedicle is encountered in its reliable position entering the muscle laterally. In this dissection the vessel loop is around the obturator nerve, and the clamp is under the vascular pedicle as it passes deep to the adductor longus.

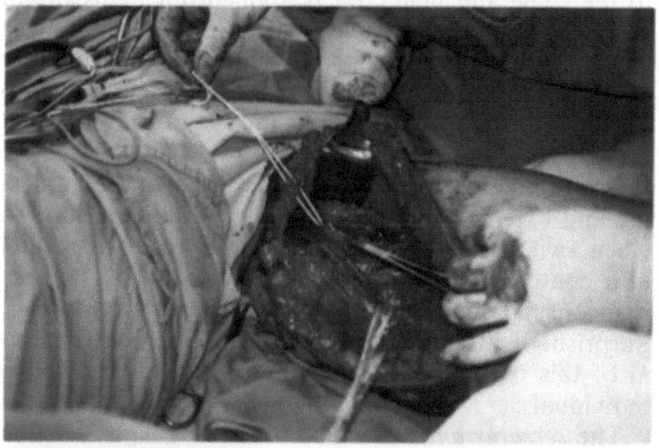

e

f. The pedicle is seen dissected. A large Richardson retractor is used to strongly retract the adductor longus muscle so that the pedicle can be dissected deep into the thigh; this provides a pedicle of 5 cm or longer. Small branches from the pedicle to the other adductor muscles are encountered which mostly travel anteriorly into the adductor longus. These branches are carefully ligated and divided to prevent troublesome bleeding as the pedicle is dissected. (Rather than "skeletonizing" the pedicle, it is easier to longitudinally incise the fascia over the adductor longus 1–2 mm away from the pedicle and let this fascia drop down toward the pedicle as increased pedicle length is dissected.)

It is not unusual for the pedicle to divide before reaching the anterior border of the gracilis. Care should therefore be taken to dissect both branches of the pedicle back to their common parent trunk. This pattern can usually be detected by noting the direction of the vessel's approach as it nears the muscle.

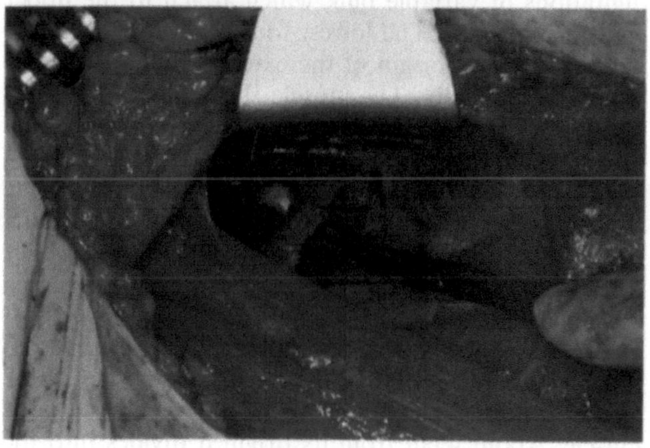

f

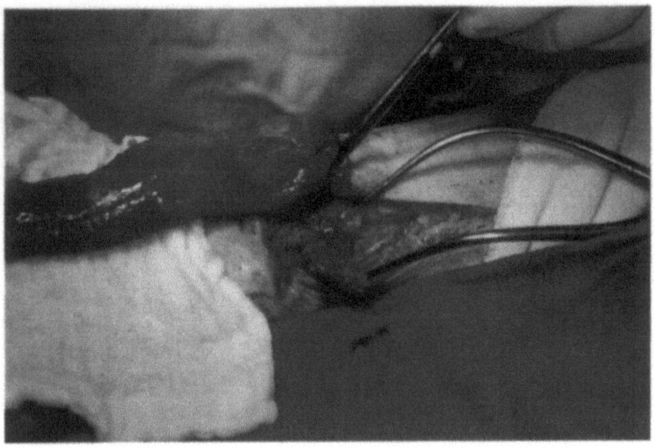

g

g. The proximal and distal tendons are divided, the pedicle is divided, and the muscle is transplanted to the recipient area. (It is important to have the recipient area completely dissected and ready for the transplant so that ischemia time is minimized.) The muscle is loosely sutured at a few points to avoid accidentally moving it during the vascular anastomoses.

1.5 Serratus Anterior and Latissimus Dorsi Muscle Transplantation

(Takayanagi and Tsukie 1982)

1.5.1 Anatomy (Plates 1-III to 1-V)

The *latissimus dorsi* is a broad, triangular muscle. It *originates* from the spinous processes of the lower six thoracic vertebrae and the posterior third of the iliac crest. Between these two attachments, it fuses with the thoracolumbar fascia, and can have muscular slips of origin from the lower three or four ribs. Its attachment to the spine and iliac crest is aponeurotic. This origin is the base of the triangle, and as the muscle passes to the apex at its insertion, it attaches to the inferior angle of the scapula. It has an elongated tendinous *insertion* into the intertubercular groove of the proximal humerus.

The latissimus dorsi is a medial rotator of the humerus, and extends the arm from the flexed position, as when swimming the crawl stroke. Its removal results in a contour defect in muscular individuals. The scar is inconspicuous but does have a tendency to spread. Surprisingly little functional deficit results from removal of this muscle, even in swimmers and other active individuals.

The *serratus anterior* muscle *arises* by eight or nine digitations of variable bulk which attach to the upper eight or nine ribs. The lowest four or five interdigitate with the slips of origin of the external oblique muscle, which pass distally. The muscle slips converge as they approach their *insertion*, passing deep to the scapula to insert into its entire medial border.

The serratus anterior keeps the scapula close to the thorax. It rotates the scapula in adduction and abduction of the arm. After removal of the lowest two or three digitations, there is very mild scapular winging but no significant functional deficit.

The *vascular supply* to both these muscles arises from the subscapular artery. This artery emanates from the axillary artery at the lower border of the subscapularis muscle. About 4 cm from its origin it divides into the circumflex scapular artery (Sec. 2.5.1) and the *thoracodorsal artery*. The thoracodorsal artery is accompanied by a single large vein. By ligating and dividing the branch to the latissimus dorsi, it can be used to vascularize the serratus anterior transplant. By ligating and dividing the branch to the serratus anterior, it vascularizes the latissimus transplant. If desired, both muscles can be transplanted simultaneously.

The thoracodorsal artery continues the general course of the subscapular artery, proceeding toward the latissimus dorsi, which it enters about 5 to 8 cm later. There, it divides into two branches running longitudinally. One travels within 2 to 3 cm of the anterior margin of the muscle, and the other runs just posterior to the midline of the muscle. The muscle can be split longitudinally between these two branches, maintaining adequate vascular supply to each (Fig. 1-30j). The latissimus dorsi is also supplied segmentally by minor pedicles from the intercostal and lumbar arteries which enter the deep surface of the posterior part of the muscle. The thoracodorsal artery has a single, patulous vena comitans.

Just before entering the latissimus dorsi, the thoracodorsal artery gives off a branch that passes onto the chest wall and runs on the *serratus anterior*. This artery travels longitudinally a few centimeters anterior to the lateral border of the scapula. The lateral thoracic artery also runs longitudinally on the serratus anterior but is more anterior, lying near where the muscle slips attach to the ribs anteriorly.

The *thoracodorsal nerve* (C7–C8), which serves the latissimus dorsi, is a branch of the posterior cord of the brachial plexus. It travels with the thoracodorsal artery.

The serratus anterior muscle is innervated by the *long thoracic nerve* (C–C7). This nerve arises from the roots of the brachial plexus in the neck, passes posterior to the plexus, and enters the axilla between the axillary artery and the serratus anterior. It then proceeds longitudinally down the muscle near the vascular pedicle. Its position may vary, but it is usually 1-2 cm anterior to the major vascular pedicle. Along its course, it sends small fascicles to each digitation as it crosses over them.

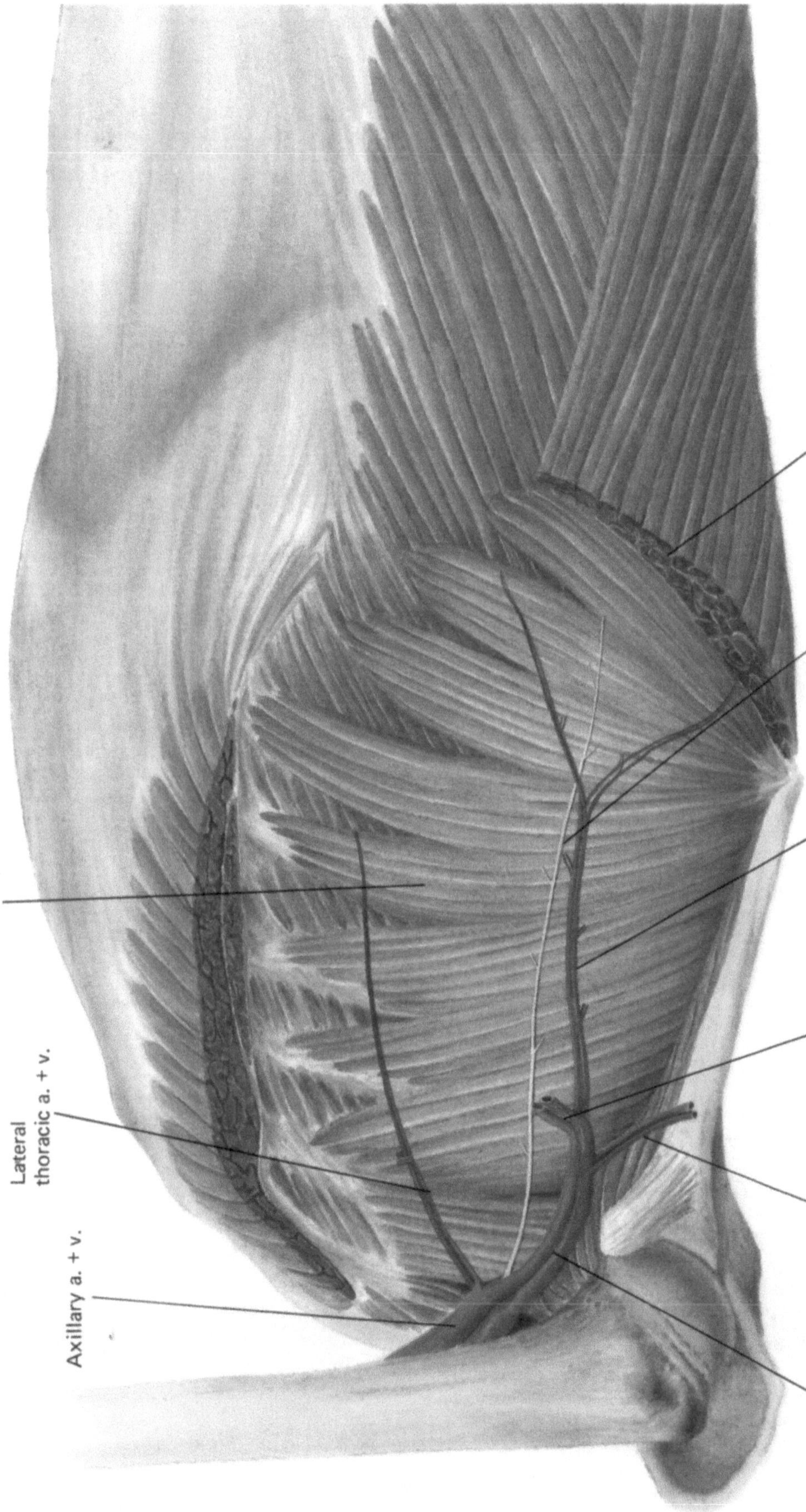

Plate 1-III. Anatomy of the serratus anterior muscle transplant.

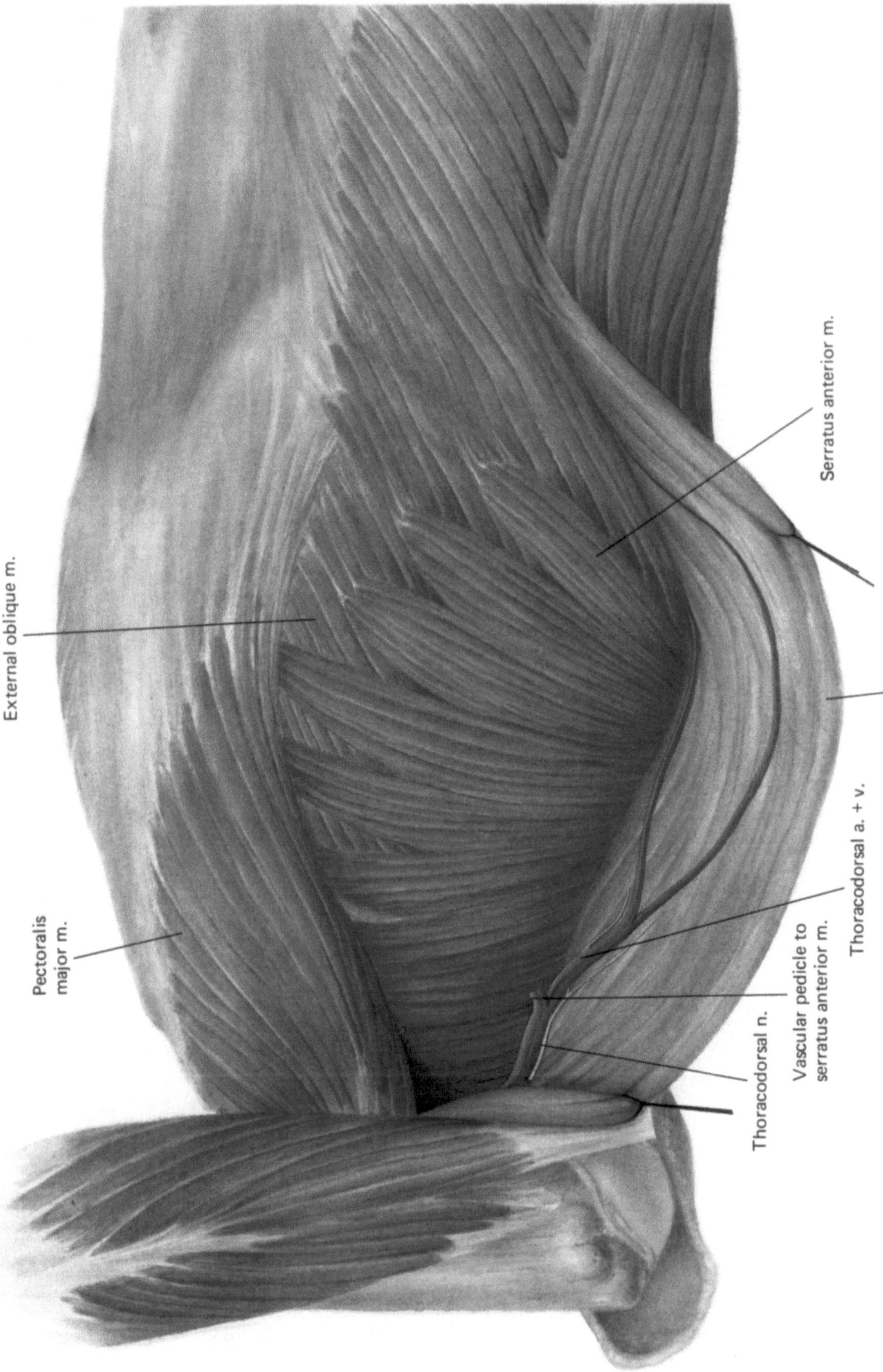

Plate 1-IV. Anatomy of the latissimus dorsi muscle transplant.

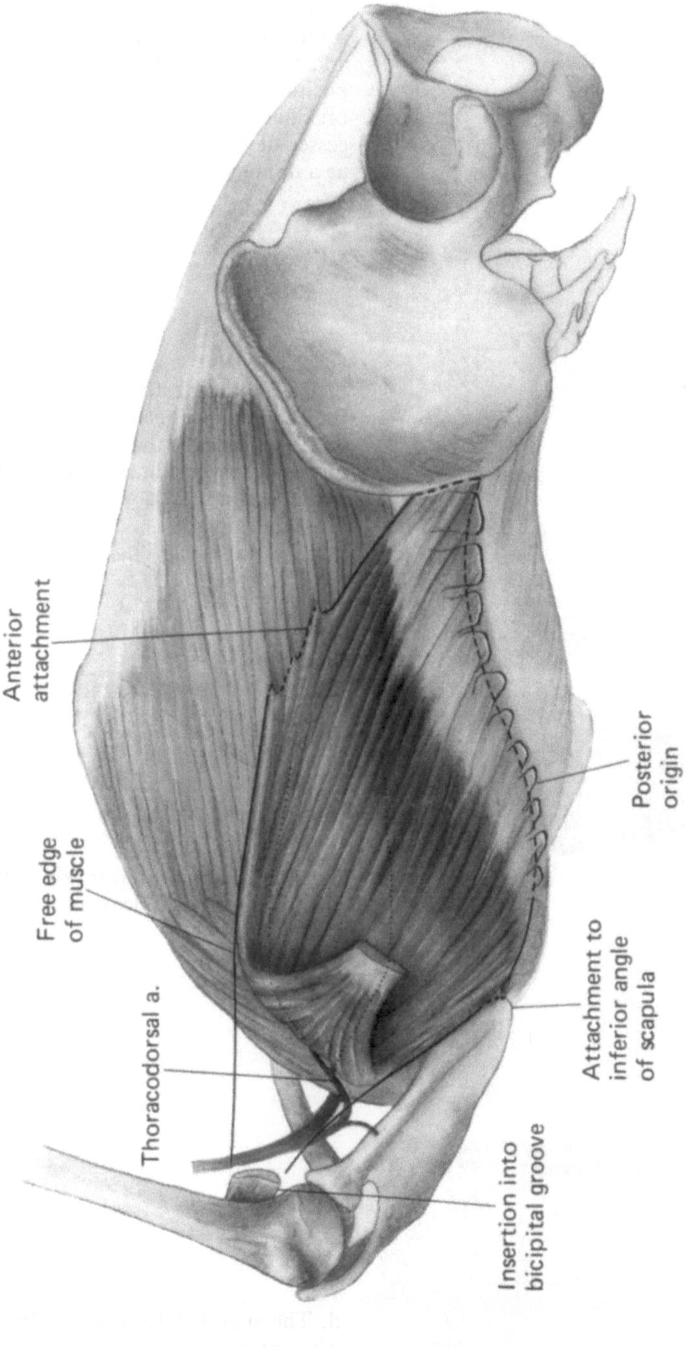

Plate 1-V. Origin and insertion of the latissimus dorsi.

1.5.2 Surgical Technique

1.5.2.1 Serratus Anterior Muscle Transplant (Takayanagi and Tsukie 1982) (Fig. 1-29; see also Fig. 1-12)

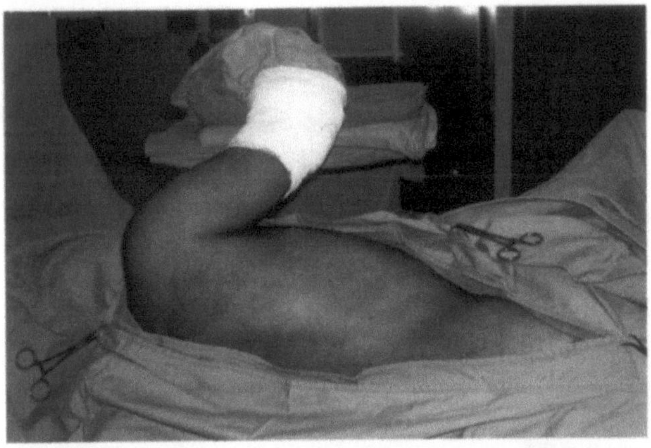
a

a. The patient is shown on the operating table in the lateral decubitus position, ready for either a serratus anterior or latissimus dorsi transplant. The entire extremity is draped free and rests on a well-padded Mayo stand. The surgeon should position the patient in a way that avoids stretching of the brachial plexus. The area prepared includes the spinous processes of the vertebrae; the thigh is included if it is needed as a donor site for a split-thickness skin graft.

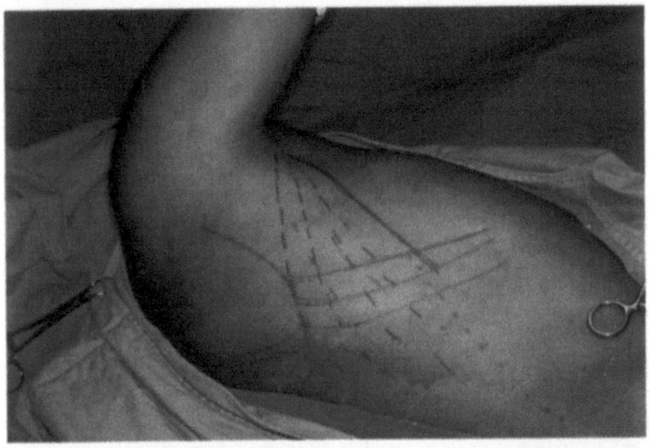
b

b. The important structures are marked. The dotted lines show the shape and direction of the fibers of the latissimus dorsi, which will overlie the lowest digitations of the serratus anterior (the transverse lines). The scapula is outlined. The incision is made about 2 to 4 cm behind the anterior margin of the latissimus dorsi.

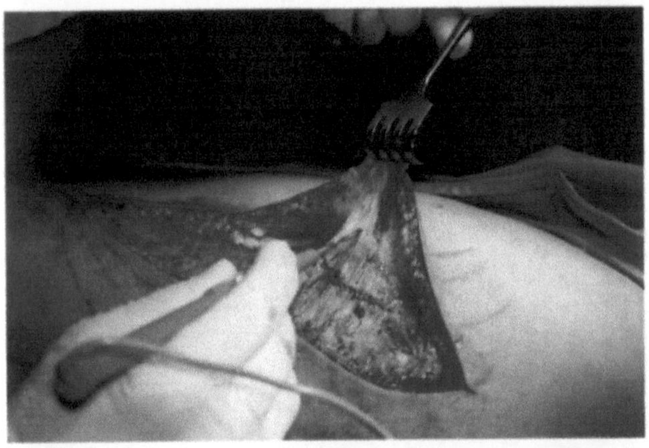
c

c. Anterior and posterior skin flaps are raised with the cutting electrocautery unit, leaving some fascia on the latissimus dorsi.

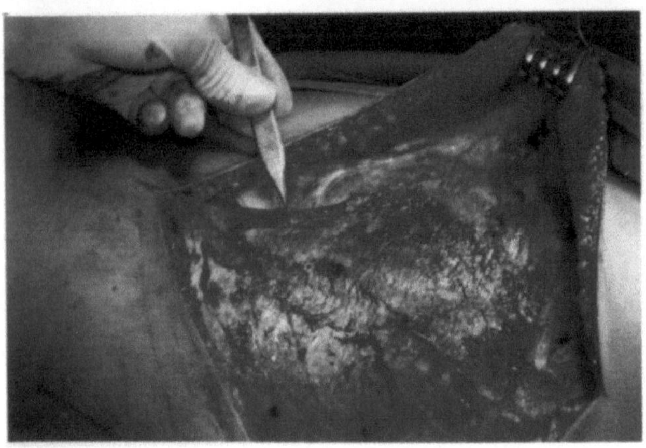
d

d. The superficial surface of the latissimus dorsi is exposed. The anterior margin of the latissimus dorsi is identified, here seen being held with the forceps.

e. Using gentle retraction, the latissimus dorsi is carefully elevated to reveal the digitations of the serratus anterior. The vascular pedicle is seen on the surface of the serratus anterior.

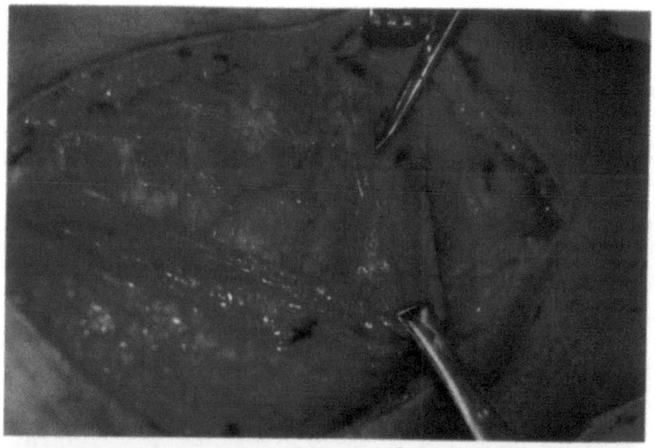

e

f. Once the lowest two or three digitations have been identified and the decision made as to how many digitations are to be included in the transplant, the muscle is carefully elevated from the surface of the ribs and chest wall. A finger is placed beneath the lowest three digitations which will be used in this patient.

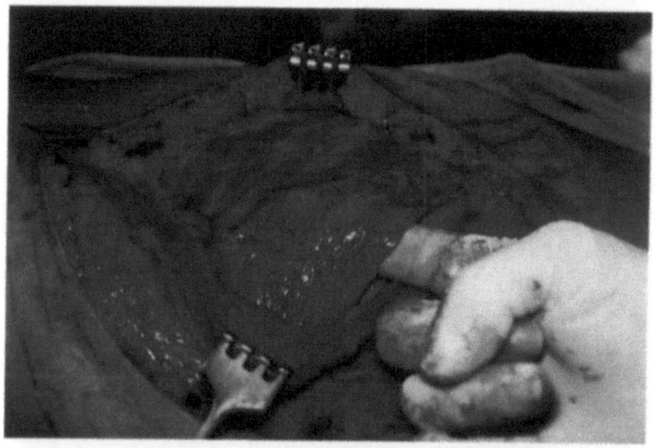

f

g. Next, the pedicle is dissected from the surface of the rest of the serratus anterior toward the axilla. As this is done, the soft tissue and fascia surrounding it are included to avoid any possibility of damaging the vessels. The pedicle is dissected proximally to the thoracodorsal artery. Additional length and larger vessel diameter can be obtained by ligating the thoracodorsal vessels which supply the latissimus dorsi. As stated earlier, the thoracodorsal artery is accompanied by a single large vein.

Care is taken in this dissection not to injure the long thoracic nerve, which usually lies 1 or 2 cm anterior to the pedicle; a nerve stimulator is useful to confirm its position. If the nerve to the lowest digitations is to be included in the transplant, the fascicles to these digitations must be separated from the rest of the nerve, leaving the supply to the remainder of the muscle intact.

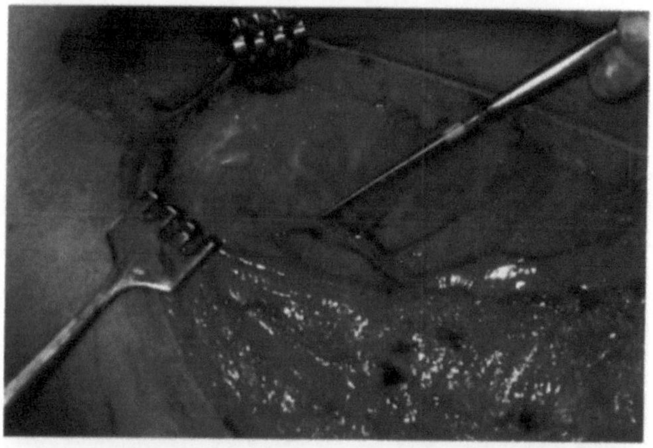

g

h. The lowest digitations are now separated anteriorly from their attachments to the ribs, and the muscle is divided posterior to the pedicle at a point which depends on the amount of tissue needed. The pedicle is dissected so that the muscle can be elevated in a cranial direction.

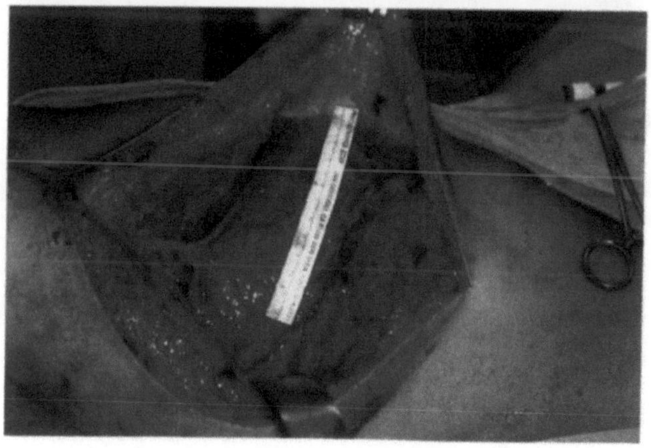

h

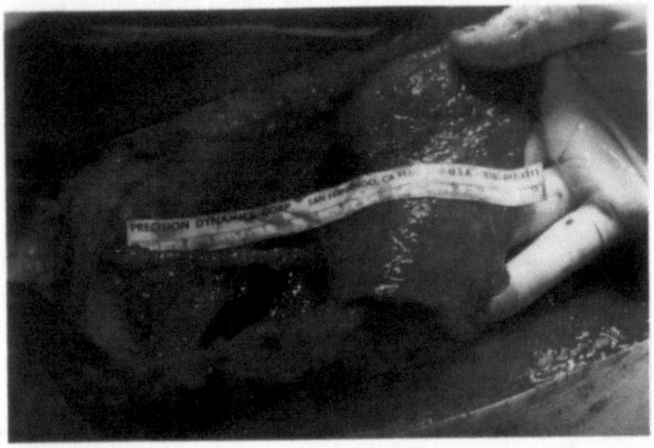
i

i. The muscle and pedicle are shown. The size of the muscle in this patient is 16 × 7 cm. The pedicle measures 8 cm in length.

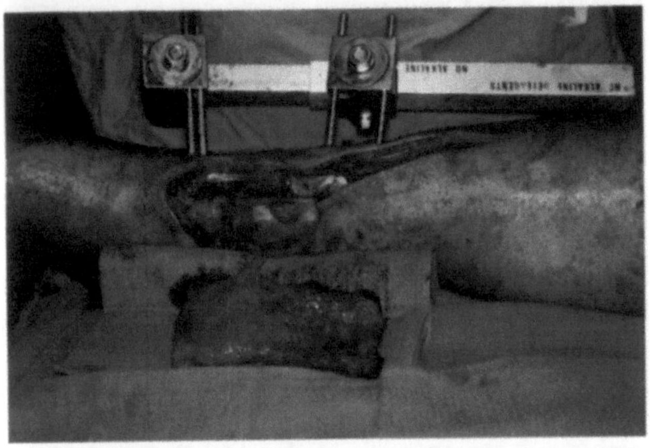
j

j. The muscle is transplanted to the leg once the anterior tibial vessels and recipient site have been prepared.

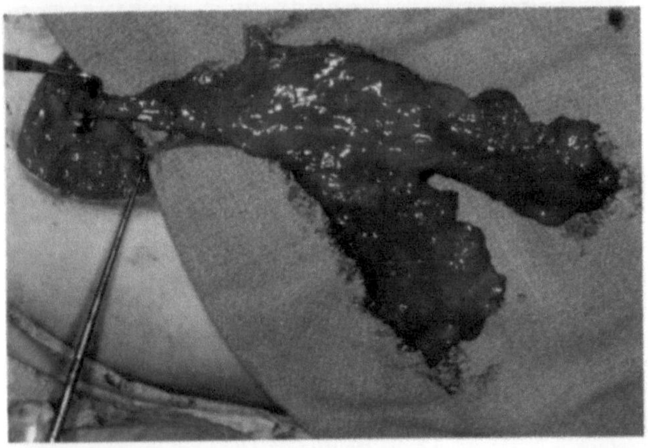
k

k. In another patient, the two digitations of the serratus anterior are shown separated. As stated earlier, this transplant is often useful in the hand where separated digitations can be placed in different locations (Fig. 1-5).

1.5.2.2 Latissimus Dorsi Muscle Transplant (Bailey and Godfrey 1982, Maxwell et al. 1979) (Fig. 1-30)

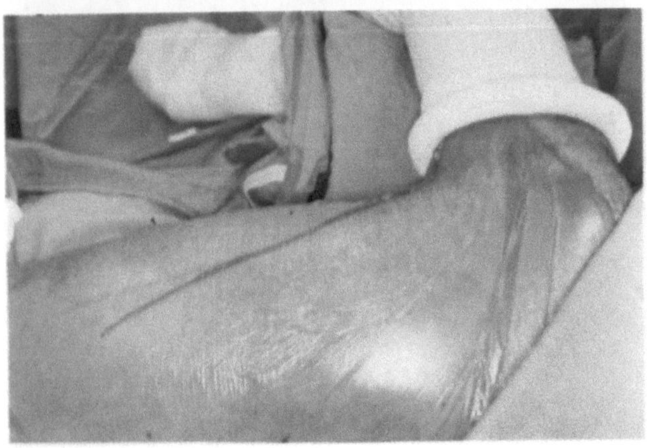
a

a. The patient is placed in the lateral decubitus position on a beanbag mattress; this position is similar to that in serratus anterior transplantation. The incision 3–5 cm posterior to the anterior margin of the latissimus dorsi is outlined.

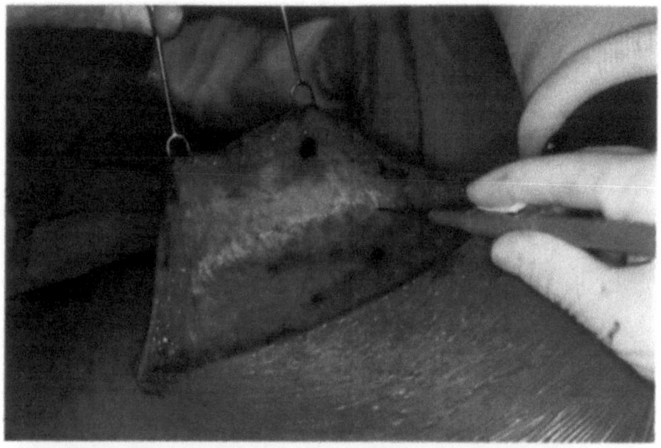

b. The incision is made, and anterior and posterior flaps are raised with the electrocautery unit.

b

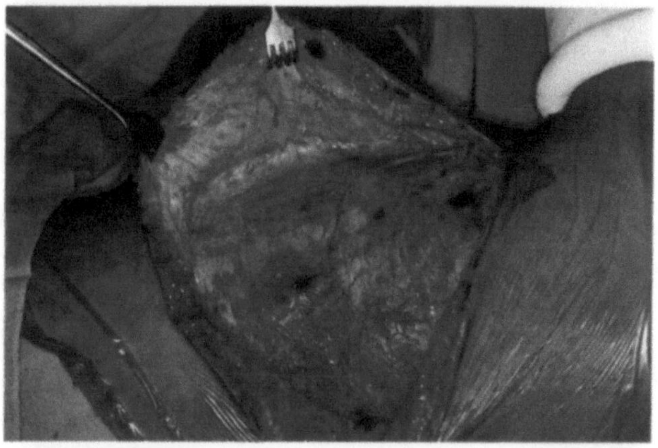

c. The superficial surface of the latissimus dorsi is seen.

c

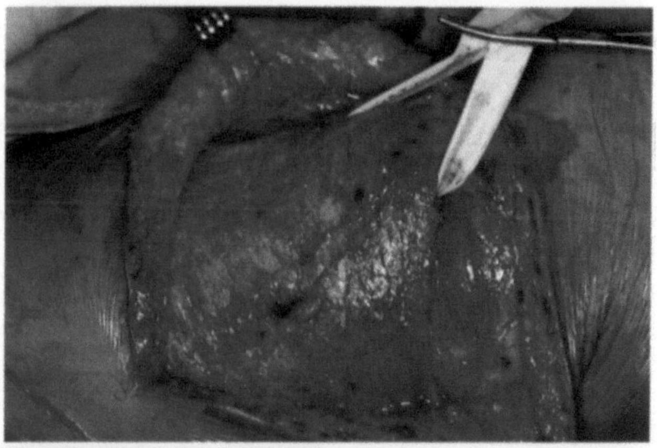

d. The anterior margin of the muscle is gently elevated, as is the posterior margin near its attachment to the tip of the scapula. Using blunt finger dissection, the deep surface of the muscle is separated from the ribs, and a Penrose drain is placed around the muscle. Defining the muscle proximally and gently elevating the Penrose drain simplifies the more distal dissection of the muscle.

d

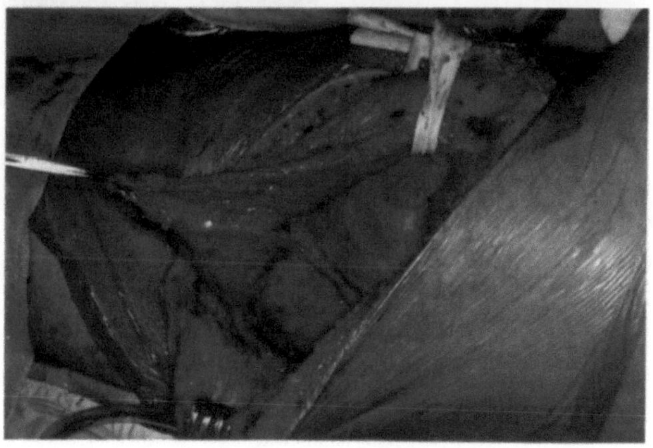

e. The anterior margin of the muscle is elevated and the distal margin is divided at a point which depends on the amount of tissue needed at the recipient site. Any bleeding vessels from the cut surface of the muscle are ligated. As the muscle is elevated from the thoracic wall in a cranial direction, several large perforating branches are encountered as they enter the deep surface of the muscle; these are ligated and divided.

e

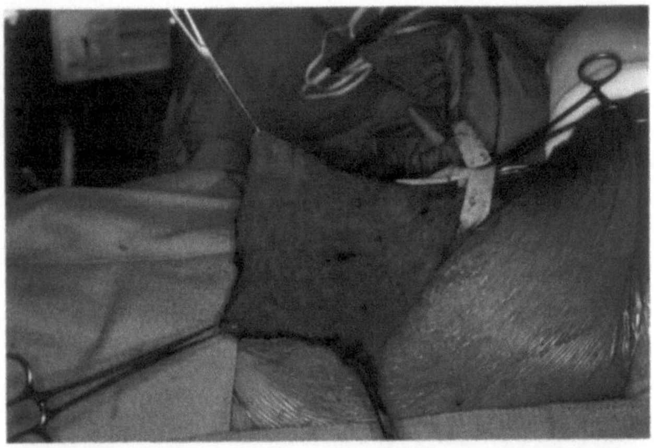

f

f. The muscle is entirely elevated and dissected anteriorly, distally, and posteriorly.

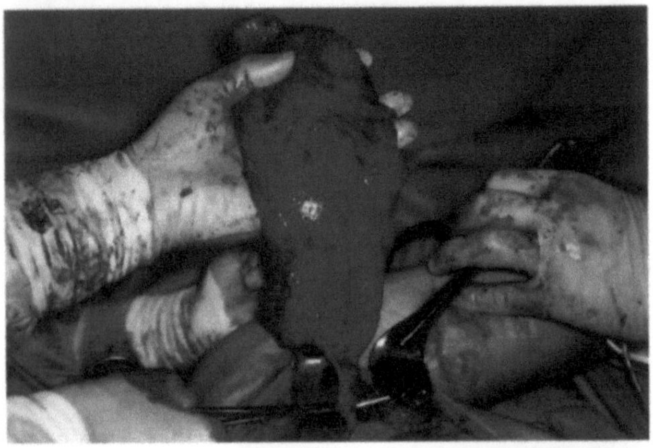

g

g. After the muscle has been elevated to the region of the axilla, the vascular pedicle is dissected (another patient, right side). Initially, the branch of the thoracodorsal vessel that supplies the serratus anterior is doubly ligated and divided. Further dissection of the pedicle into the axilla is then possible and provides a pedicle of 6–8 cm or longer. This pedicle contains a large artery approximately 2 mm in external diameter, a single vein, and the thoracodorsal nerve (the clamp is seen under the pedicle). The muscle attachments are divided proximally so that the muscle is now seen attached only by the neurovascular pedicle. This pedicle is divided once the recipient site has been completely prepared and the recipient vessels are ready for the transplant.

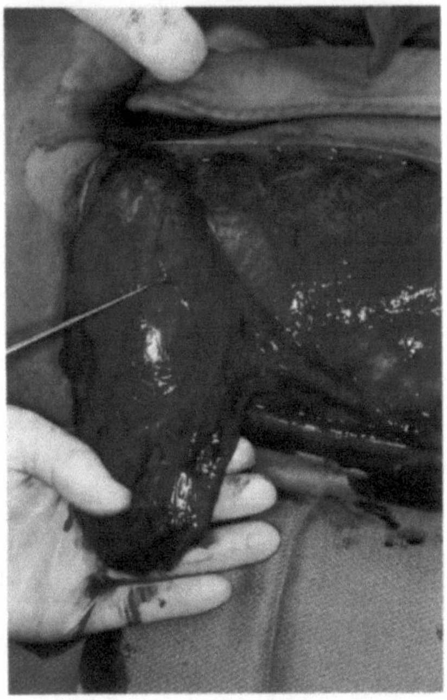

h

h. This same procedure in another patient (right side) shows the dissection of the neurovascular pedicle.

This dissection shows the deep surface of the latissimus dorsi with the vasculature on the deep surface of the muscle. The vessel enters the hilus of the muscle and then bifurcates into branches which run longitudinally. One branch supplies the anterior and the other the posterior segment of the muscle. The branch to the serratus anterior can be seen on the chest wall.

i. A close-up of this vascular pattern.

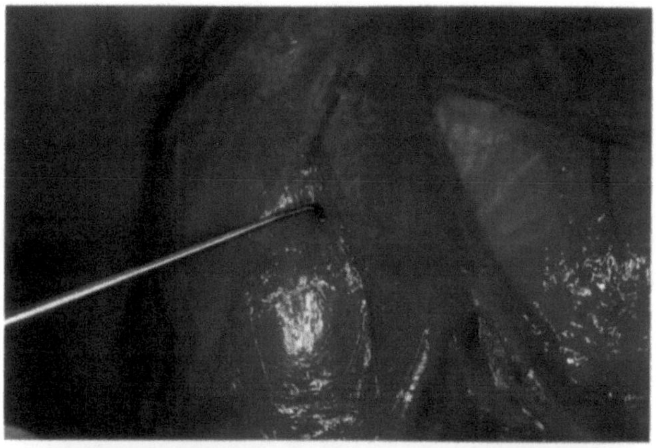

i

j. The latissimus dorsi can be divided into two parts, as long as care is taken to maintain one of the vascular branches in each of the divisions.

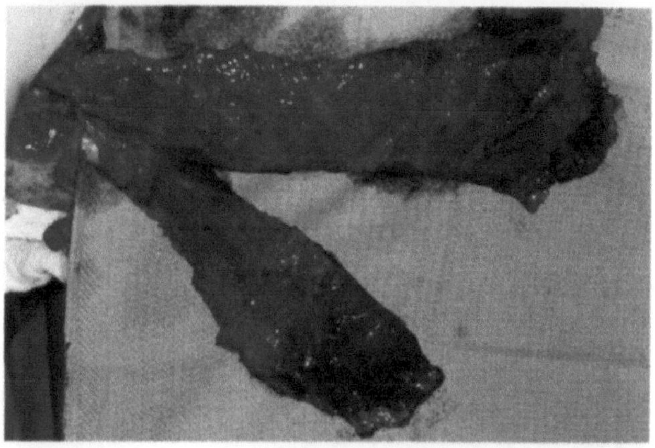

j

1.5.2.3 Latissimus Dorsi Musculocutaneous Transplant (Bailey and Godfrey 1982, Fisher and Cooney 1983, Maxwell et al. 1979) (Fig. 1-31; see also Fig. 1-26)

a. The cutaneous portion of the musculocutaneous transplant is outlined behind the anterior margin of the muscle.

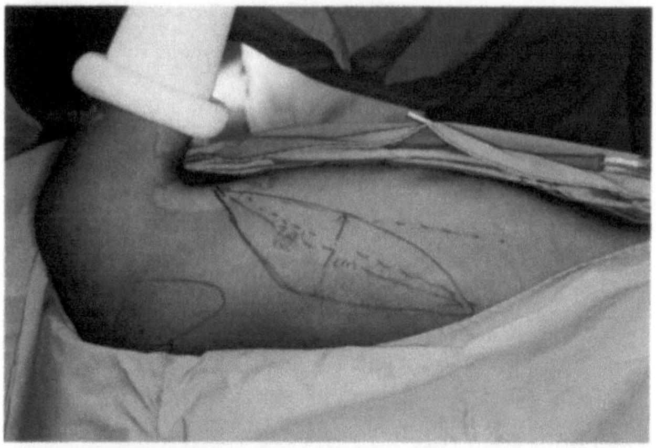

a

b. The anterior and posterior skin incisions are made. The margins of the cutaneous portion of the transplant are sutured to the muscle fascia; this is done to prevent damage to the cutaneous vessels which course into the skin from the underlying muscle through shearing of the skin away from the muscle. The anterior and posterior skin flaps over the rest of the latissimus dorsi are then raised.

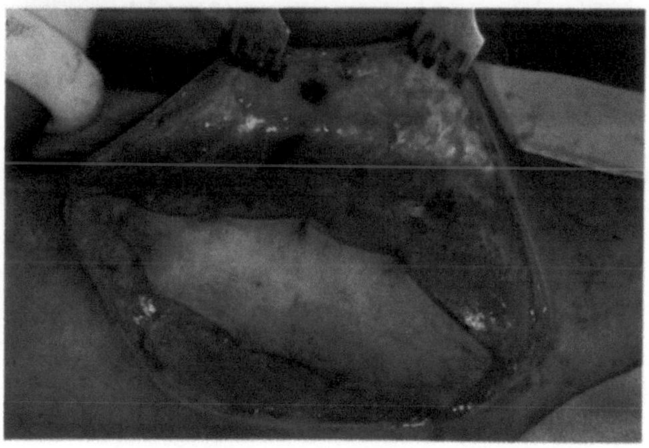

b

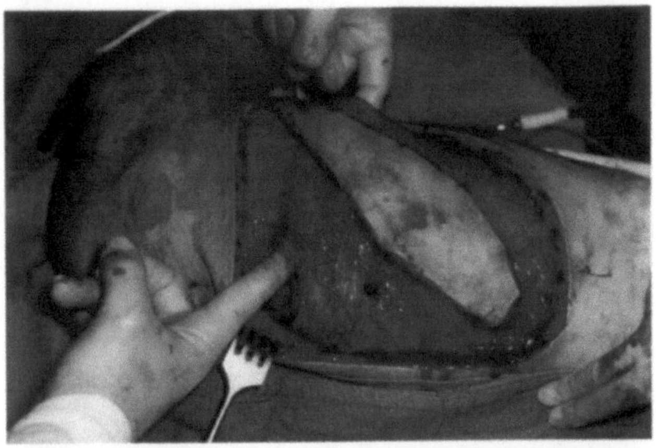

c

c. The anterior and posterior margins of the latissimus dorsi are dissected in the fashion described in Section 1.5.2.2.

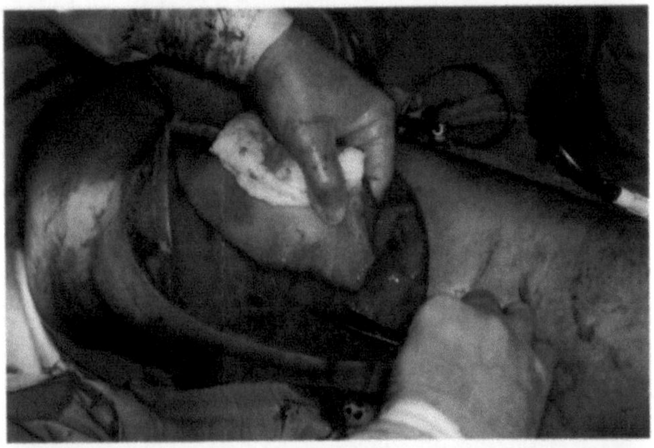

d

d. The anterior margin is elevated and the muscle can be divided distally and posteriorly, depending on the amount required. It is important to ligate the vessels on the cut surface as the muscle is divided. If the entire muscle is taken, there will be less bleeding as the aponeurotic attachments are divided.

The remainder of the dissection is similar to that in Section 1.5.2.2.

1.5.2.4 Combined Latissimus Dorsi and Serratus Anterior Transplant (Harii et al. 1982) (Fig. 1-32)

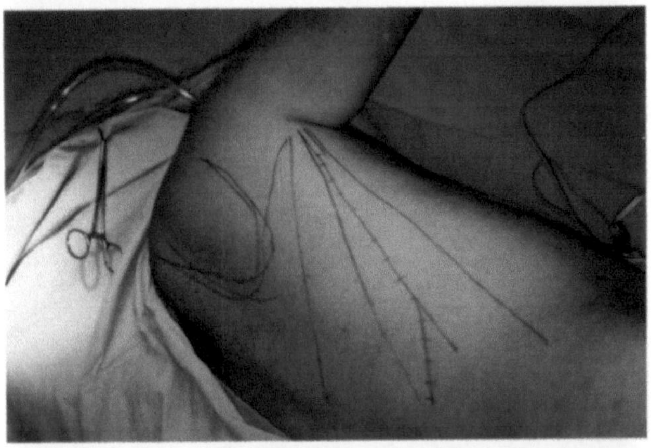

a

a. The position used is similar to that described in Section 1.5.2.1. The incision is made approximately 4 cm posterior to the anterior margin of the latissimus dorsi.

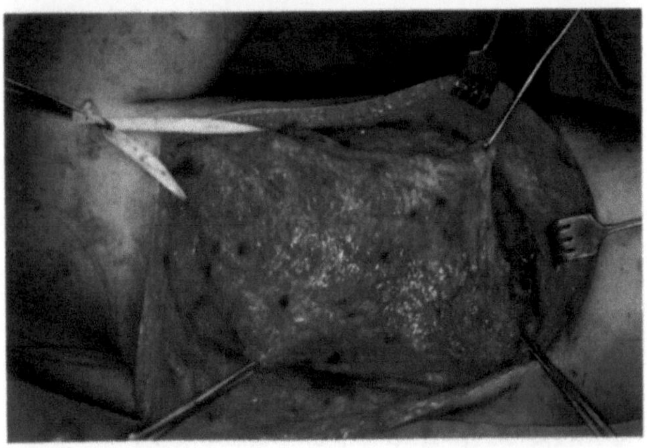

b

b. The latissimus dorsi is dissected as described in Section 1.5.2.2, but the branch to the serratus anterior is *not* ligated.

c. The latissimus dorsi is elevated and the vessels are dissected back to the thoracodorsal vessels, which supply both muscles. The lowest digitations of the serratus anterior are then dissected as described in Section 1.5.2.1.

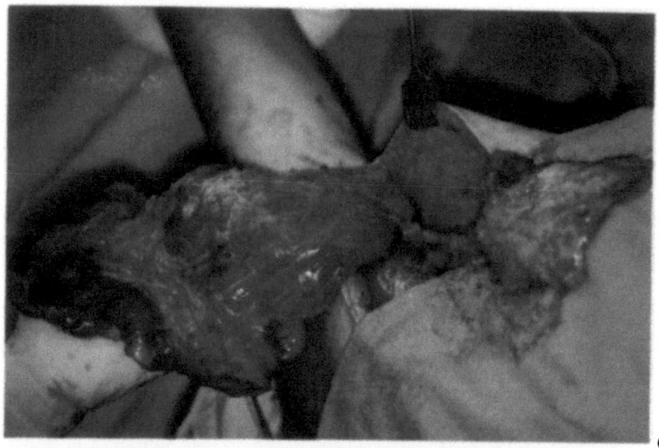

c

d. Further dissection proceeds into the axilla, dissecting the thoracodorsal vessels. Both muscles are then removed and are shown here, connected only by their vascular supply.

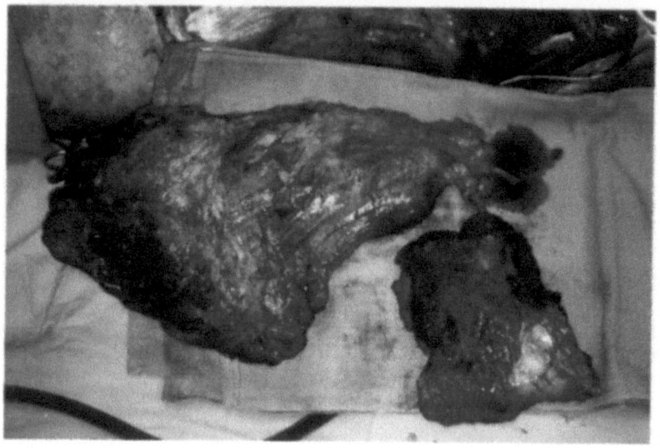

d

1.6 Tensor Fasciae Latae Musculocutaneous Transplant

(Cafee and Asokan 1981, Hill et al. 1978, Nahai et al. 1979)

1.6.1 Anatomy (Plate 1-VI)

The tensor fasciae latae muscle *arises* from the anterior part of the outer lip of the iliac crest and the outer surface of the anterior superior iliac spine. It is enclosed between the two layers of the fascia lata as it passes distally to *insert* into the iliotibial tract at the junction of the proximal and middle thirds of the thigh. Its *function* is that of a flexor, abductor, and medial rotator of the thigh, but its most important function is maintaining the extended knee in the erect position by keeping the iliotibial band taut.

The *vascular supply* to the muscle is from the lateral circumflex artery. This artery is a short vessel measuring a few centimeters in length and emanates from the profunda femoris artery. Thereafter, it gives off an ascending, a descending, and a transverse branch which becomes the pedicle to the tensor fasciae latae. This pedicle lies between the vastus lateralis and rectus femoris muscles approximately 8 cm distal to the iliac crest. It travels into the tensor fasciae latae muscle and divides into ascending, transverse, and descending branches which lie between the fascia and the muscle. It is the single dominant vessel to the muscle and is accompanied by two large venae comitantes. The artery rarely measures less than 1.5 mm in external diameter.

Perforating vessels pass from the muscle and fascia into the skin and allow a greater *cutaneous territory* to be supplied. This territory is distal to the muscle insertion and can reach approximately 8 cm from the lateral knee joint line (Mathes and Nahai 1979).

The lateral femoral cutaneous nerve is the *sensory supply* to the skin of the region (L2–L3). This nerve enters the area under the lateral end of the inguinal ligament. It can be superficial or deep to the sartorius. It lies deep to the fascia lata and becomes subcutaneous about 8 to 10 cm distal to the anterior superior iliac spine. There, it divides into anterior and posterior branches. A less important sensory supply proximally comes from the lateral cutaneous branch of T12, which enters the posterior aspect of the cutaneous flap.

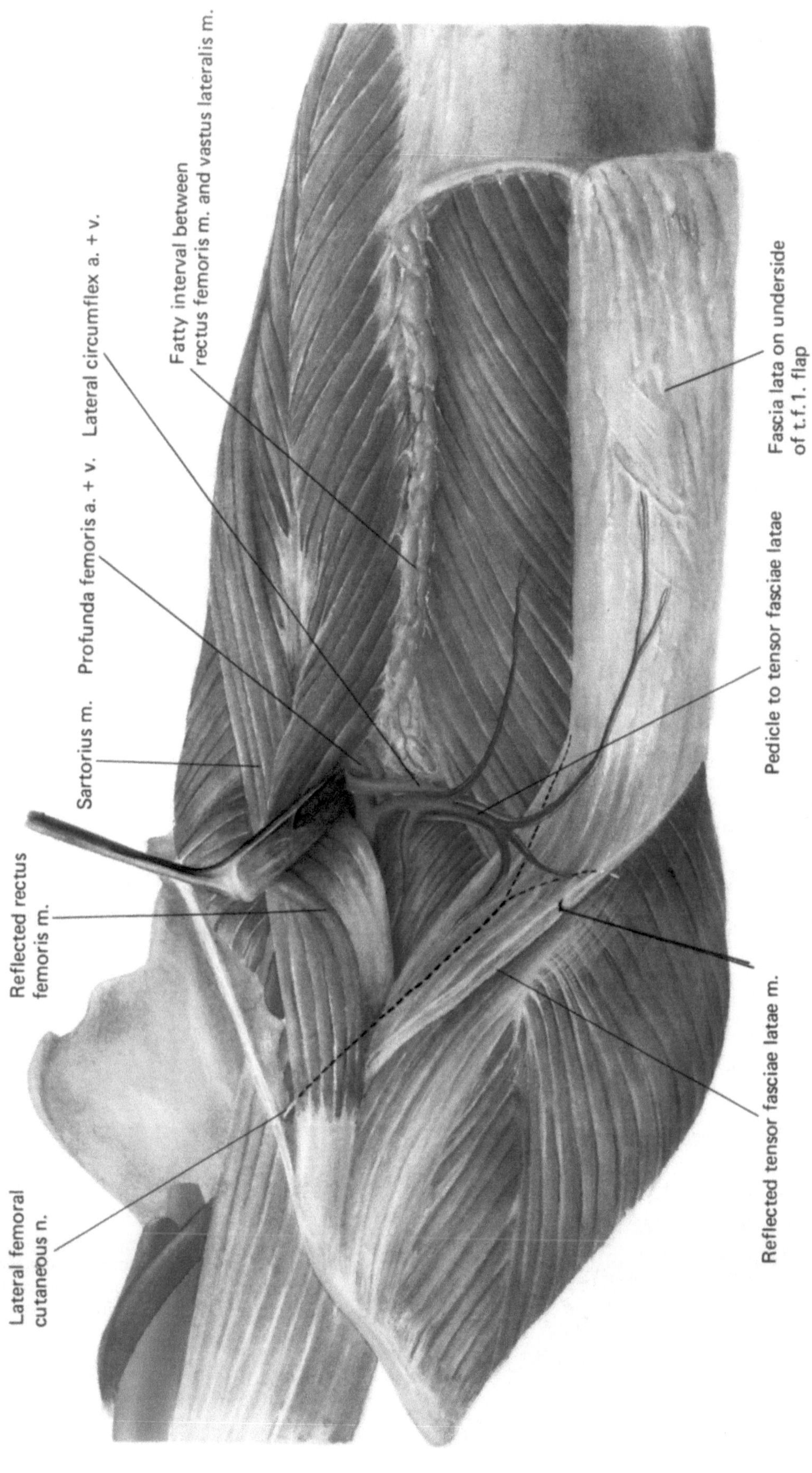

Plate 1-VI. Anatomy of the tensor fasciae latae muscle transplant.

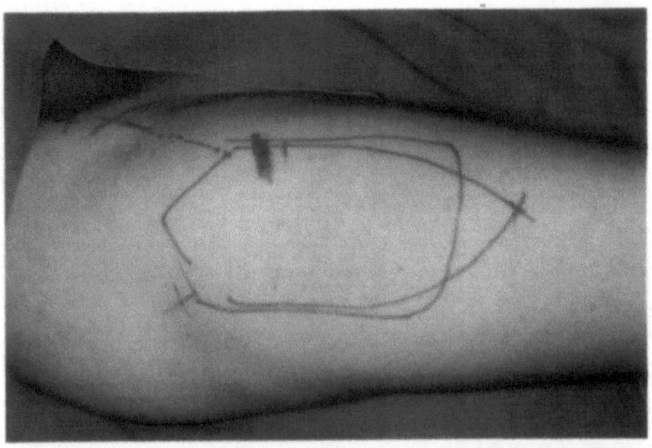

a

1.6.2 Surgical Technique
(Fig. 1-33; see also Fig. 1-21)

a. The skin incision which is outlined is centered proximally over the tensor fasciae latae, and distally along the anterolateral surface of the thigh. The anterior margin of this transplant runs from the anterior superior iliac spine to the lateral femoral condyle. The posterior margin parallels this line from the greater trochanter distally. If primary closure of the donor site is required, a narrower flap should be planned. Also, if the flap is not carried proximally to the iliac crest, donor site closure is easier. Distally, the flap can be extended to a point about 8 cm from the lateral knee joint line.

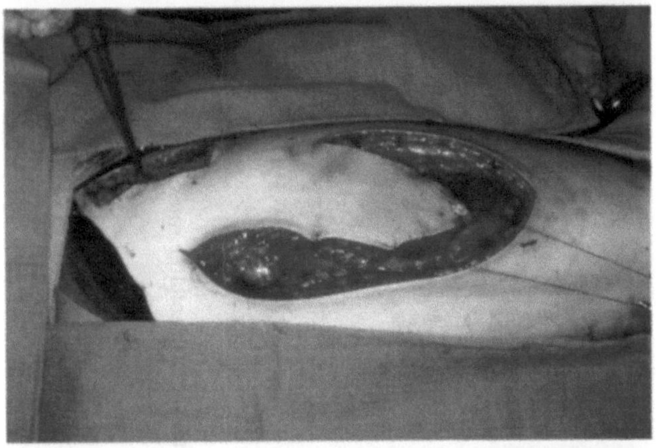

b

b. The lateral femoral cutaneous nerve is identified through a transverse incision that is made just distal to the lateral extent of the inguinal ligament. This nerve is then followed into the region of the proposed transplant. (Making an incision along the posterior and proximal margin of the flap, the lateral cutaneous branch of T12 can be dissected. This branch supplies the most proximal part of the flap and may sometimes be included.)

The skin incision is made laterally, medially, and distally down to the fascia lata. The skin is sutured to the fascia lata laterally, medially, and distally to prevent shearing of vessels between the skin superficially and the muscle and fascia.

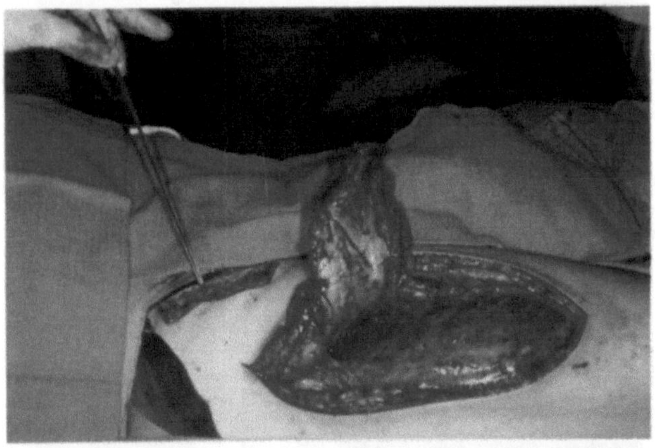

c

c. The fascia lata is then incised, and the fascia and skin are elevated proximally as a unit.

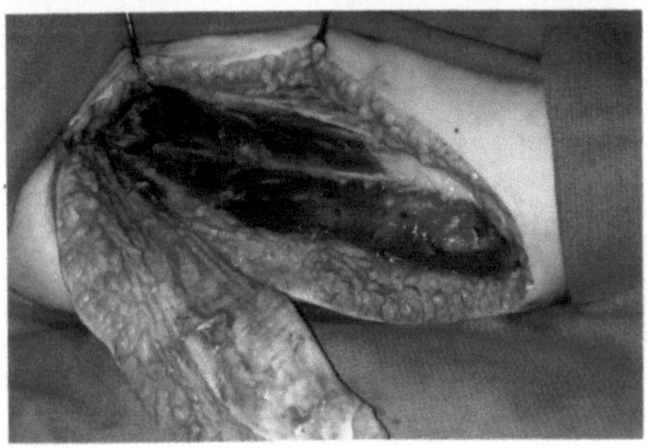

d

d. As this flap is elevated, a fatty interval between the vastus lateralis and the rectus femoris becomes apparent. This fatty interval is shown in a cadaver dissection.

e. The pedicle is found within this interval 6–8 cm from the iliac crest. The vascular pedicle is dissected back to the origin from the lateral circumflex artery. The pedicle consists of two large venae comitantes and an artery.

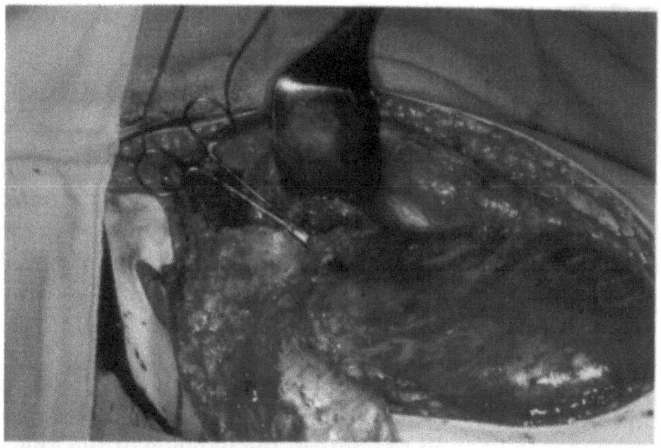

e

f. The pedicle is shown in this cadaver dissection.

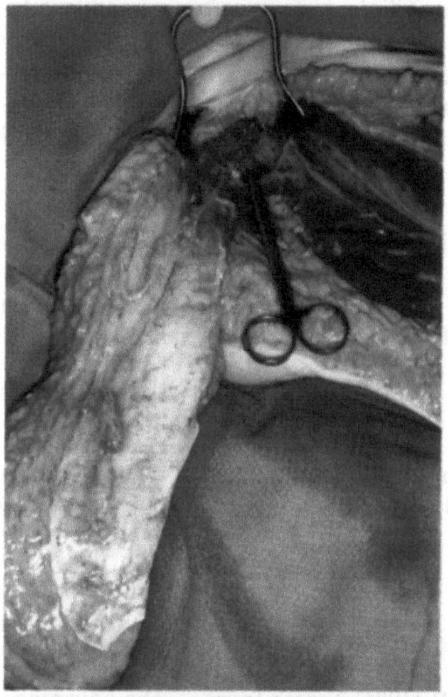

f

g. The proximal dissection is then completed by either dividing the tensor fasciae latae proximally or separating the muscle from its origin at the outer border of the iliac crest. Care must be taken to find the plane that separates the gluteus minimus proximally and anteriorly.

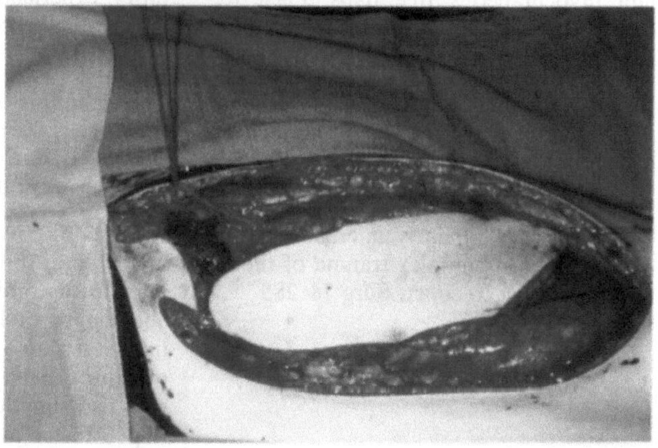

g

1.6.3 Donor Site Closure

a. If a flap 6–8 cm wide is taken, the donor site can usually be closed primarily. Closing the donor site too tightly may be dangerous because of the possibility of vascular compromise and consequent muscle necrosis.

b. If primary closure is not possible, a split-thickness skin graft is used on the muscle bed. Such skin grafting often has a poor cosmetic result because of a contour defect. If cosmetically unacceptable, the site can be treated secondarily with tissue expansion and subsequent graft removal.

1.7 Postoperative Care

Especially when split-thickness skin grafts have been used to cover a muscle transplant, it is important to apply *dressings* that contour the muscle well. Petroleum gauze followed by strips of cotton soaked in mineral oil will make such a dressing. Next, bulky gauze sponges are placed, followed by a plaster splint. A small opening is made in the skin graft to enable viewing of the muscle directly, and a window is left in all layers of the dressing for the same reason (Fig. 1-18).

No reliable surface *monitor* is currently available to monitor muscle tissue, but implanted temperature probes may be used to confirm the patency of the anastomoses (Fig. 8-2e). *Clinical observation* is usually adequate to assess whether the muscle is healthy and beefy red, or whether there is a vascular problem. Fortunately, it is unusual for a muscle transplant to develop vascular problems if vascularity has been adequate and muscle color has been good during the first 12–18 hours after surgery.

Low-molecular-weight dextran (30 cc/hour for approximately 3 days) is used as an *anticoagulant*. Particular attention is devoted to ensuring that *hydration* is good and that body and ambient *temperature* are warm. Heparin should not be used, as it will often result in a hematoma at the donor site, probably because of the extensive raw surface area following this kind of procedure. The suction drain placed in the donor site should not be removed for 24 hours after the dextran has been discontinued – a precaution which is also aimed at preventing hematoma formation.

Continuous elevation for two weeks is imperative. This requisite is followed by a slow program of progressive dependency, starting with 10–15 minutes at a time. For 3 months an elastic bandage is worn whenever the extremity is dependent. If the transplant becomes congested or blue, the periods of dependency must be reduced.

1.8 Selected Bibliography

Bailey BN, Godfrey AM (1982) Latissimus dorsi muscle free flaps. Br J Plast Surg 35:47

Uses of the latissimus dorsi free flap in nine patients (in the lower extremity in seven cases, and one case each in the hand and head) are described. The benefits at the donor and recipient sites of using the muscle without overlying skin are discussed.

Byrd HS, Spicer TE, Cierney G III (1985) Management of open tibial fractures. Plast Reconstr Surg 76:719

A prospective, nonrandomized study of 73 type III and type IV open fractures treated with open-wound techniques or muscle flaps is reported. Early acute flap coverage provided the best results and had a lower complication rate than did open-wound techniques. Aggressive and repeated debridement is emphasized with the goal of flap coverage before wound colonization. Subacute wounds – those colonized and infected within 1 to 6 weeks of the injury – did relatively poorly with flap coverage, whereas chronic wounds with granulation fared better with this technique.

Cafee HH, Asokan R (1981) Tensor fascia lata myocutaneous free flaps. Plast Reconstr Surg 68:195

The advantages and disadvantages of this flap are described, based on the authors' experience with 12 transplants. The territory of the cutaneous flap, the problem of excessive bulk, and other technical aspects of the procedure are discussed.

Fisher J, Cooney WP III (1983) Designing the latissimus dorsi free flap for knee coverage. Ann Plast Surg 11:554

The technique of using the latissimus dorsi musculocutaneous free flap for knee coverage is described. The superficial femoral artery and vein are used as recipient vessels, and excess muscle is used to pack into the knee defect while cutaneous cover distally and over the knee is achieved.

Godina M (1986) Early microsurgical reconstruction of complex trauma of the extremities. Plast Reconstr Surg 78:285

A series of 532 patients who had undergone microsurgical reconstruction was divided into three groups: "early", "delayed", and "late" – designations which refer to the timing of the procedure. Flap failure, infection, bone healing time, and length of hospital stay were criteria used in evaluating the results. The infection rate among the free flaps that had been performed within 72 hours of injury (early) was only 1.5%. The flap failure rate in this group (0.75%) was also significantly lower than in the groups of patients who had undergone flap transfer at later stages (72 hours to 3 months later [delayed] –12%; 3 months to 12.6 years later [late] – 9.5%). Godina attributes this superior success rate to the absence of fibrosis, which makes procedure planning easier. Thorough wound debridement is emphasized.

Godina M, Bajec J, Baraga A (1986) Salvage of the mutilated upper extremity with temporary ectopic implantation of the undamaged part. Plast Reconstr Surg 78:295

Temporary "banking" of the hand in the axilla is described.

Gordon L, Buncke HJ, Alpert BS (1982) Free latissimus dorsi muscle flap with split-thickness skin graft cover: A report of 16 cases. Plast Reconstr Surg 70:173

This report describes using the latissimus dorsi muscle covered with a split-thickness skin graft instead of a musculocutaneous flap. Using split-thickness skin graft results in less bulk at the recipient site and superior donor site appearance.

Gordon L, Chiu E (1988) Treatment of infected nonunions and segmental defects of the tibia with staged microvascular muscle transplantation and bone grafting. J Bone Joint Surg 70-A:377

Most cases of chronic osteomyelitis combined with soft-tissue wounds can be controlled by appropriate bone and soft-tissue debridement, antibiotics, and microvascular muscle transplantation. The bone reconstruction that follows carries substantial risk of recurrent infection. In the humerus, femur, or where both bones have a segmental defect, vascularized bone transplantation should follow the muscle procedure after an infection-free interval. If the fibula is intact, however, a tibiofibular synostosis should be considered.

Gordon L, Rosen J, Alpert BS, et al (1984) Free microvascular transfer of second toe ray and serratus anterior muscle for management of thumb loss at the carpometacarpal joint level. J Hand Surg 9A(5):642

The second toe was used to reconstruct a thumb that had been previously amputated at the trapezium level. Absent thenar muscles were reconstructed with the serratus anterior.

Harii K, Ohmori K, Torii S (1976) Free gracilis muscle transplantation with microneurovascular anastomosis for the treatment of facial paralysis. A preliminary report. Plast Reconstr Surg 57:133

The anatomy and technique of gracilis transplantation are described.

Harii K, Yamada A, Ishihara K, et al (1982) A free transfer of both latissimus dorsi and serratus anterior flaps with thoracodorsal vessel anastomoses. Plast Reconstr Surg 70:620

The vascular anatomy of the two muscles as well as the surgical technique of flap elevation are described. This technique is useful in extremely large wounds where either the size of the latissimus dorsi is inadequate or dead space needs to be filled with muscle at the same time cover is provided. Donor site function is discussed.

Hill H, Nahai F, Vasconez L (1978) The tensor fascia lata myocutaneous free flap. Plast Reconstr Surg 61:517

Details of the anatomy and elevation of the flap are described. Six patients in whom this transplant was used are featured; three of the flaps contained a nerve, and four required debulking. Other advantages and disadvantages of this flap are discussed.

Manktelow RT, McKee NH (1979) Free muscle transplantation to provide active finger flexion. J Hand Surg 3:416

This article describes two patients who sustained traumatic loss of the long flexors to the digits. In both, flexor function was restored using free muscle transplantation – with the gracilis in one patient and the pectoralis major in the other. The *details* of each operative procedure are given and the functional results of the full range of flexion and grip strength are described. Also included is a discussion of some guidelines for performing the procedure.

Mathes SJ, Alpert BS, Chang N (1982) Use of the muscle flap in chronic osteomyelitis. Experimental and clinical correlation. Plast Reconstr Surg 69:815

This article reviews 11 patients with chronic osteomyelitis of the distal tibia and foot who were treated with debridement and gracilis muscle transplantation. An experimental model in the dog was used to compare musculocutaneous flaps with random-pattern cutaneous flaps. Possible reasons for the success of muscle flaps are given. The advantages of gracilis transplantation are discussed and operative technique is described.

Mathes SJ, Nahai F (1979) Clinical Atlas of Muscle and Musculocutaneous Flaps. St. Louis, C.V. Mosby

This outstanding volume presents the gamut of muscle flaps available for local or distant transfer.

Mathes SJ, Nahai F (1981) Classification of the vascular anatomy of muscles: Experimental and clinical correlation. Plast Reconstr Surg 67:177

This article is important reading for those involved in muscle transplantation. An anatomic study of the vascularity of different muscles is given with classification into five types of arterial supply. The importance of the vascular supply is correlated with clinical considerations in muscle transplantation.

Maxwell GP, Manson PN, Hoopes JE (1979) Experience with 13 latissimus dorsi myocutaneous free flaps. Plast Reconstr Surg 64:1

The vascular anatomy of the latissimus dorsi is described and the details of surgical technique are outlined. The possibility of "delay" of the flap and preliminary ligation of intercostal perforators are mentioned. Five cases are described in detail. The uses are listed and the donor site is discussed.

May JW Jr, Gallico GG III, Jupiter J, et al (1984) Free latissimus dorsi muscle flap with skin graft for treatment of traumatic chronic bony wounds. Plast Reconstr Surg 73:641

This use of the latissimus dorsi microvascular transplant is described. Indications and technique are outlined.

Nahai F, Hill HL, Hester TR (1979) Experience with the tensor fascia lata flap. Plast Reconstr Surg 63:788

The anatomy and vascular supply of the muscle along with the large cutaneous territory associated with it are described in this article. The sensory innervation is discussed. A variety of local uses are described, and a section on neurovascular uses is also included.

Nahai F, Mathes SJ (1984) Musculocutaneous flap or muscle flap and skin graft? Ann Plast Surg 12:199

This article discusses six factors to consider when choosing muscle only versus a musculocutaneous flap: size, bulk, donor deformity, durability, pliability, and sensitivity. The advantages and disadvantages of each muscle flap are discussed for different defects and donor sites.

O'Brien BMcC, Morrison WA, MacLeod AM, et al (1982) Free microneurovascular muscle transfer in limbs to provide motor power. Ann Plast Surg 9:381

The cases of seven patients who underwent muscle transplantation to the upper limb are described in detail. The defects were the result of severe crush and avulsion injuries to the upper limb, Volkmann's contracture, or pressure necrosis of muscle. Details of the procedure, including donor nerve and tension of the muscle, are presented. Selection of donor muscle is discussed and postoperative therapy and problems encountered are briefly mentioned.

Swartz WM, Mears DC (1985) The role of free-tissue transfers in lower-extremity reconstruction. Plast Reconstr Surg 76:364

The authors analyze a series of 76 patients treated with microvascular transfers for lower-extremity soft-tissue defects. Twenty-eight flaps were performed as emergencies after traumatic soft-tissue loss. Forty-six flaps were reconstructive, correcting defects created by the sequelae of trauma. A classification of wounds based on reconstructive requirements is described and used to help define the role of free tissue transplantation in severe leg wounds. Radical debridement of all devitalized tissue is emphasized. The difficulty of treating segmental bone defects is discussed.

Takayanagi S, Tsukie T (1982) Free serratus anterior muscle and myocutaneous flaps. Ann Plast Surg 8:277

The anatomy and elevation procedure for this transplant are described. Details of the vascularity to the slips and the possibility of including a rib with the muscle are discussed. In two cases, donor site morbidity is addressed and the benefit of variable muscle size and a large vascular pedicle is emphasized.

Terzis JK, Sweet RC, Dykes RW, et al (1978) Recovery of function in free muscle transplants using microneurovascular anastomoses. J Hand Surg 3:37

The functional capacity of transplanted muscles in the rabbit was only 25% of normal with regard to maximum working strength. (Clinically, the strength of the transplanted gracilis appears to be better than this, and is adequate for finger flexion, grasp, and pinch.)

Weiland AJ, Moore JR, Daniel RK (1984) The efficacy of free tissue transfer in the treatment of osteomyelitis. J Bone Joint Surg 66-A:181

Thirty-three patients with osteomyelitis of various bones were treated with free tissue transfer. The procedures consisted of muscle transplantation, cutaneous flaps, and vascularized bone grafting with a fibula or osteocutaneous transplant. Six patients had recurrent sepsis at follow-up.

2 Cutaneous Transplantation

2.1 Overview

The first microvascular cutaneous transplant, a groin flap, was performed in 1972 by Daniel and Taylor. Over the next decade, the free groin flap gained acceptance and was used as an alternative to pedicle flaps. The free groin flap was only used when a pedicle flap was impractical, this policy being due to certain difficulties with the former. The superficial circumflex iliac vessels are small, and although the deep circumflex iliac vessels are larger (Taylor et al. 1979, Sec. 3.7), the arterial anatomy is variable and dissection is tedious and difficult compared with other cutaneous transplants. In addition, the flap is often too bulky and sometimes hair-bearing.

In recent years, a great many different microvascular cutaneous transplants with larger, more reliable vessels have been introduced. Because these flaps do not have the disadvantages of the groin flap, their benefits relative to pedicle flaps can be fully realized. The free groin flap has come to be used relatively rarely, and in its place, other flaps are now used to provide skin cover.

When compared with pedicle flaps, these microvascular procedures have the following advantages:

1. They permit immediate or early elevation of the extremity – a feature that is particularly important after major trauma, where there is a tendency toward edema and joint stiffness.
2. They permit immediate or early joint mobilization and hand therapy.
3. A transplant can be chosen that is non-hair-bearing and has a size and thickness that match the recipient problem.
4. A composite flap can be used to treat loss of both soft tissue and bone or joint. Occasionally, tendons can also be included in the transplant.
5. The procedure can be performed in a single operation (Freedlander et al. 1986).

Cutaneous transplantation is indicated when cosmetic considerations make cutaneous cover desirable. Such situations are encountered less often when treating extremity defects than when reconstructing the face. More frequently, cutaneous transplants are performed for the accompanying subcutaneous fatty tissue they provide, particularly when subsequent tendon reconstruction will be needed. Cutaneous transplants are also indicated when sensation in the transplant is important (Fig. 2-1). As discussed in Chapter 1, *muscle transplantation* is preferable where infection has been a problem, for extremely large wounds, to fill dead space, or to provide cover where shearing movement of the transplant on the deeper structures is a problem.

2.2 Indications

a. For covering wounds of the forearm, hand, or leg in which nerves, tendons, vessels, bone, or hardware is exposed (Figs. 2-2 and 2-3).

b. For cover on the *dorsum of the hand.* Cutaneous flaps can mimic the thin mobile skin of this region. Cutaneous transplants are best in this area because the subcutaneous fat provides the best tissue for subsequent tendon reconstruction (Figs. 2-4 and 2-5).

c. For cover in areas where *sensation is important*, such as the sole of the foot (Fig. 2-6) or the palmar surface of one or more fingers (Figs. 2-1 and 2-7). These flaps can be used to provide cover for several digits by syndactylizing them. (If this procedure is done, later separation of the fingers is required.) The flaps that provide sensation are the lateral arm flap (lower lateral cutaneous nerve of the arm), dorsalis pedis flap (superficial peroneal nerve), radial forearm flap (lateral cutaneous nerve of the forearm), and deltoid flap (upper lateral cutaneous nerve of the arm). The tensor fasciae latae musculocutaneous flap (lateral femoral cutaneous nerve) also provides sensation, but only in the half of the flap nearest the pedicle.

d. For cover over *major flexion creases*, such as the antecubital and popliteal fossae. In these regions,

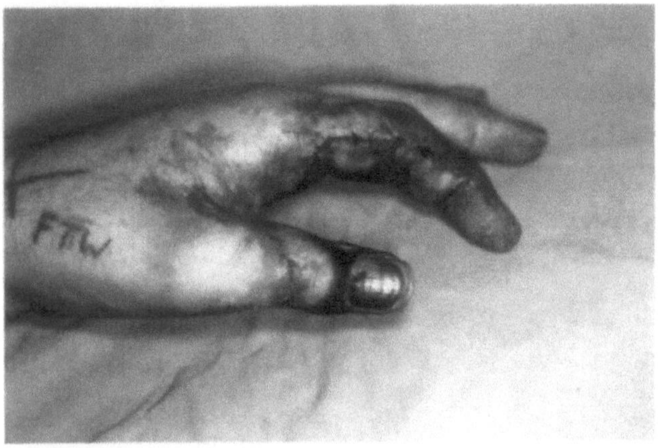

a

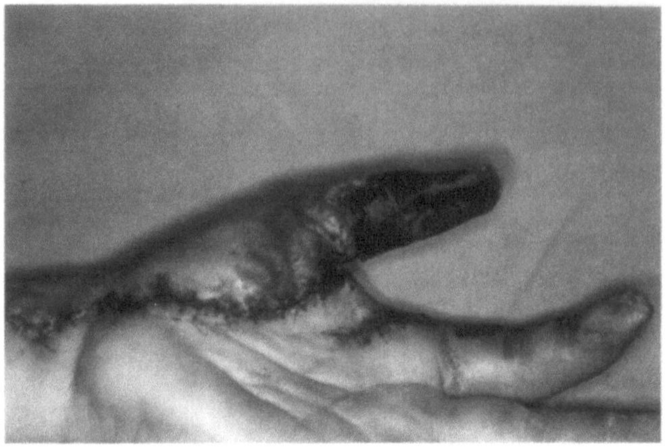

b

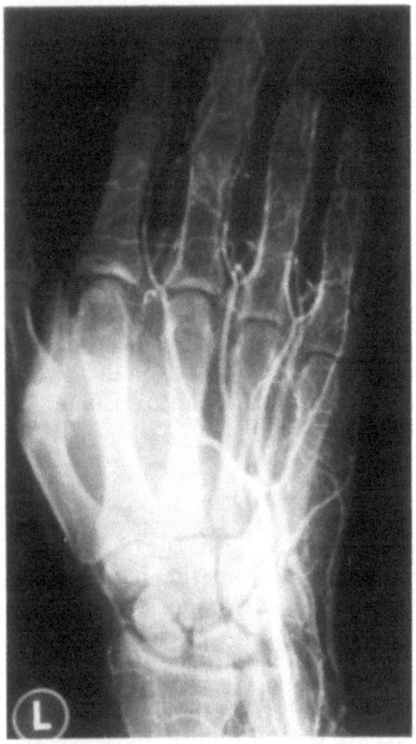

c

Fig. 2-1. a and **b.** A 19-year-old boy injected methylphenidate HCl into his radial artery at the midforearm level. Necrosis of the thumb and part of the radial aspect of the index finger resulted, along with inflammation on the dorsal aspect of the hand. Thin skin was needed to resurface the thumb and retain as much of its length as possible. It was also important to use a flap with good sensory innervation. Neither a radial forearm flap nor a rotation flap from the dorsum of the hand was possible in this patient because of the injury to the radial artery. A dorsalis pedis flap was used, as it best suited the patient's complex needs. **c.** Arteriography revealed an ulnar artery that supplied the ulnar three fingers and the ulnar aspect of the index finger. (It is important to recognize that the radial artery sometimes provides the only circulation to the thumb, index, and long fingers.) In light of this finding, the palmar arch was felt to be the safest recipient vessel. **d.** The necrotic tissue was removed, and the mummified portion of the thumb was amputated at the interphalangeal joint. The digital nerve was dissected to the base of the thumb where it had become necrotic. The superficial palmar arch was dissected as well as the median nerve, preserving the recurrent branch. The dorsalis pedis artery was sutured end-to-side into the superficial palmar arch, the vein was sutured end-to-end into the venae comitantes of the palmar arch, and the digital nerve was sutured to the superficial peroneal nerve. **e.** The flap is shown in place. A skin graft has been used on the radial aspect of the thumb. (Compared with skin grafting at the dorsalis pedis flap donor site, which can produce long-term healing problems, it is preferable to use a skin graft in the hand; this is especially true in this region of the thumb which is not directly involved in pinch or grip.) At 3 months, good sensation has been restored in the flap.

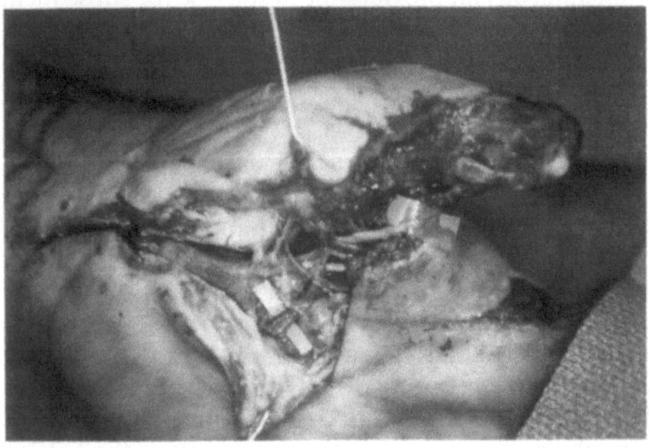

d

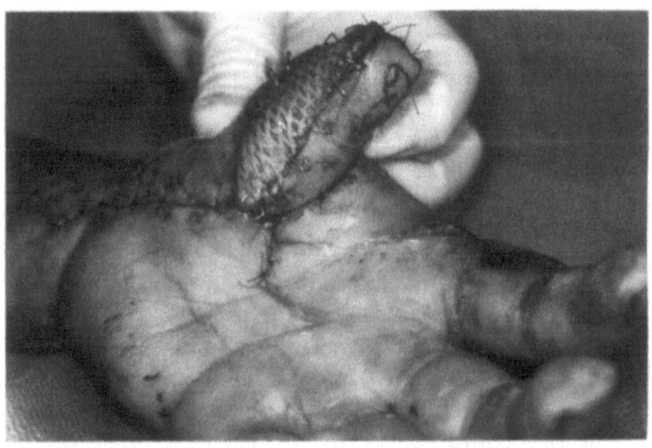

e

a b c d

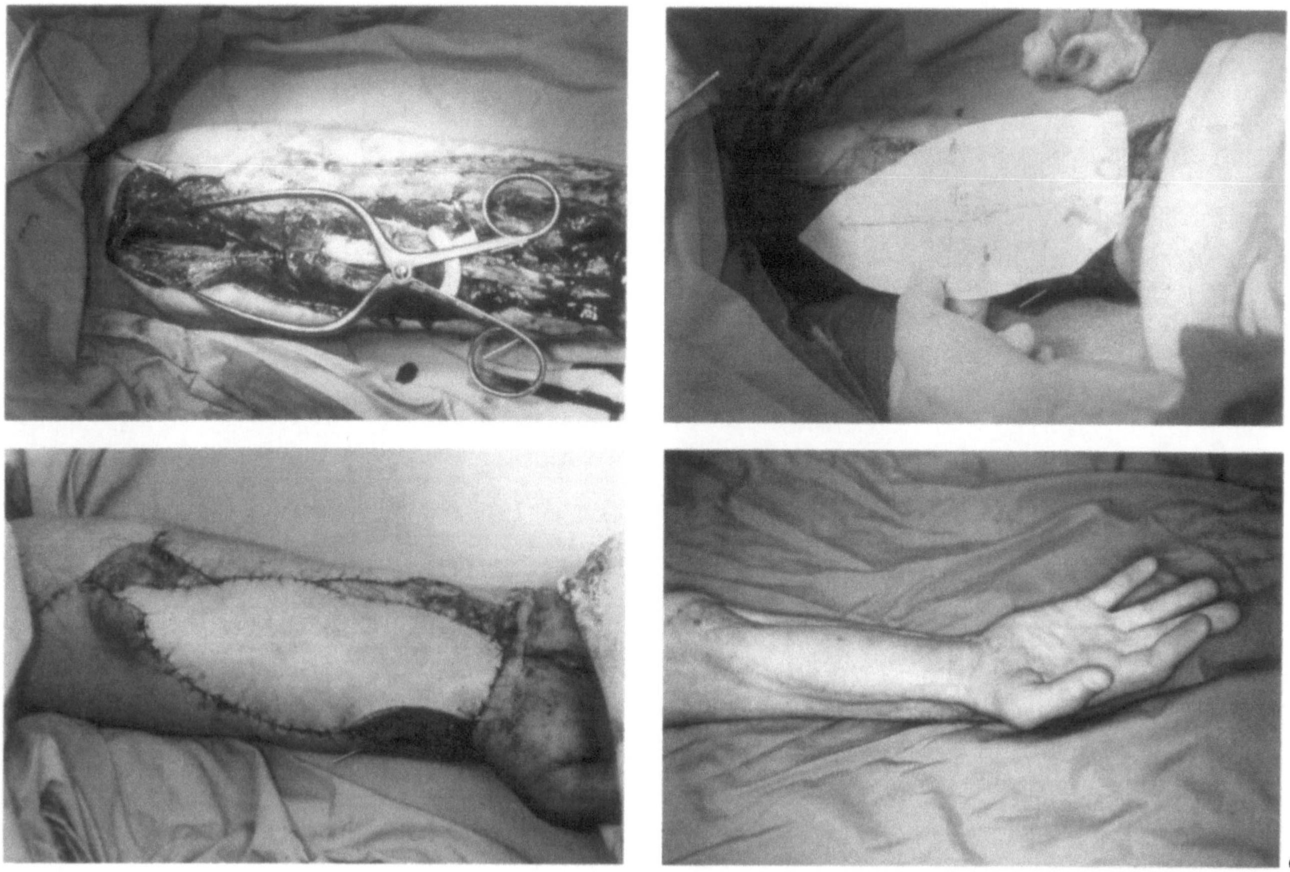

Fig. 2-2. a. Replantation was performed after an avulsive injury that involved amputation of the hand. Subsequently, a large cutaneous flap was needed to cover this extensive defect of the forearm which exposed the median nerve, radial artery, and many tendons of the flexor compartment. The radial vascular bundle was dissected proximally in order to provide the recipient vessels. **b.** A template of the wound was made so that a flap of appropriate dimensions could be harvested. **c.** Although the flap was shaped carefully to fit the defect, a small amount of skin graft was needed distally. **d.** The flap provided excellent cover and restored good function.

muscle coverage with a split-thickness skin graft tends to break down, and excessive scarring is often a problem. Musculocutaneous flaps can also be used in these areas (Fig. 1-26).

2.3 Choice of Transplant

A good microvascular cutaneous transplant must meet several criteria. For most defects, the skin should be thin (no excess subcutaneous fat) and large enough to cover the defect without excessive tension. The pedicle should be easy to dissect and have reliable anatomy, and its external diameter should be 1.5 mm or larger. The need for a long vascular pedicle will depend on the recipient site. In general, however, a pedicle at least 5 cm in length will allow the anastomosis to be performed more simply, away from the transplant, and with recipient vessels that are outside of the zone of injury. In addition, the donor site should be located in an inconspicuous area that can be closed primarily and not require skin grafting.

Skin flaps from almost every part of the body (the deltoid region; posterior, medial, and lateral arm; radial forearm; posterior and medial thigh; posterior and lateral calf; dorsum of the foot; instep; groin; and even the temporoparietal region) have been used to provide cutaneous soft-tissue cover. The two flaps that have achieved widespread acceptance because of the best overall combination of assets are the **lateral arm flap** (Figs. 2-3, 2-5, and 2-6) and the **scapular flap** (Figs. 2-2 and 2-4). When cutaneous soft-tissue cover is required, these two flaps can address any clinical contingency. The lateral arm flap provides some sensation and consists of thinner skin. The choice of cutaneous flap depends also on the *size of the defect*, as follows:

1. Defects measuring 2–3 cm × 6–8 cm – dorsalis pedis flap
2. Defects measuring up to 6–8 cm × 10–12 cm – lateral arm flap
3. Defects measuring 8–10 cm × 14–16 cm – scapular flap
4. Defects larger than 10 cm × 16 cm – latissimus dorsi musculocutaneous flap.

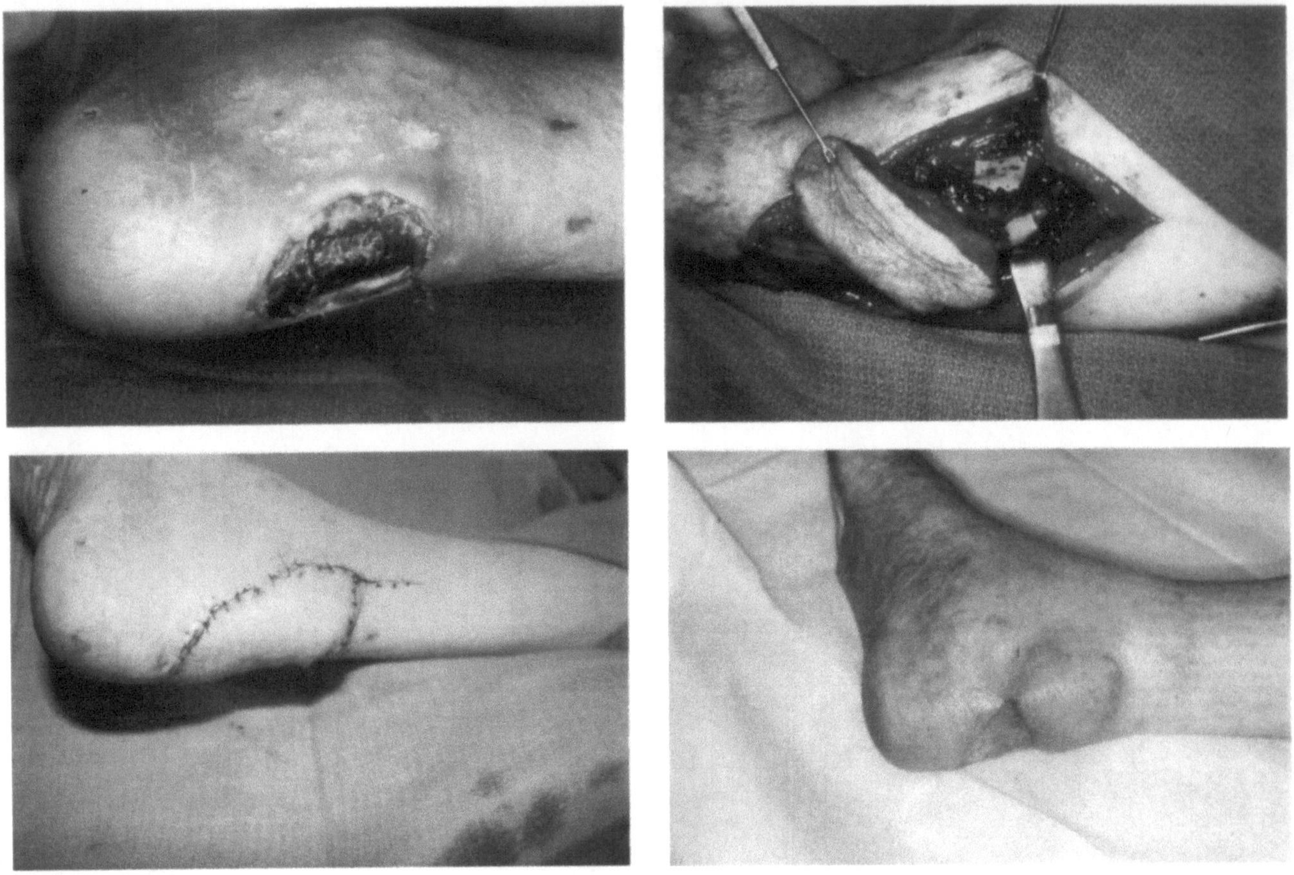

Fig. 2-3. a. An 80-year-old man with severe peripheral vascular disease developed this ulcer over his Achilles tendon. Loss of the Achilles tendon was imminent and the wound was not amenable to a local flap procedure. **b.** A lateral arm flap was harvested. The pedicle can be seen under the blue background. **c.** The vessels were anastomosed to the posterior tibial artery and vein. (Vessels in patients with diabetes and peripheral vascular disease must be sutured very carefully, passing the needle from the inside to the outside of the vessel so that the intima is not separated.) The flap of skin is thin and can be seen placed in the defect. **d.** The flap provided good cover 1 year later.

The lateral arm flap can be taken with an extension of the triceps fascia. This approach extends the area that can be covered with this flap, but the fascial extension requires split-thickness skin grafting. Some sensation in the flap is made possible by transplanting the lower lateral cutaneous nerve of the upper arm with it, but in my experience, the sensation restored is generally only fair. An insensate area over the lateral aspect of the elbow can be expected.

Katsaros and Schusterman (1984) have described the possible addition of bone or the use of the triceps fascia alone without overlying skin. The modification of taking fascia alone and using it for reconstruction in the lower extremity is appealing. Use of the humerus as part of an osteocutaneous transplant carries the risk of fracture at the donor site. These considerations must be carefully evaluated in relation to the many other options for bone transplantation.

Care should be taken not to close this wound too tightly. Katsaros and Schusterman (1984) have described one case in which the wound was extended distal to the elbow and closed tightly. Postoperatively, the patient was found to have radial nerve compression which resolved once the sutures were released.

The scapular and lateral arm flaps are compared in Table 2-1.

Table 2-1. A comparison of the lateral arm and scapular flaps.

	Lateral arm flap	Scapular flap
Size	6–8 × 10–12 cm	8–10 × 14–16 cm
Vascular anatomy	Dependable	Dependable
Skin characteristics	Thin	Slightly thicker
Subcutaneous tissue	Little	Moderate (depends on body fat)
Pedicle length	6 cm	6 cm (with difficulty, can be extended to 10 cm)
Patient position	Supine	Prone or lateral
Donor site result	Linear scar; slight contour defect	Linear scar; tends to spread

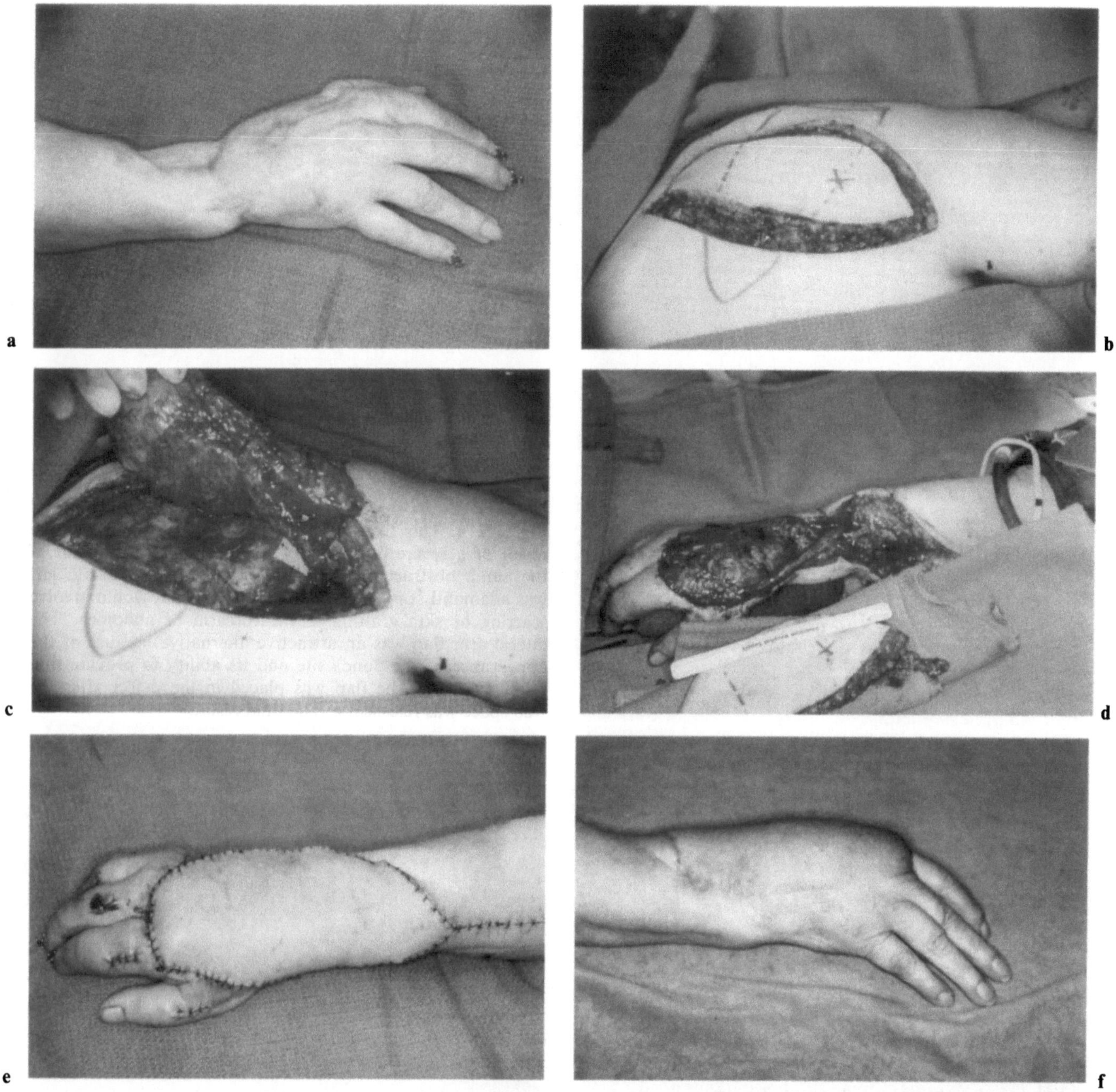

Fig. 2-4. a. A car rolled over onto this patient's hand and wrist, resulting in severe bone and soft-tissue loss at the wrist level. Wrist fusion was needed in addition to tendon reconstruction, and adequate soft-tissue cover was lacking. The patient is shown approximately 1 year after the accident. A flap was needed which would be wider than the lateral arm flap and contain more subcutaneous tissue so that it would fill the defect. It was felt that skin with subcutaneous tissue would allow for subsequent tendon gliding better than would muscle or fascial cover. For these reasons, the scapular flap was chosen. **b.** The scapula was outlined and the flap incised. The Doppler signal was marked. **c.** The flap was elevated; the blue background is beneath where the pedicle curves around the lateral border of the scapula through the triangular space. **d.** The defect was prepared and the proximal radial artery dissected as the recipient vessel. The flap measured 15 cm × 9 cm and had a 5-cm vascular pedicle. **e.** The flap was sutured into place, providing good cover. **f.** Improved contour was achieved with adequate cover for subsequent tendon reconstruction and wrist fusion.

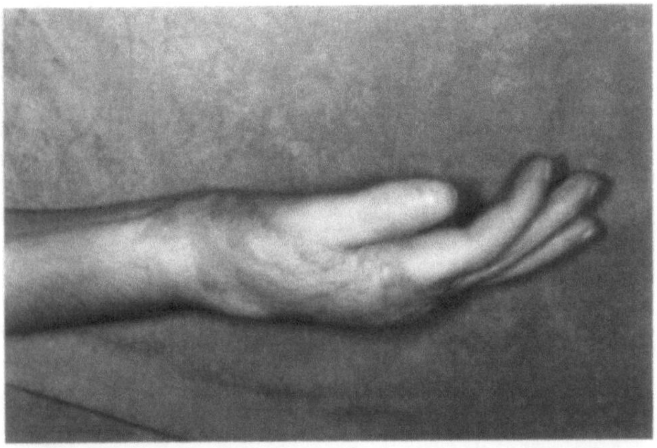
a

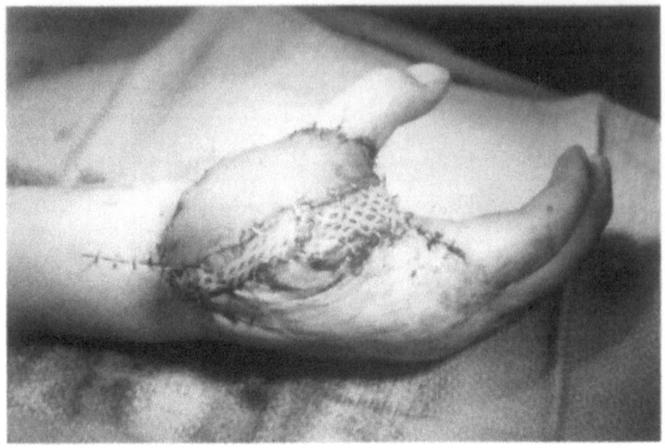
b

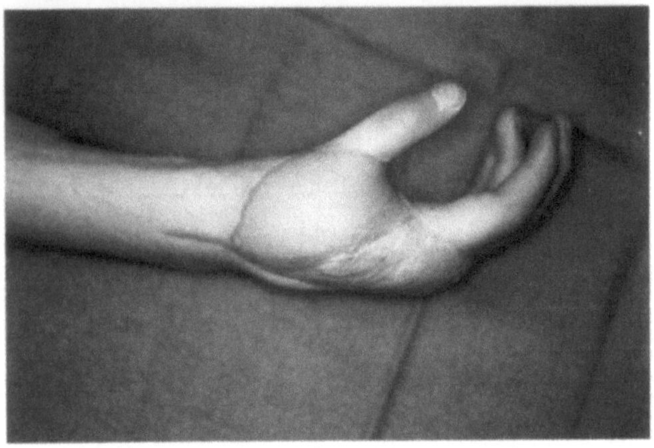
c

Fig. 2-5. **a.** This fixed adduction deformity, which was the result of a severe crush injury to the dorsum and palm of the hand, obstructed thumb function. This 12-year-old girl was adamantly opposed to any procedure that would involve scarring or skin grafting in the forearm or abdomen. The lateral arm flap was an attractive alternative because of the appearance of the donor site and its ability to provide thin pliable skin. **b.** The flap was placed in the defect after the web space was released. **c.** The final result.

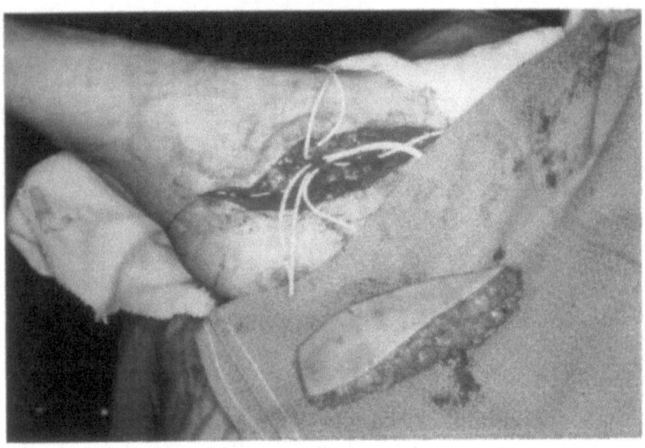
a

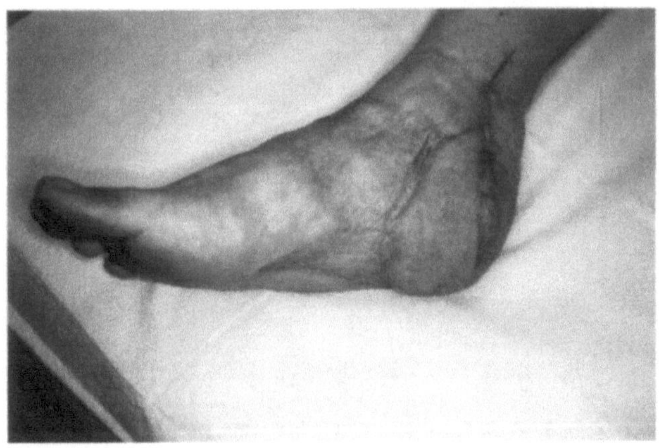
b

Fig. 2-6. a. The lateral arm flap is useful where sensation is important, such as on the sole of the foot. In this patient, a split-thickness skin graft had been performed to cover the entire heel after an injury there. Subsequently, intermittent breakdown occurred in the region. **b.** A lateral arm flap was used to provide sensation and good full-thickness cover.

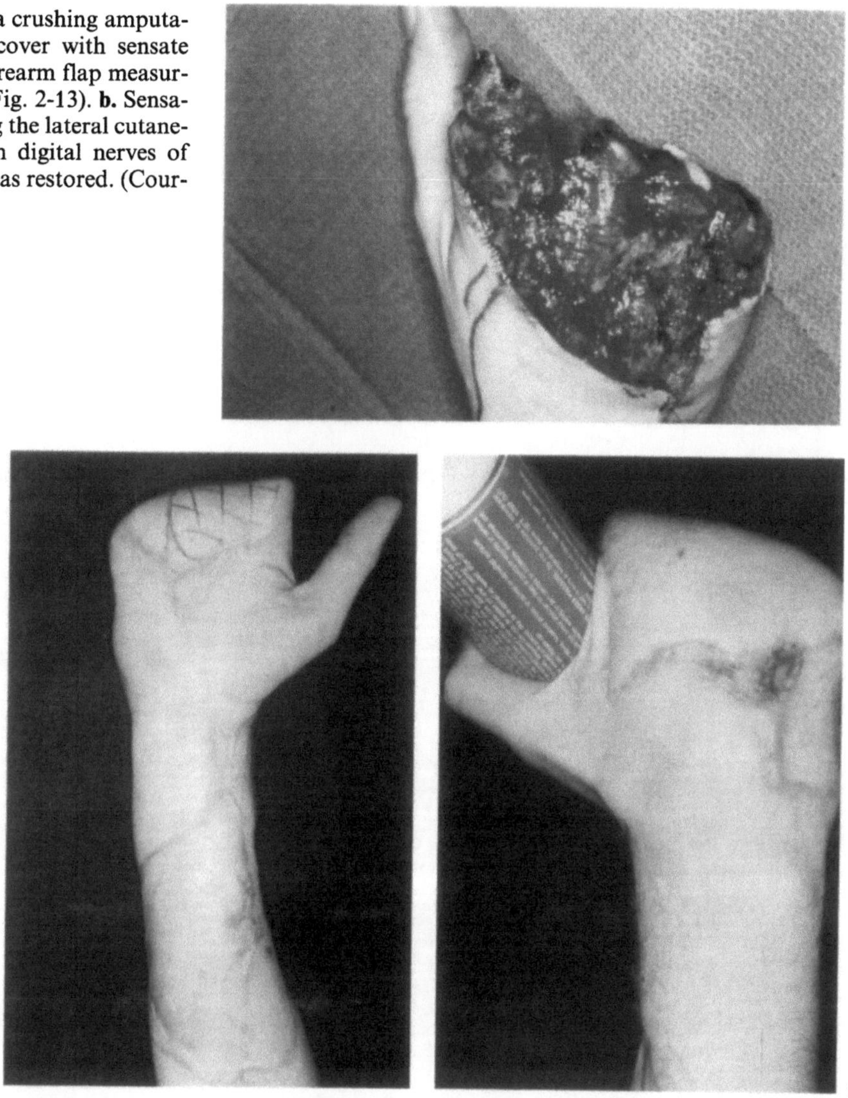

Fig. 2-7. a. A 24-year-old laborer suffered a crushing amputation of all his fingers. Good soft-tissue cover with sensate skin was needed. A "retrograde" radial forearm flap measuring 12 cm × 10 cm was indicated (see also Fig. 2-13). **b.** Sensation was restored (*shaded areas*) by suturing the lateral cutaneous nerve of the forearm to the common digital nerves of the index and long fingers. **c.** Good grasp was restored. (Courtesy of Hill Hastings II.)

a b c

The **dorsalis pedis flap** (McCraw and Furlow 1975, Zuker and Manktelow 1985) (Fig. 2-1) provides good thin skin but is quite small. Its main advantage is that it includes a nerve and can provide sensory return. Skin grafting is required if a flap wider than 3 cm is taken, in which case the donor site can present problems with discomfort and breakdown. If a flap wider than 3 cm is needed, donor site problems make this flap undesirable compared with other skin flaps that allow primary donor site closure in less critical areas (Fig. 2-8).

The utility of this flap is greatest when it accompanies the metatarsophalangeal joint or the metatarsal and tendon as a composite tissue transplant (Fig. 4-19). In this circumstance, a narrow flap is usually sufficient and primary closure of the donor site is possible. The dorsalis pedis flap may be tailored to specific problems in the hand (Fig. 2-1) and may include skin from the dorsum of the foot with extensions distally on one or both sides of the first web space (Fig. 2-9); this may be useful in some hand defects (Doi and Hattorii 1980). This flap is particularly indicated where sensation is important.

In 3–7% of patients, the dorsalis pedis artery emanates from the peroneal artery (Fig. 1-23; Plate 4-V). Also, the first dorsal metatarsal artery is variable (Plate 4-IV). Arteriography and Doppler studies should confirm the anatomy of the dorsalis pedis and first dorsal metatarsal arteries (Man and Acland 1980, see comments by Banis in Zuker and Manktelow 1985).

The **radial forearm flap** (Mühlbauer et al. 1982, Song et al. 1982) (Fig. 2-7) is based on the radial artery, and provides thin pliable skin. This flap is relatively large and the anatomy of the vessels is constant, making dissection easy. However, the donor site requires skin grafting and may be unsightly because of its location in an exposed region. By including the lateral and/or the medial cutaneous nerve of the forearm, a flap with sensation can be achieved. In rare circumstances, a part of the radius, the brachioradialis, or flexor carpi radialis can also be included. Removal of a corticocancellous

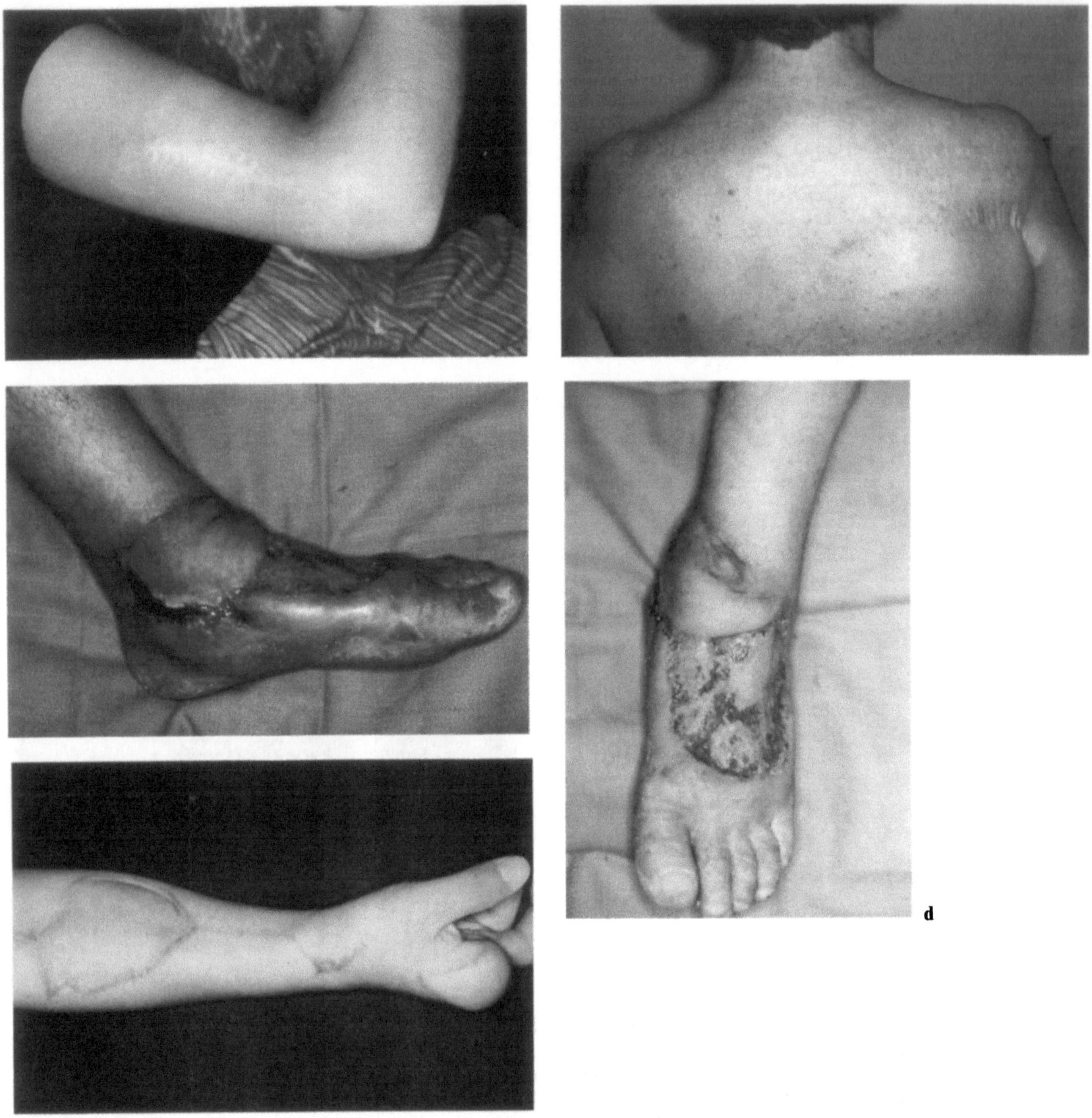

a b c d e

Fig. 2-8. a. The lateral arm flap. For flaps measuring 6–7 cm or less in width, an inconspicuous scar can be expected with primary closure. There may be a minor contour deficit on the lateral aspect of the upper arm. **b. The scapular flap.** The donor site is closed primarily, but there is usually a moderate amount of tension on the suture line which frequently results in a spread scar. **c and d. The dorsalis pedis flap.** The donor site cannot be closed primarily if it is wider than 3 cm. Skin grafting in this area can produce problems with healing, breakdown, and swelling. This patient was referred for consultation after a dorsalis pedis rotation flap had been harvested. There is marked swelling distally and the skin graft provided inadequate cover; such conditions may subsequently result in chronic discomfort and intermittent breakdown. If the skin grafting at this donor site is done with meticulous precision, these problems can usually be avoided. Continuous elevation for 2–4 weeks and patient cooperation are imperative. If possible, a narrow flap should be used with primary closure of the donor site (Fig. 2-12). Wider dorsalis pedis flaps should only be used very rarely. **e. The radial forearm flap.** The donor site is relatively conspicuous, even in this patient who had a small flap.

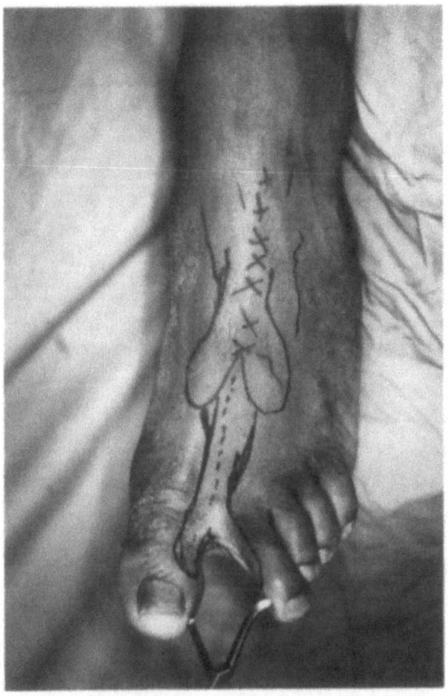

Fig. 2-9. A flap which is based on either the dorsalis pedis artery (*indicated with an "x"*) or the first dorsal metatarsal artery (*dotted line*) can include the adjacent sides of the first web space to resurface adjacent fingers. If no first dorsal metatarsal artery is present, a dorsalis pedis flap can be fashioned, depending on the shape of the recipient site; however, the flap should be proximal to the deep plantar artery (Sec. 4.5).

segment of the radius, however, carries the risk of subsequent fracture and may otherwise have no substantial benefit over a nonvascularized bone graft. The radial artery is sacrificed, although some surgeons reconstruct this artery with a vein graft. Even if the ulnar artery is present and supplies the hand, there is some question about the wisdom of sacrificing the radial artery if other flaps with more benign donor sites will suffice. If the Allen test does not provide an unequivocal result, then a preoperative arteriogram is advisable to confirm that the ulnar artery supplies the palmar arch; even with a strong ulnar pulse, the ulnar and radial vessels may supply separate sides of the hand with little communication (Figs. 2-1 and 1-26) (Coleman and Anson 1961, Jones and O'Brien 1985).

The **temporoparietal fascial flap** (Upton et al. 1986) is based on the superficial temporal vessels, and consists of temporoparietal fascia on which a split-thickness skin graft is placed. This flap is described here because it is sometimes used as an alternative to a cutaneous flap. It is used for small defects, especially those in the hand. Because the deep surface of this flap is smooth and lined, it has been suggested that tendon gliding can occur beneath it. Despite this layer, the fascia often adheres to the deeper tissues, making subsequent tendon reconstruction difficult. In addition, the ultimate cover is inferior to full-thickness skin with a mobile subcutaneous fatty layer – characteristics that are desirable for the dorsum of the hand.

The **deltoid flap** (Franklin 1984, Russell et al. 1985) can also provide skin cover. This flap can include a branch of the axillary nerve, i.e., the upper lateral cutaneous nerve of the arm; this nerve will provide some sensation in the part of the flap above the deltoid-triceps groove. The donor site is often unsightly, having a spread scar, and sometimes requires split-thickness skin grafting. This flap does not display particular benefits when compared with those described above.

Dissection of the **groin flap** (Daniel and Taylor 1973) is difficult compared with other cutaneous transplants, and the vascular anatomy is variable. The superficial circumflex iliac vessel is small. If the deep circumflex iliac vessel is used, the dissection requires elevation of abdominal muscles, which can cause subsequent hernia. The flap is hair-bearing and often too bulky, requiring repeated defatting procedures. However, the flap is used as part of an osteocutaneous transplant.

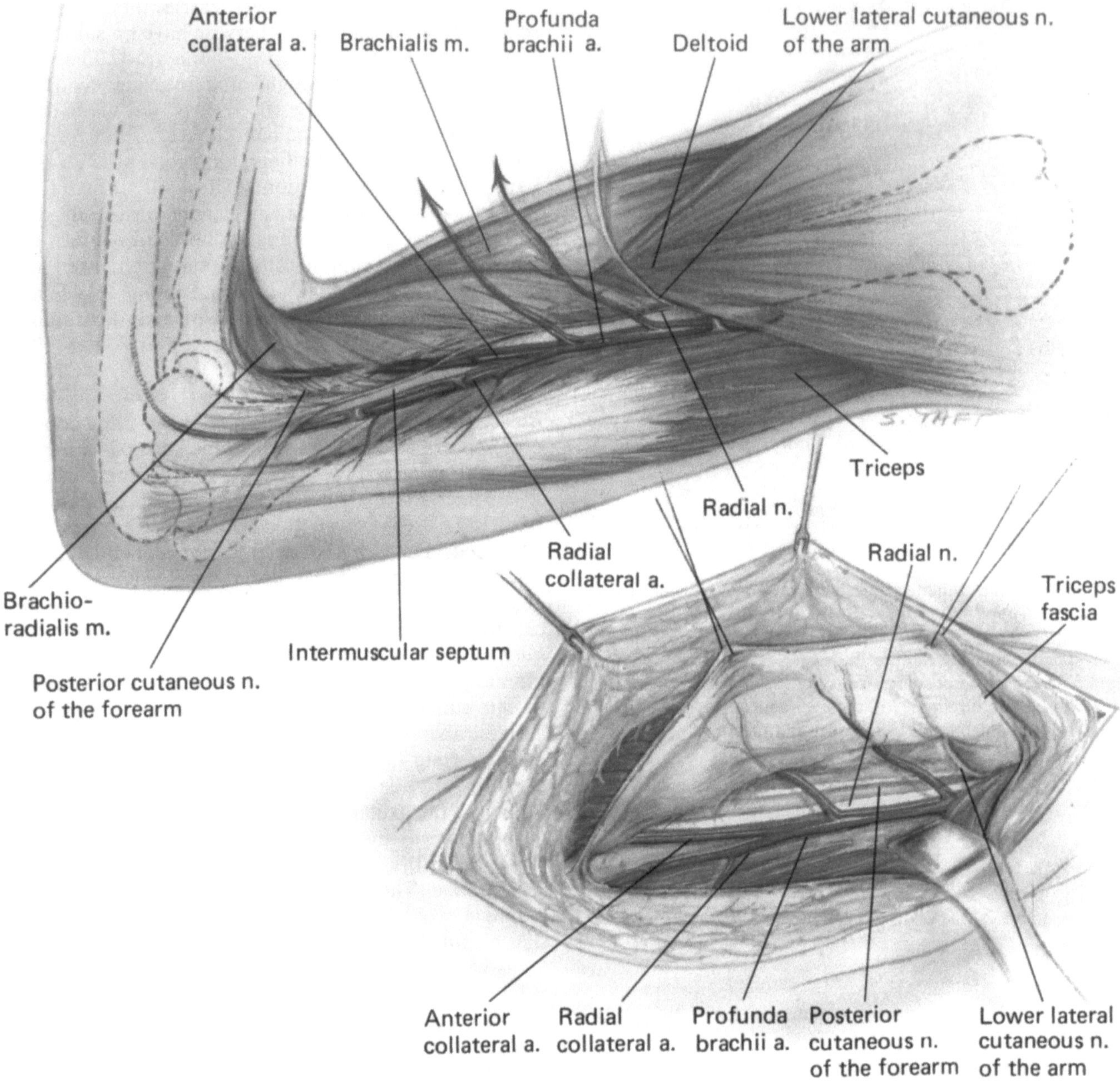

Plate 2-I. Anatomy of the lateral arm flap.

2.4 Lateral Arm Flap (Katsaros and Schusterman 1984)

2.4.1 Anatomy (Plate 2-I)

The *profunda brachii artery* accompanies the radial nerve in its course around the humerus, lying between the deltoid insertion anteriorly and the triceps posteriorly. Its continuation is the *radial collateral artery* (sometimes called the posterior radial collateral artery), which travels distally at the base of the lateral intermuscular septum between the triceps posteriorly and the brachialis anteriorly. It has several *cutaneous branches* which supply the skin of the lateral arm. It gives off the *anterior collateral artery* which proceeds distally with the radial nerve, but is a small and less constant vessel. The radial collateral artery then proceeds to the lateral epicondyle to take part in the arterial anastomosis around the elbow by connecting with a recurrent branch from the interosseous or radial artery.

The *sensory supply to the region, the lower lateral cutaneous nerve of the arm*, is a branch of the radial nerve which usually arises in the spiral groove. Some sensation in this area may also be provided by the *proximal branch of the posterior cutaneous nerve of the forearm*, which emanates from the radial nerve more distally. Because two nerves supply this region, sensation in this flap varies in quality from patient to patient.

2.4.2 Surgical Technique (Fig. 2-10)

a. The lateral arm flap is a fasciocutaneous flap harvested from the lower lateral portion of the arm. It consists of a thin layer of skin, subcutaneous tissue, and upper-arm fascia. The cutaneous portion can extend from the deltoid insertion to the lateral epicondyle. The width is limited to approximately 6 cm if the donor site is to be closed primarily. The cutaneous flap can be extended with fascia, which is then skin-grafted at the recipient site.

The dissection is easiest performed with the arm draped free, lying across the chest, and with the elbow flexed. In lean arms, a sterile tourniquet can be used. The axis of the flap lies along a line that runs from the deltoid insertion to the lateral epicondyle of the humerus. This line represents the surface landmark of the intermuscular septum between the anterior and posterior brachial compartments. The flap is outlined 3 cm anterior and 3 cm posterior to this axis.

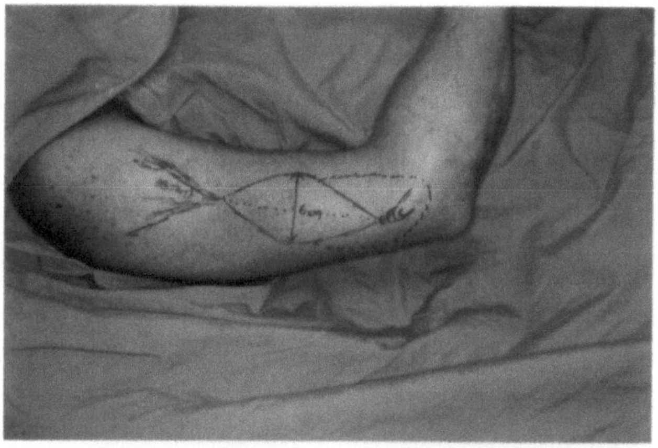
a

b. The posterior incision is made initially and carried down to the triceps fascia. The triceps fascia is incised. Dissection is continued deep to this fascia toward the intermuscular septum, elevating the fascia with the flap.

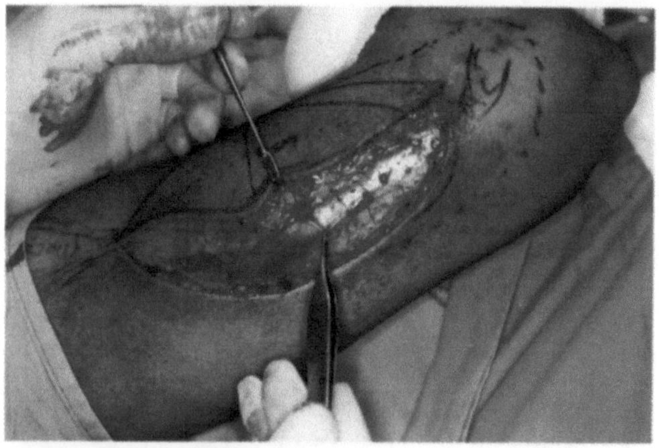
b

c. When the intermuscular septum is reached, dissection is done carefully and slowly, identifying the radial nerve, lower lateral cutaneous nerve (*in the hook*), profunda brachii artery, and radial collateral artery in the process. The radial collateral vessel can be seen traveling toward the skin in this region.

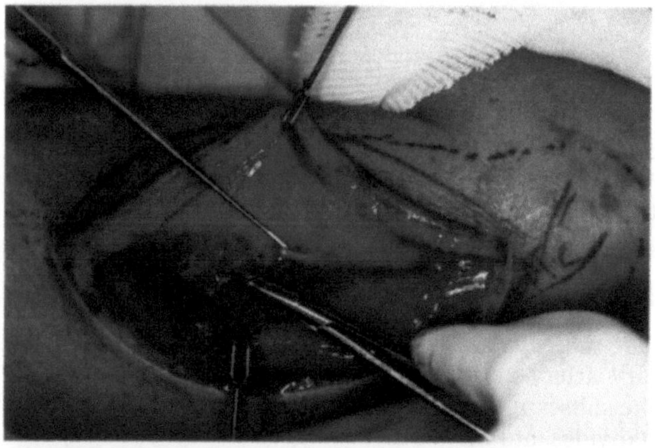
c

d. The neurovascular bundle (*in the nerve hook*) and radial nerve are dissected. At times the profunda brachii and its branches can divide around the radial nerve, which may make dissection in this region somewhat tedious. However, once this region has been dissected and the various branches identified and divided, the pedicle can then be followed proximally for 4 to 6 cm.

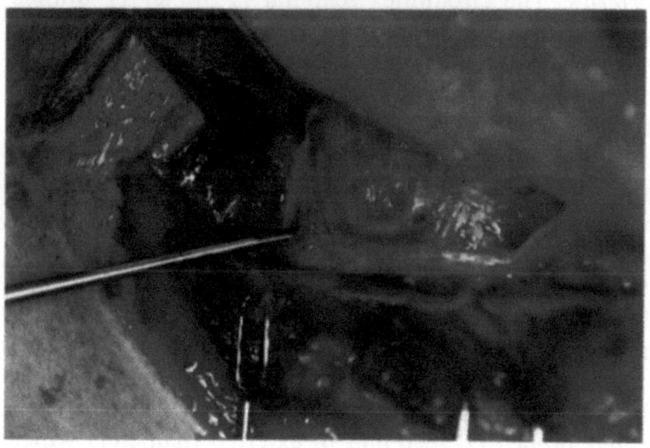
d

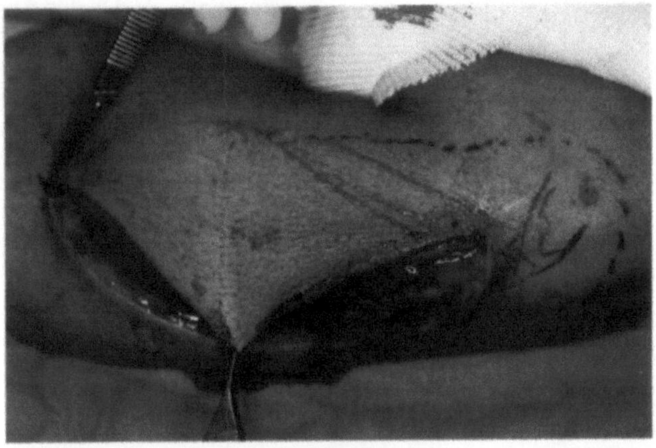

e

e. The anterior incision is then made and dissection is similarly carried out beneath the deep fascia, once again toward the intermuscular septum. Once the anterior incision meets the posterior incision, the flap is raised and the pedicle can be dissected further. A vessel loop placed around the vessels helps to identify them when the intermuscular septum is approached anteriorly.

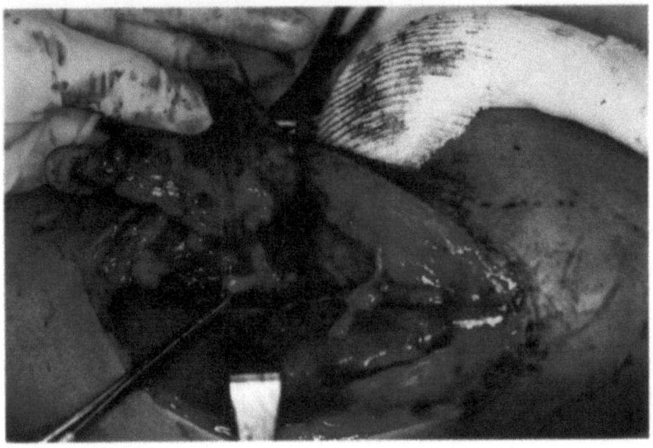

f

f. The proximal and distal parts of the flap are then raised, making sure that the vessel is included. If a longer pedicle is required, an extension of the skin incision may be necessary. This incision is carried up from the proximal apex of the flap to a point approximately 1 cm posterior to the deltoid muscle insertion. As the pedicle is dissected proximally, branches from the pedicle to the triceps muscle are carefully ligated and divided. The radial nerve is protected (*seen in the clamp*).

2.5 Scapular Flap (Barwick et al. 1982, dos Santos 1980, Gilbert and Teot 1982, Hamilton and Morrison 1982, Mayou et al. 1982, Urbaniak et al. 1982)

2.5.1 Anatomy (Plate 2-II)

The *subscapular artery* is the largest branch of the axillary artery and descends along the axillary border of the subscapularis muscle. Three to 4 cm from its origin, it divides into the thoracodorsal and *circumflex scapular arteries*. The circumflex scapular is the larger branch passing posteriorly through the *triangular space*. This space is bounded by the subscapularis and teres minor above, the teres major below, and the long head of the triceps laterally. It then turns under the teres minor onto the dorsum of the scapula, ramifying in the infraspinous fossa and taking part in the rich arterial anastomosis around the scapula. In the triangular space, it gives off one branch to the subscapularis muscle, and the *parascapular branch*, which runs along the medial border of the scapula between the teres minor and teres major muscles toward the inferior angle of the scapula.

As the circumflex scapular artery courses around the lateral border of the scapula, it gives off a sizeable *cutaneous branch* (1.5-2.0 mm in external diameter) which supplies the skin over the scapula; this area is the territory of the scapular flap, and the branch supplying it is a constant cutaneous vessel. A *pedicle* of 5–6 cm can be dissected, with an additional 3–4 cm of length if dissection is taken back to the origin of the circumflex scapular vessels. Two *venae comitantes* accompany the circumflex scapular artery and its major branches.

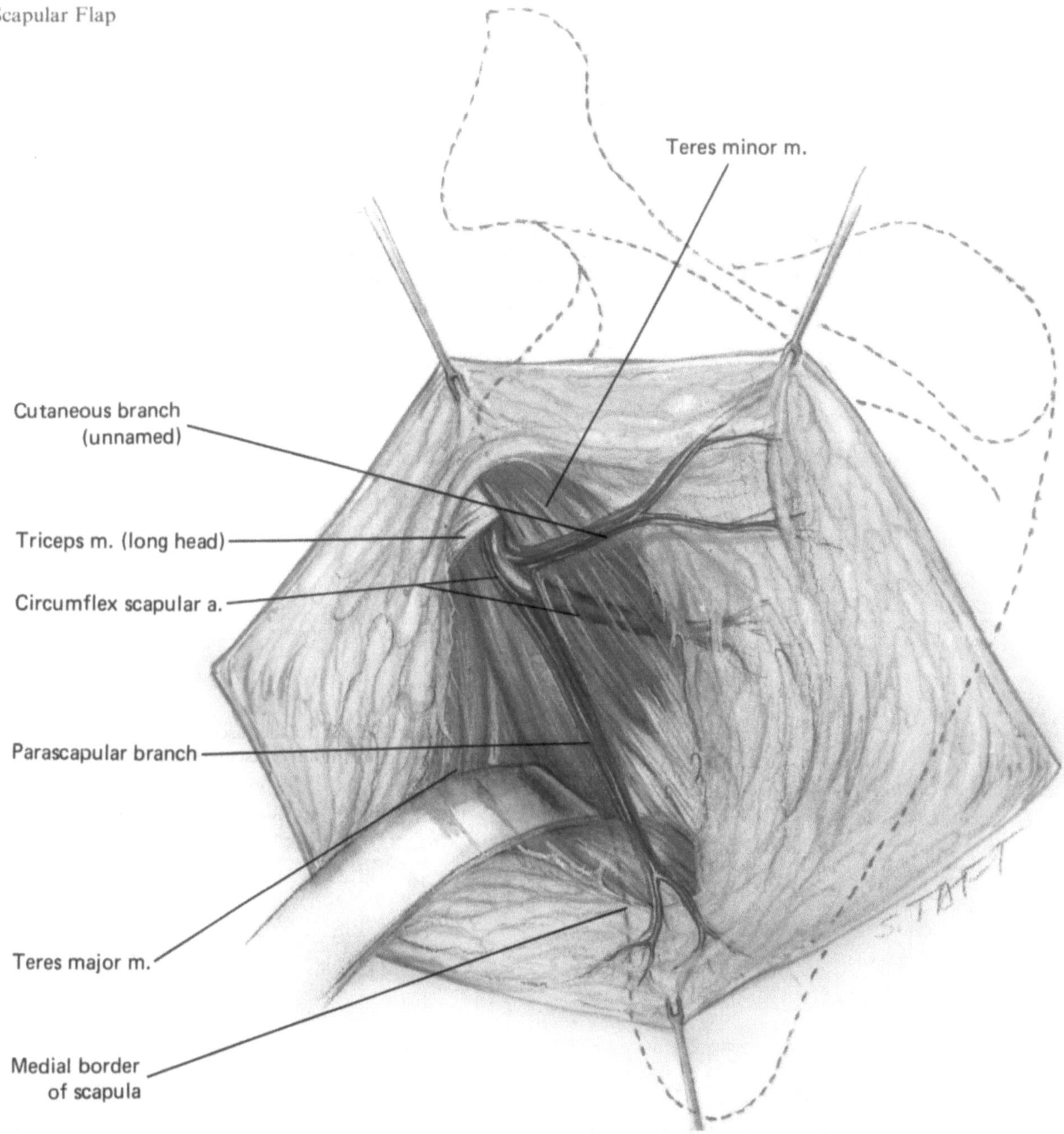

Plate 2-II. Anatomy of the scapular flap.

2.5.2 Surgical Technique (Fig. 2-11)

a. The scapular flap can be dissected with the patient in the prone or lateral decubitus position, allowing access to the dorsal or palmar surfaces of both upper extremities. The position used when covering the dorsum of the hand is shown. (Either the dorsum or palm of each upper extremity, or the medial or lateral aspect of each lower extremity can be approached if the side of the flap and position of the patient are carefully chosen.)

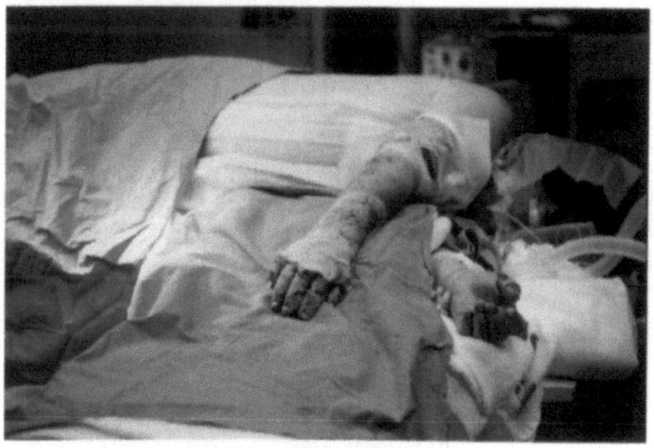

a

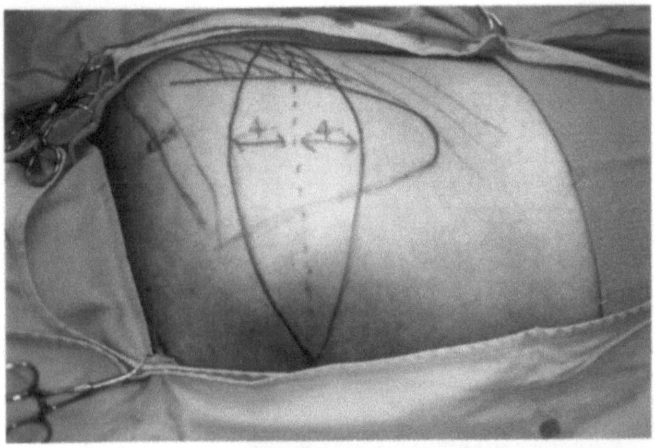

b

b. The scapula and the muscles bordering the triangular space are outlined. The flap axis is perpendicular to the midpoint of the long axis of the scapula. The flap can extend from the posterior axillary fold to the midline, and from the spine to the tip of the scapula. For primary donor site closure, the width of the flap should not exceed 10 cm.

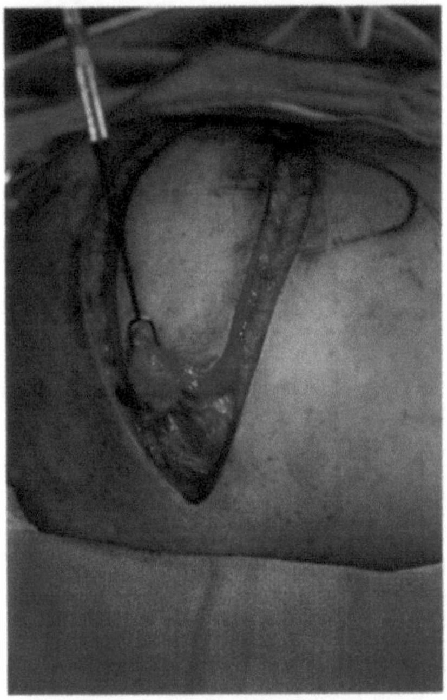

c

c. Incision is made down to the fascia circumferentially. The fascia is incised, exposing the musculature beneath.

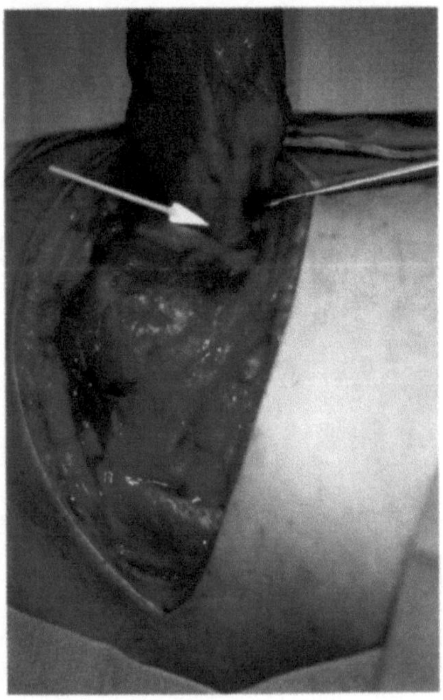

d

d. The flap is now elevated from the medial to the lateral side. Full-thickness skin is elevated, including both the fascia over the infraspinatus muscle and the more lateral fascia. The vessels can be identified curving around the lateral border of the scapula (*arrow*). The lateral dissection should be done carefully because the vascular pedicle is encountered in this region.

e. The flap has now been elevated. There is fascia on its deep surface. The vascular pedicle (one artery, two veins) is now dissected in the triangular space. The teres major and teres minor are retracted. There is a rich anastomotic network around the scapula which connects the circumflex scapular vessel with the suprascapular vessels. These branches and the parascapular branch are ligated and divided. A pedicle about 5 cm long can be obtained with ease. The diameter of the artery is generally greater than 1.5 mm. If a longer pedicle is needed, dissection can be continued deep into the triangular space to the thoracodorsal branch, which can be divided to provide an additional 3–5 cm of pedicle length.

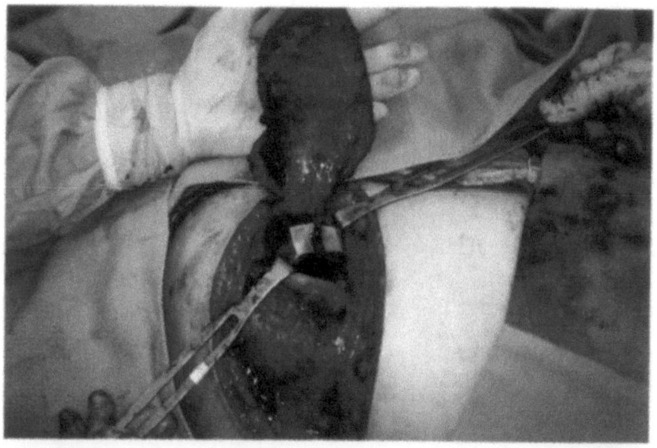
e

2.6 Dorsalis Pedis Flap (McCraw and Furlow 1975, Zuker and Manktelow 1985)

2.6.1 Anatomy (Plate 4-I)

2.6.2 Surgical Technique (Fig. 2-12)

a. The axis of this flap lies along the course of the dorsalis pedis and first dorsal metatarsal arteries. The pulse of these vessels is mapped out on the skin. The flap may be eccentric, i.e., larger on the lateral side, as long as these vessels lie well within the flap. If taken distally, confirmation of the course of the first dorsal metatarsal artery either by arteriography or Doppler study is important. The course of the superficial veins in the foot is marked, as is the anticipated position of the superficial peroneal nerve. A flap less than 3 cm wide will allow primary closure of the donor site.

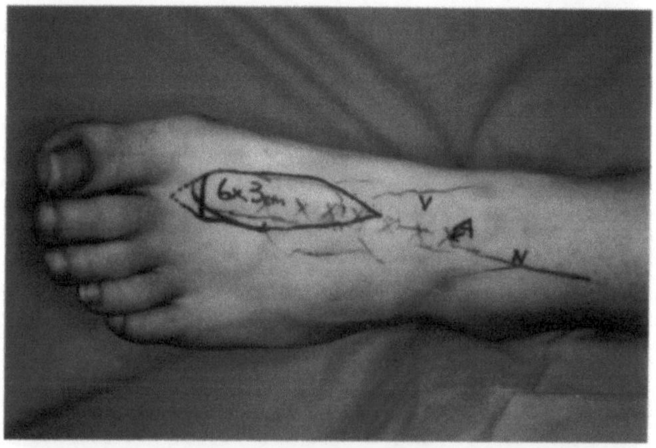
a

b. The dissection is done under tourniquet control. The venous dissection is easier if elevation alone is used for exsanguination; this leaves the veins moderately filled. A superficial vein emanating from the flap is dissected, depending on the diameter and length needed at the recipient site (*blue background*). The superficial peroneal nerve is located and dissected, taking special care to protect any branch that travels toward the flap (*yellow background*).

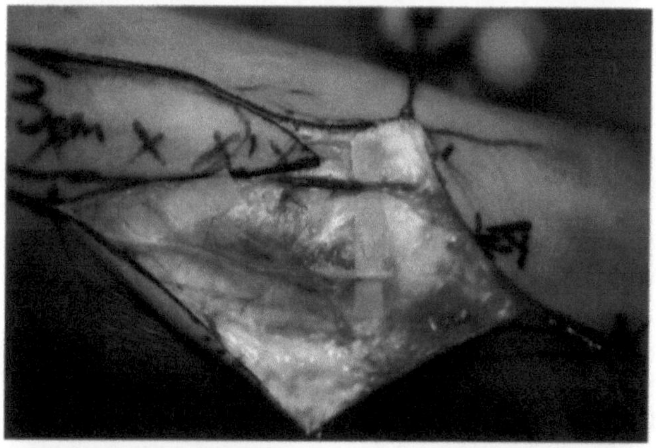
b

c. At the ankle, the neurovascular bundle lies between the extensor hallucis longus medially and the extensor digitorum longus laterally. Distally, it is found under the tendon of the extensor hallucis brevis. This tendon, which crosses superficial to the neurovascular bundle, is divided and left in the flap. The deep peroneal nerve lies lateral to the vessels but may cross from the medial side proximally (as in this patient). This nerve is important if skin from the first web space is taken. The dorsalis pedis artery is dissected *proximal* to the flap.

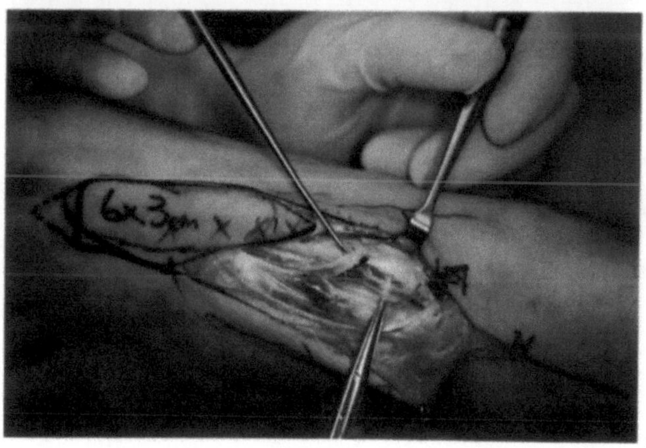
c

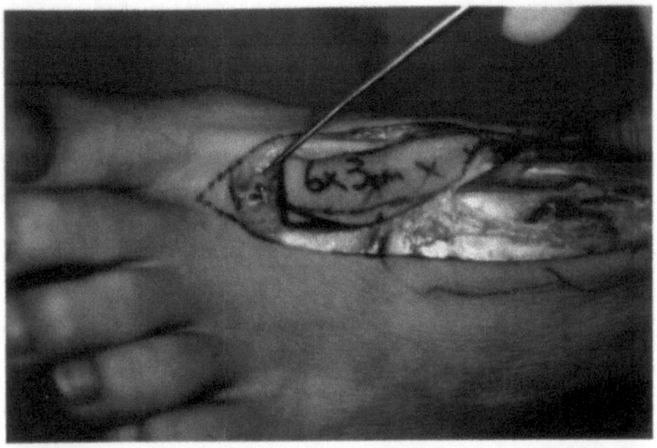

d

d. The rest of the incision is made, and the first dorsal metatarsal artery is located distal to the flap, ligated, and divided.

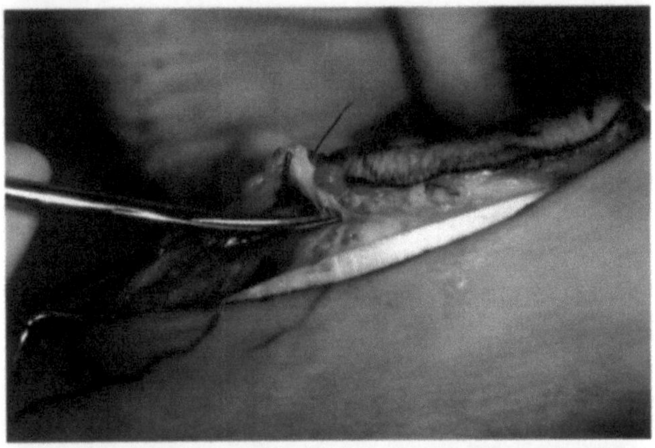

e

e. The next step is the key to dissecting the dorsalis pedis flap. It involves separating the flap from the periosteum and paratenon. This dissection may be done from the proximal or distal aspect, but must be *deep to the vessels* so that communications between these vessels and the skin are *not* disturbed. If a skin graft is anticipated, it is important to leave the periosteum and paratenon intact. As the perforating branch of the dorsalis pedis artery is approached, great care must be exercised and the anatomy of the region kept in mind (Plates 4-I and 4-IV). The continuity between the dorsalis pedis artery and the first dorsal metatarsal vessel must be maintained, even if the latter emanates from the plantar surface. This dissection can be a difficult one. If the first dorsal metatarsal artery originates from the plantar system, a dorsalis pedis flap proximal to the perforating branch should be planned. In cases where a plantar vessel has not been identified by the preoperative arteriogram, the first dorsal metatarsal artery can be sutured to the dorsalis pedis vessel either end-to-end or by using a short vein graft, thereby restoring vascularity to the distal flap.

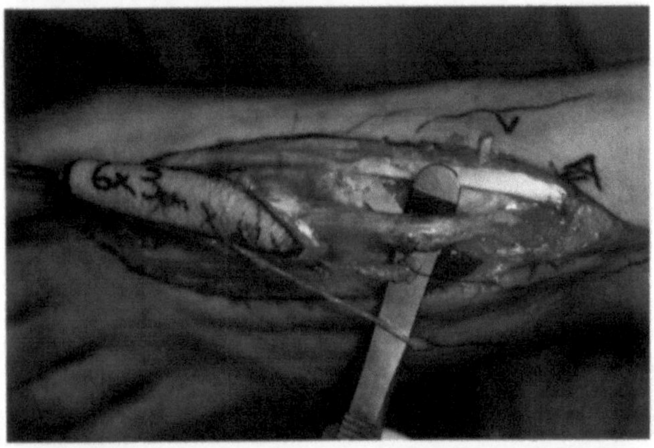

f

f. The *dorsalis pedis artery*, *two venae comitantes*, and *superficialis veins* can be dissected as far proximally as needed. The *superficial peroneal nerve* is dissected proximally and included if sensation is desired. The tourniquet is released and bleeding from the margins of the flap and good capillary return are demonstrated.

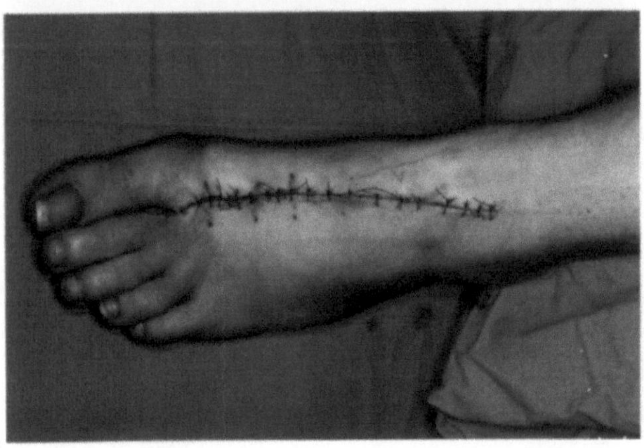

g

g. The donor site was closed primarily without tension.

2.6.3 Foot Closure

Foot closure is accomplished by one of three methods.

1. For narrow flaps, *primary closure* seldom produces a problem.
2. For wider flaps, a *split-thickness skin graft* is meshed and sutured to the margins of the defect. Careful hemostasis is important after tourniquet release prior to graft placement. The graft must be placed on paratenon and have contact with the bed in all areas, especially in the first web space; pledgets of cotton soaked in mineral oil can be helpful in accomplishing this. Continuous elevation for 14 days is imperative.
3. Following an osteocutaneous transplant or a joint transplant, the second metatarsal is removed near its base and a ray amputation of the second toe is done, taking care to plan the skin flaps for perfect closure once the first and third metatarsals are approximated. The intermetatarsal ligament is repaired. The closure is then similar to that following a second-toe transplant (Fig. 4-3). An excellent cosmetic and functional outcome can be expected.

2.7 Radial Forearm Flap

2.7.1 Anatomy

The skin of the radial volar forearm is thin and pliable. This fasciocutaneous flap receives its *vascular supply* via the radial artery. A constant fasciocutaneous perforator is found approximately 8 cm proximal to the radiocarpal joint, with many smaller perforators proximally. Venous drainage is through the two venae comitantes. Tributaries of the cephalic vein are usually abundant and also drain this area. The flap can be used as a retrograde island flap. If the proximal radial artery and venae comitantes are then ligated, the venae comitantes will still allow adequate retrograde flow of blood from the flap. The flap can also be used as a free flap, anastomosing the proximal vessels at the recipient site, or as a "flow-through flap," in which case arterial reconstruction is possible by anastomosing the artery both proximally and distally. Pedicle length of 15–20 cm can be obtained without difficulty.

The *nerve supply* consists of the lateral and medial cutaneous nerves of the forearm. The musculocutaneous nerve pierces the deep fascia just proximal to the elbow and lateral to the biceps tendon where it becomes the *lateral cutaneous nerve of the forearm.* As this nerve crosses the elbow, it passes deep to the cephalic vein and divides into volar and dorsal branches. The volar branch runs along the radial aspect of the forearm to the wrist and is used in this flap. If a large flap is taken, the *medial cutaneous nerve of the forearm* can be included. It crosses the anteromedial surface of the elbow running on the volar aspect of the forearm, slightly on the ulnar side of the midline. The superficial branch of the radial nerve lies deep to the brachioradialis, but becomes superficial 8–10 cm proximal to the wrist. This nerve is not included in the radial forearm flap.

2.7.2 Surgical Technique (Fig. 2-13; see also Fig. 2-7)

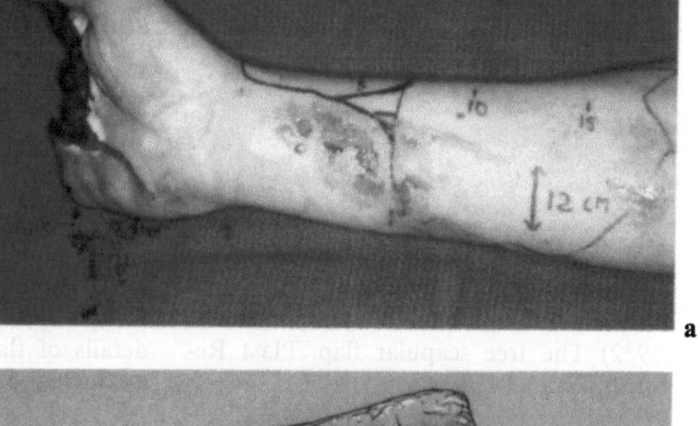

a

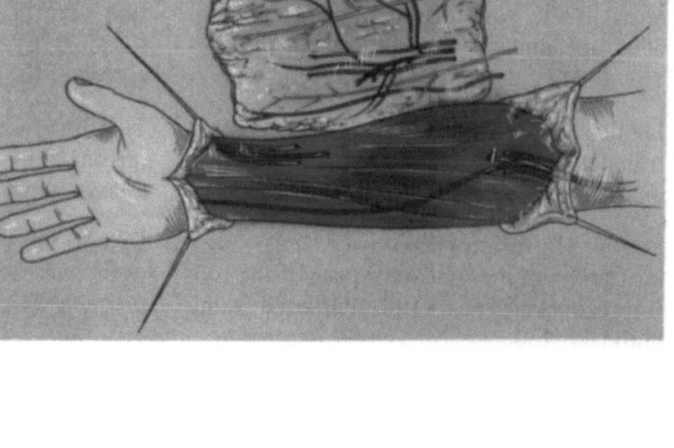

b

a. Before beginning the procedure, it is imperative to confirm that the ulnar artery supplies the entire hand (Fig. 2-1c) (Jones and O'Brien 1985). An Allen test as well as a Doppler study of the thumb and index finger arteries are performed while the more proximal radial artery is compressed. If there is any doubt that the ulnar artery does not supply the entire hand, an arteriogram should be done. The axis of the radial artery is marked, as are the superficial veins. The shape of the proposed flap conforms to the defect and is outlined, centered on the axis of the radial artery. The flap can extend from the elbow to the wrist and include most of the volar surface of the forearm. Large flaps, however, will have unsightly donor sites. A flap measuring 15 cm × 10 cm can be taken. (Courtesy of Hill Hastings II.)

b. Under tourniquet control, the radial artery, venae comitantes, superficial veins, and lateral and/or medial cutaneous nerve of the forearm are dissected proximally. These structures are ligated at a point determined by the requirements of the recipient site. The vessels can be dissected and ligated both proximally and distally, creating a "*flow-through flap*" for arterial reconstruction. The flap is elevated in a plane that lies between the deep fascia and the muscle, taking care to not disturb communications between the radial artery and the flap. Distally, the superficial radial nerve is identified and protected. (Illustration by Gary Schnitz.)

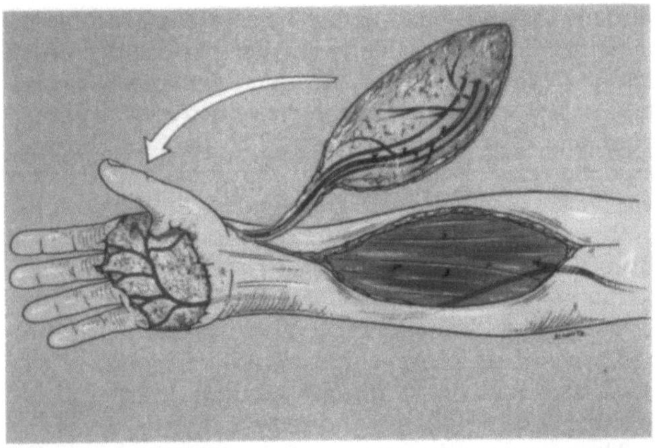

c

c. The vessels can be ligated proximally, creating a retrograde *island flap*. The proximal nerves can be sutured to nerves in the hand, providing sensory return.

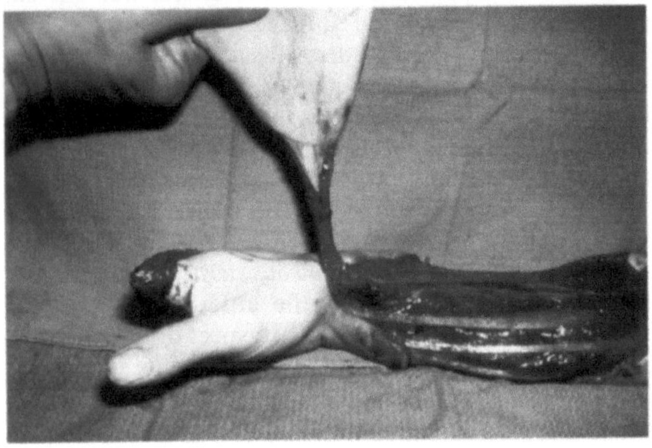

d

d. The retrograde flap has been elevated and is based on the radial artery and venae comitantes. The donor defect is extensive and requires split-thickness skin grafting.

2.8 Postoperative Care

A monitor is extremely helpful in assessing the vascularity of skin flaps (Chapter 8). Vascular problems may arise as late as 7–10 days after operation, but are most frequently encountered within 48–72 hours. The usual attention to *hydration*, warm ambient *temperature*, and *elevation* is essential. Low-molecular-weight dextran (30 cc/hour) is used for 5 days as an *anticoagulant*, after which aspirin (325 mg daily) is taken for 2 weeks.

2.9 Selected Bibliography

Barwick WJ, Goodkind DJ, Serafin D (1982) The free scapular flap. Plast Reconstr Surg 69:779

Early experience with the free scapular flap is described in 14 patients. The details of flap dissection and a discussion of the indications and advantages are included.

Coleman SS, Anson BJ (1961) Arterial patterns in the hand based upon a study of 650 specimens. Surg Gynecol Obstet 113:409

The supply to the hand originating from the radial and ulnar arteries is described. In a significant number of specimens, all or a particular part of the hand is supplied by one of the arteries or the other – not both. The authors do not correlate the supply of the deep and superficial palmar arches.

Daniel RK, Taylor GI (1973) Distant transfer of an island flap by microvascular anastomoses. Plast Reconstr Surg 52:111

This historical case report of the first distant transfer of an iliofemoral island (groin) flap outlines the anatomy, method, and ultimate success of covering a large wound of the distal medial leg.

Doi K, Hattorii S (1980) Free neurovascular flap from the first web space of the foot for reconstruction of the mutilated hand. Hand 12:130

Extensions of the dorsalis pedis flap to include one or both sides of the first web space are described. This technique can provide a Y-shaped flap for resurfacing a web space and the adjacent sides of two digits.

dos Santos LF (1980) The scapular flap: A new microsurgical free flap. Bol Chir Plast 70:133

This article is the first to elucidate the anatomy and use of the free scapular flap.

Franklin JD (1984) The deltoid flap: Anatomy and clinical applications. In Buncke HJ, Furnas DW (eds): Symposium on Clinical Frontiers in Reconstructive Microsurgery, Vol. 24. St. Louis, Mosby pp 63–70

The deltoid flap is an option for cover if a sensate cutaneous flap is needed. This article outlines the pertinent anatomy and surgical technique.

Freedlander E, Dickson WA, McGrouther DA (1986) The present role of the groin flap in hand trauma in the light of a long-term review. J Hand Surg 11-B:187

In many cases requiring full-thickness cover of the hand, the choice between the pedicle groin flap and a microvascular flap must be made. The characteristics of the microvascular groin flap in the hand are similar to those of the pedicle groin flap in the long term. This article analyzes the late results of 73 pedicle groin flaps. Partial necrosis occurred in 20% and debulking was necessary in most cases. Although good cover and appearance resulted on the dorsum of the hand, results were less successful on the palm, where creases did not develop and bulk remained a problem. Microvascular flaps provide better early mobility of the hand and allow immediate elevation.

Gilbert A, Teot L (1982) The free scapular flap. Plast Reconstr Surg 69:601

The anatomy of the circumflex scapular artery and its cutaneous branch to the scapular flap is described. This cutaneous branch ranges in diameter from 0.8 mm in infants to 2 mm in adults, and ranges in length from 4 to 9 cm. Of the two venae comitantes, one was dominant and large. These statistics were obtained from cadaver dissections. Four clinical cases involving the heel and ankle are described. The fullest cutaneous size possible was not used in these early cases.

Hamilton SG, Morrison W (1982) The scapular free flap. Br J Plast Surg 35:2

The anatomy of the scapular flap is described in lucid detail. A description of the cutaneous territory, which measures 24 cm × 12 cm, is included.

Jones BM, O'Brien CJ (1985) Acute ischemia of the hand resulting from elevation of a radial forearm flap. Br J Plast Surg 38:396

After harvesting a radial forearm flap, acute ischemia of the hand resulted. Saphenous vein grafting was required, emphasizing the risk of losing the hand. (It is important to note that even in the presence of an ulnar artery, different areas may be independently supplied by the radial or ulnar artery, as described by Coleman and Anson [1961]. Ischemia may result from injury to the radial artery due to trauma, surgery, or radial artery catheter placement [Figs. 1-26 and 2-1].)

Katsaros J, Schusterman M (1984) The lateral arm flap: Anatomy and clinical applications. Ann Plast Surg 12:489

Katsaros and Schusterman note the inconsistent vascular anatomy of the medial aspect of the upper arm, and describe the details of the vascular supply to the lateral arm flap after studying cadavers. A number of points are emphasized: the cutaneous territory (8 cm × 10 cm to 15 cm × 14 cm), the constancy of the vessels, and the dimensions of the vessels. Clinical aspects are discussed along with details of the operative technique. The results in 23 patients, including complications, are given. The option of performing a neurosensory flap by including the posterior cutaneous nerve of the arm is mentioned. (I have included the lower lateral cutaneous nerve of the upper arm.) Including more fascia than skin is another option discussed. The advantages of the flap are reviewed and a comparison with the scapular flap is made. The lateral arm flap is smaller, the skin is thinner, and it is dissected with the patient supine.

Man D, Acland RD (1980) The microarterial anatomy of the dorsalis pedis flap and its clinical applications. Plast Reconstr Surg 65:419

Familiarity with the anatomy of the dorsalis pedis artery is important for the dissection of this flap and also for toe transplantation. In injected specimens, three of 23 did not have a first dorsal metatarsal artery, and 14% had inadequate vasculature for skin survival in the distal third of the flap territory.

Mayou BJ, Whitby D, Jones BM (1982) The scapular flap. An anatomical and clinical study. Br J Plast Surg 35:8

The surgical technique of raising the scapular flap is outlined, and nine cases are discussed. This flap is based on the descending branch of the circumflex scapular vessel. The option of placing the flap obliquely (parascapular flap) is described, and a case combining the scapular flap with the latissimus dorsi musculocutaneous flap based on a single pedicle is mentioned.

McCraw JB, Furlow LT Jr (1975) The dorsalis pedis arterialized flap. Plast Reconstr Surg 55:177

The detailed anatomy and surgical technique of this flap are described and clinical examples given.

Mühlbauer W, Herndl E, Stock W (1982) The forearm flap. Plast Reconstr Surg 70:336

The history, surgical technique, and clinical uses of the radial forearm flap are described. These authors prefer immediate reconstruction of the radial artery with a reversed vein graft.

Nassif TM, Vidal L, Bovet JL, et al (1982) The parascapular flap. A new cutaneous microsurgical free flap. Plast Reconstr Surg 69:591

The axis of this flap, which is based on the descending branch of the circumflex scapular artery, follows the lateral border of the scapula. This flap demonstrates the versatility of the tissue supplied by the subscapular artery, and the article emphasizes combinations of the scapular flap, parascapular flap, and latissimus dorsi transplant. The anatomy and surgical technique are described in detail.

Russell RC, Guy RJ, Zook EG, et al (1985) Extremity reconstruction using the free deltoid flap. Plast Reconstr Surg 76:586

The detailed anatomy and technique of raising this flap are given. The area of sensation averages 15 cm × 10 cm. Results in ten clinical cases where the flap measured 4 cm × 6 cm to 33 cm × 13 cm are described. The authors emphasize that inclusion of a sensory nerve is an advantage, and they used this flap on the palm and dorsum of the hand as well as in the heel.

Song R, Gao Y, Song Y, et al (1982) The forearm flap. Clin Plast Surg 9:21

This paper discusses the anatomic basis of the forearm flap, and provides the details of dissection.

Upton J, Rogers C, Durham-Smith G, et al (1986) Clinical applications of free temporoparietal flaps in hand reconstruction. J Hand Surg 11A:475

Vascularized temporoparietal fascia was used for defects in the hand or fingers that measured up to 14 cm × 12 cm. Technique and clinical applications are discussed. The variations in anatomy of the superficial temporal artery are important.

Urbaniak J, Koman LA, Goldner RD, et al (1982) The vascularized cutaneous scapular flap. Plast Reconstr Surg 69:772

The anatomy and surgical technique are explained in detail, and five clinical cases involving the lower extremities are described.

Zuker RM, Manktelow RT (1985) The dorsalis pedis free flap. Technique of elevation, foot closure, and flap applications. Plast Reconstr Surg 77:93

The dorsalis pedis flap is described for reconstruction of the heel and the hand where innervation is important. Anatomy and technique are outlined clearly and in detail. In this series of 45 patients, the vascular anatomy was found to be reliable. The primary disadvantage of this procedure lies in the donor site if too broad a flap is taken for primary foot closure. The details of skin grafting and care of the donor site are included. (Further analysis of this flap is found in the accompanying discussion of the article by Dr. Joseph C. Banis, who addresses the anatomic variability of the dorsalis pedis artery.)

3 Vascularized Bone Transplantation

3.1 Overview

The many bone grafting methods which surgeons have used over the years have utilized a graft that serves primarily as a matrix with relatively few surviving osseous cells. Ostrup and Fredrickson (1974) were the first to scientifically investigate the fate of bone cells in grafts when circulation to the grafted bone could be maintained. Later, others confirmed experimentally that, under such conditions, osteocytes will survive, obviating the slow process of creeping substitution whereby dead bone is replaced by living bone (Berggren et al. 1982). The applicability of this experimental work to clinical cases continues to be a subject of spirited investigation.

This chapter deals with situations where nonvascularized bone grafts are likely to fail because of slow or absent bone healing. When faced with such problems, vascularized bone grafting provides an attractive alternative. To a great extent, bone healing relies on the ingrowth of vascularity from the surrounding bed. A nonvascularized graft may fail when used in a poorly vascularized bone graft bed or in abnormal bone, which is why vascularized bone grafts are advocated for irradiated or infected areas and areas with extensive fibrosis. In these situations, better healing is likely with the use of bone that has an independent vascular supply.

3.2 Indications

3.2.1 Congenital Problems – Inherent Bone Pathology (Gordon et al. 1986, Pho et al. 1985, Weiland et al. 1987)

Congenital pseudarthrosis of the tibia is a poorly understood problem in which healing of the tibia is difficult to secure and maintain. There is strong clinical evidence that *healing can be achieved earlier* (usually within 3 months of transplantation) and *hypertrophy attained more rapidly* with vascularized bone transplantation than with other techniques (Fig. 3-1); in several centers, 5- to 10-year results are now available, confirming the usefulness of this technique (Weiland et al. 1987). The operation takes 4–5 hours and is straightforward and reliable. The sole disadvantage is that the *donor leg* is left with a single bone. (A synostosis between the tibia and what remains of the distal fibula will prevent ankle valgus in the donor leg.) Patients with this condition must be followed to skeletal maturity to ensure that pseudarthrosis does not recur.

3.2.2 Traumatic Bone Defects

(Taylor 1983, Weiland et al. 1979, Wood 1986)

In treating *extensive traumatic bone defects*, healing and hypertrophy can often be obtained earlier with vascularized bone transplantation than with nonvascularized grafting. However, other treatment options such as allograft replacement or conventional (nonvascularized) bone grafting must also be considered.

The disadvantages of bone allografts are their high rate of infection, fatigue fracture, and nonunion (Mankin et al. 1983). This is especially true where there has been prior infection, fibrosis, or poor blood supply – conditions under which healing is also likely to be slow. Allografts have been used extensively after tumor resection. The remaining tissues are generally of better quality in these cases than they are following trauma. Fatigue fractures of allografts generally heal poorly, whereas similar fractures of vascularized bone tend to heal rapidly.

Conventional bone grafts from the iliac crest and other, more recently developed bone substitutes can sometimes achieve osseous integrity for *short defects*. The difficulty arises in establishing a cut-off length above which vascularized bone transplantation is preferable, but below which conventional bone grafting techniques will suffice. Clearly, no absolute cut-off ex-

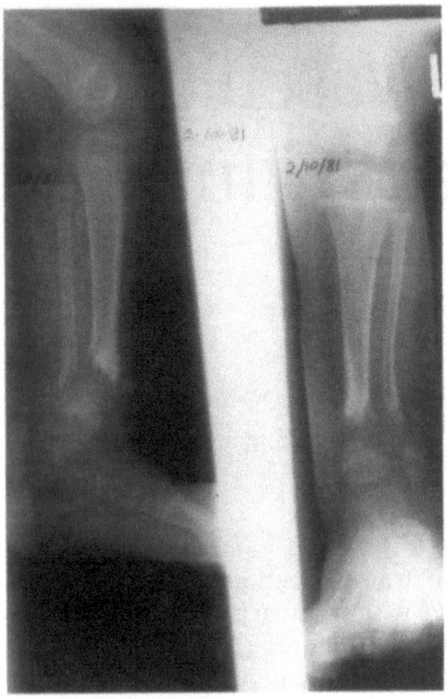

a

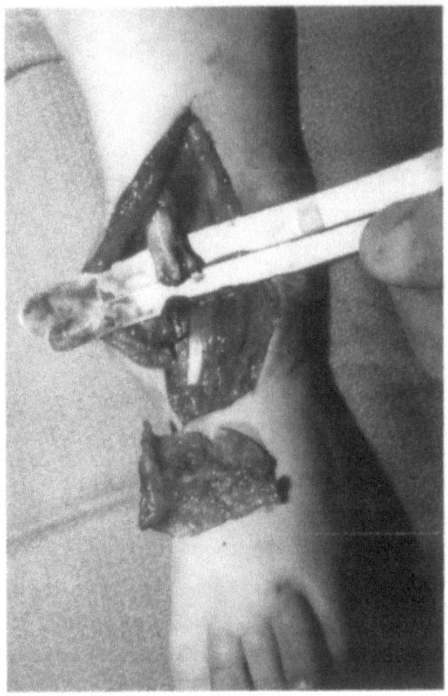

b

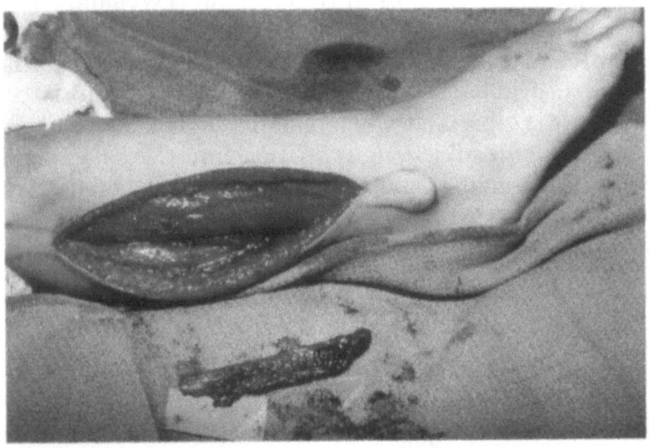

c

Fig. 3-1. a. A 26-month-old girl had been diagnosed with congenital pseudarthrosis of the tibia (Boyd, type 2) at 2 weeks of age. The pseudarthrosis was near the ankle joint, and the unfavorable radiographic appearance is shown. **b.** It is important to debride the abnormal bone and soft tissue in the region of the pseudarthrosis. The tibia was resected back to healthy, bleeding bone where a medullary cavity was present. The anterior tibial vessels were dissected (they are easy to expose on the lateral aspect of the tibia). **c.** The donor fibula was dissected. The vascular pedicle is seen under the blue background.

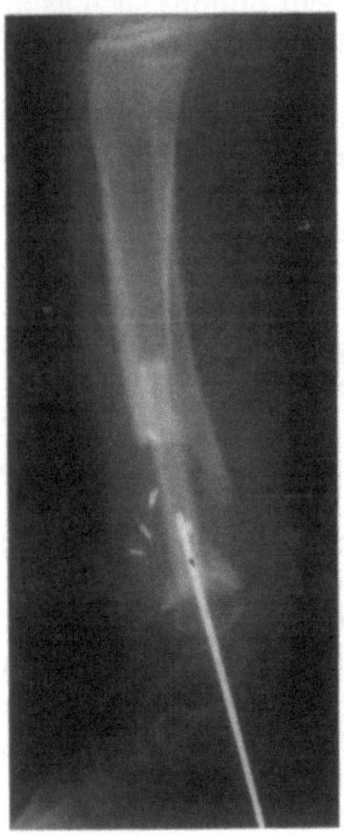

d

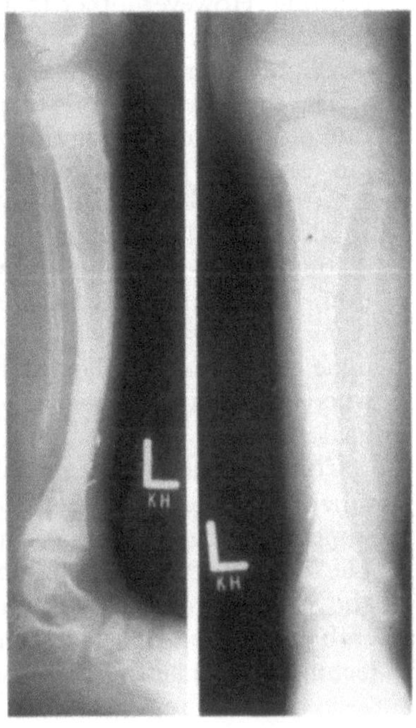

e

Fig. 3-1. d. The vascularized fibula transplant was placed in the medullary canal of the tibia proximally. Because fixation to the very soft distal tibial fragment was difficult, an intramedullary Kirschner wire was used to hold the transplant in place. **e.** Solid healing and good hypertrophy of the transplant were achieved by 5 months. In an incident 2 years after the transplant, the patient discarded her brace and jumped from a 6-foot height, fracturing her tibia; the fracture healed uneventfully in an interval similar to that expected for a normal bone. At follow-up 5 years later, solid healing had been maintained.

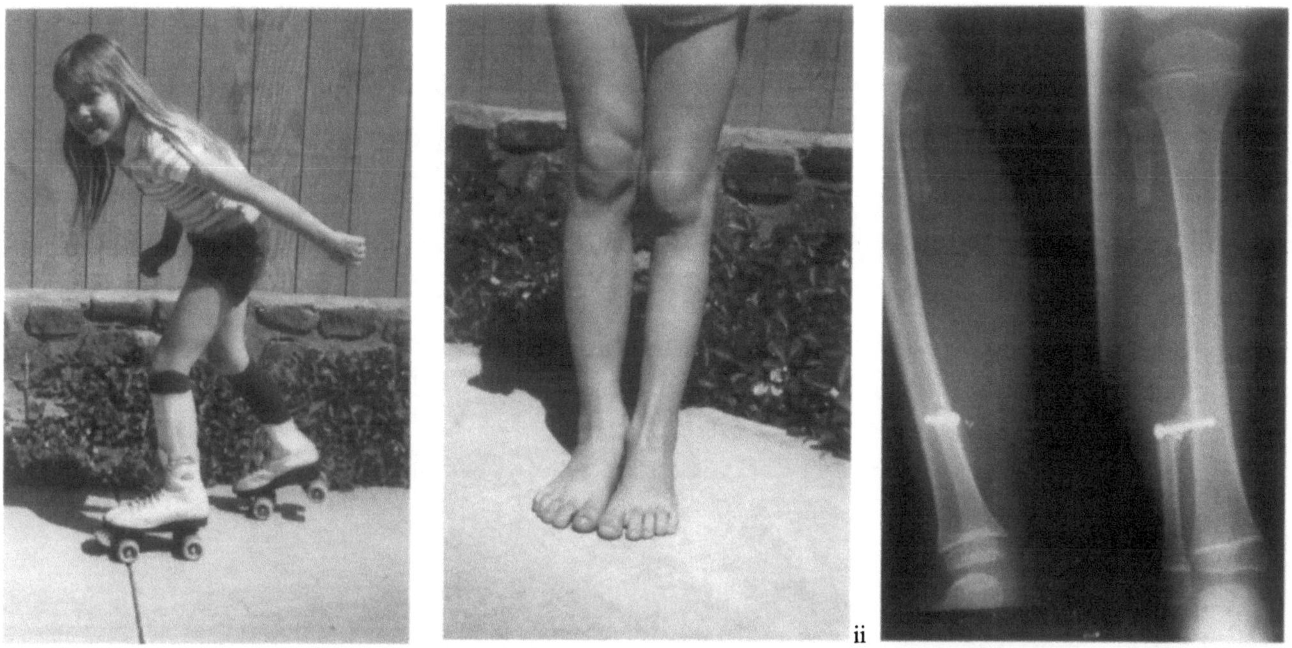

fi ii g

Fig. 3-1. f. i and ii. At the time of this photograph, the patient was 7 years old and fully active. Her left knee was slightly more distal than her right. A brace will be worn until she reaches skeletal maturity. **g.** In the donor leg, a tibiofibular synostosis was done between the remaining fibula and the tibia. (At least the distal fourth of the fibula should be retained.) (I thank Dr. Harry Jergesen for his expert orthopaedic care of this patient.)

ists, and this length varies, depending on the philosophy, expertise, and training of the surgeon. The condition of the recipient bed and the demands on the recipient bone must be evaluated. These factors require that an individualized decision be made for each patient.

It is important that each surgeon establish clear indications for vascularized bone transplantation. The following discussion outlines my protocol.

3.2.2.1 Extensive Bone Defect: No Intact Bone

For defects of the humerus (Fig. 3-2), femur (Fig. 3-3), or both bones of the forearm or leg (Fig. 3-4) that are longer than approximately 5 cm, vascularized fibula transplantation may be indicated, depending on the graft bed (Jupiter et al. 1987). Allografts should be considered if there has not been previous infection, but most posttraumatic defects have a great deal of fibrosis and the condition of the soft tissue is poor. Vascularized fibula transplantation has the advantage of early healing and rapid hypertrophy. The worse the bone graft bed, the more attractive vascularized bone transplantation becomes.

A similar philosophy applies to very long tibial defects in which there has been previous infection, even if the fibula is intact, because the additional support of the transplanted fibula may be important. An infection-free interval of 3–6 months is required following debridement if bone grafting is to be done relatively safely (Fig. 3-5).

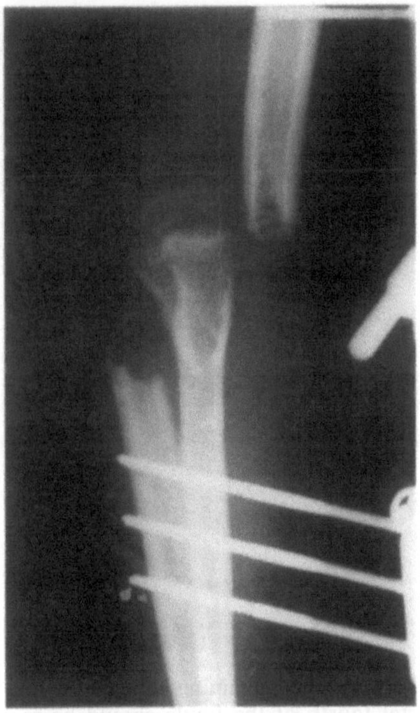

a

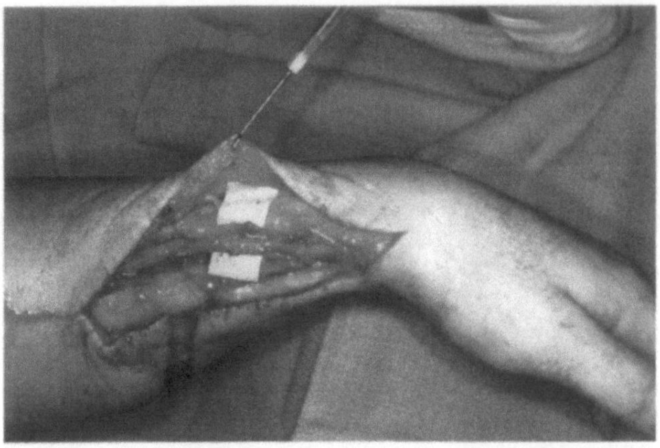

b

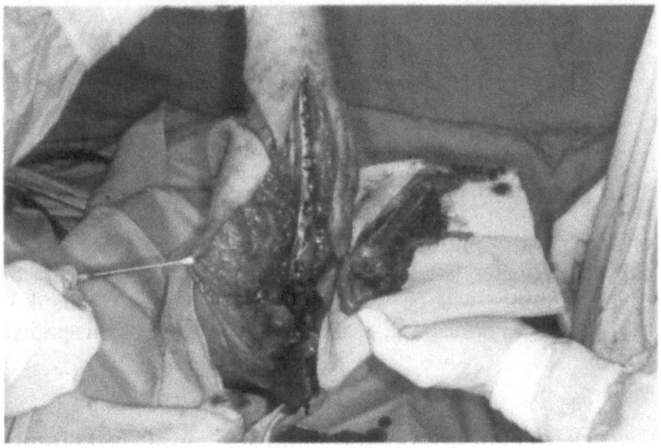

c

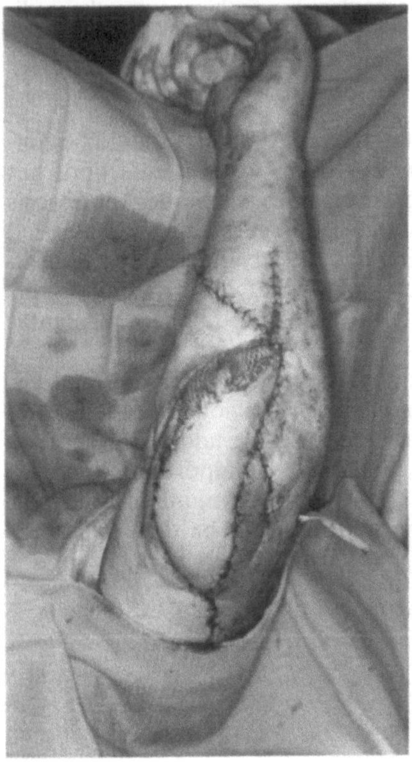

d

Fig. 3-2. a. A 36-year-old man lost his distal humerus, elbow joint, and proximal radius in a car accident. There was severe muscle damage, *soft-tissue cover* posteriorly was inadequate for extensive bone grafting, and the surrounding area was fibrotic. In addition to the *cortical bone defect*, there was poor cancellous bone. An elbow fusion was planned. Both corticocancellous bone and soft-tissue cover were needed. After considering these deficiencies and the fact that vascularized bone can enable the earliest healing possible, an iliac crest osteocutaneous transplant made the most attractive treatment option. **b.** The radial artery and venae comitantes were dissected distally, divided near the wrist, and swung across the volar surface of the forearm to be used as the recipient vessels; this was preferable to using the brachial artery, the proximal radial artery, or the ulnar artery. Not only would these options have required extensive vein grafting, but use of the brachial or ulnar artery involves greater risk to the hand circulation. **c.** The plate was placed to provide stability, but a bone defect remained between the ulna and humerus, and the soft-tissue defect with the exposed plate was evident. This photograph shows the flap, which is based on the deep circumflex iliac vessel and contains a portion of the iliac crest and overlying groin skin. **d.** Two lagged cortical screws were used to fix both ends of the bone transplant, and the cutaneous flap was sutured into place.

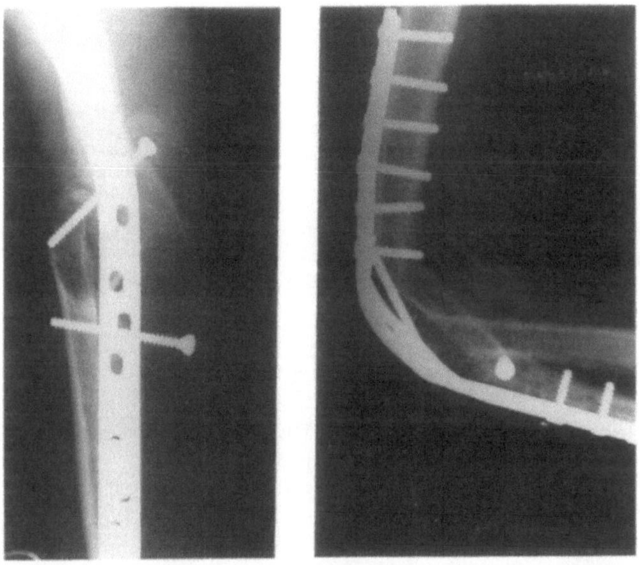

e

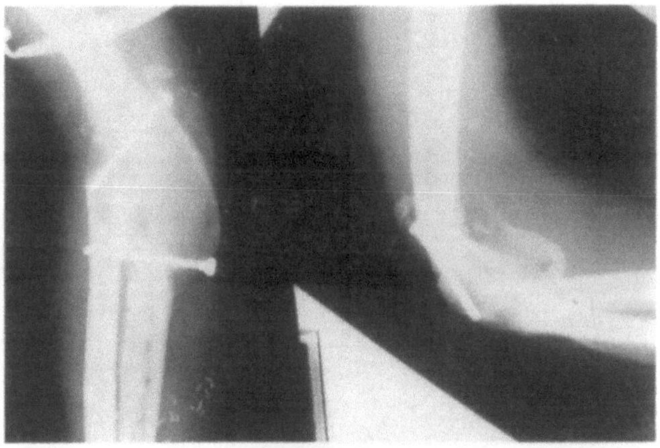

f

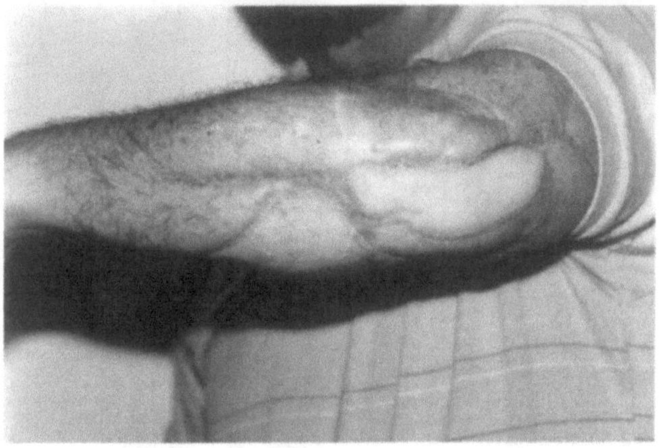

g

Fig. 3-2e. Postoperative radiographs. **f.** Final result. Radiographs show the position of the bone graft, which was well healed by 3 months and allowed plate removal at 7 months. **g.** The cutaneous portion of the transplant provides good cover.

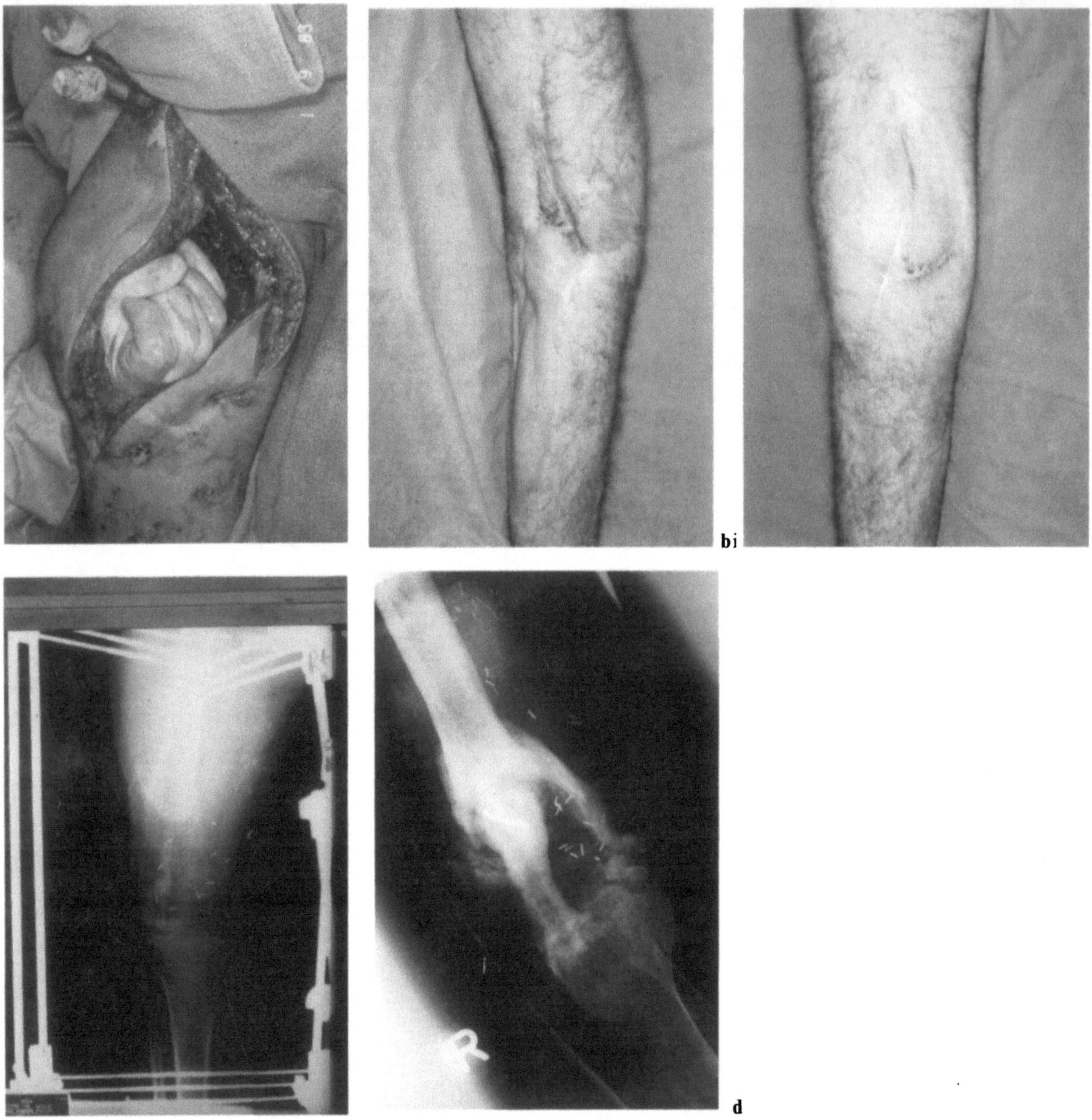

a bi bii c d

Fig. 3-3. a. Four months after a motorcycle accident in which this patient lost a substantial amount of his distal femur, he developed a gram-negative infection. The wound was thoroughly debrided, leaving an extensive through-and-through soft-tissue defect in the distal thigh and knee region. **b.** i and ii. A latissimus dorsi muscle transplant was used to fill the through-and-through soft-tissue defect and provide cover medially and laterally. **c.** The initial bone defect is shown. A fibula transplant was chosen over an allograft because of the extensive fibrosis and previous infection. **d.** Eighteen months later, marked hypertrophy of the bone graft with solid healing at both ends was demonstrated on radiography; this degree of healing allowed the patient to be fully weight bearing in a brace.

Fig. 3-4. a. A segmental defect of the tibia and fibula resulting from a gunshot wound was combined with a severe soft-tissue wound. A muscle transplant was used to provide soft-tissue cover. **b.** The bone defect is shown here. A single vessel, the posterior tibial, was present in this leg, necessitating an end-to-side anastomosis. **c.** A vascularized fibula transplant was placed in the intramedullary position proximally and distally in the tibia. **d** and **e.** Fourteen months later, solid healing and hypertrophy of the vascularized fibula transplant allowed the patient to be fully weight bearing.

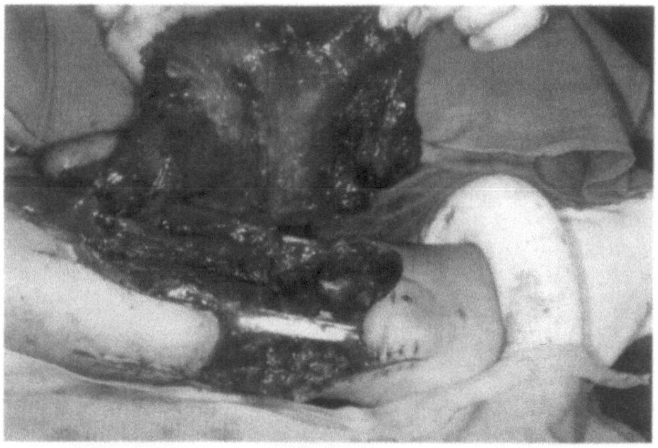

a

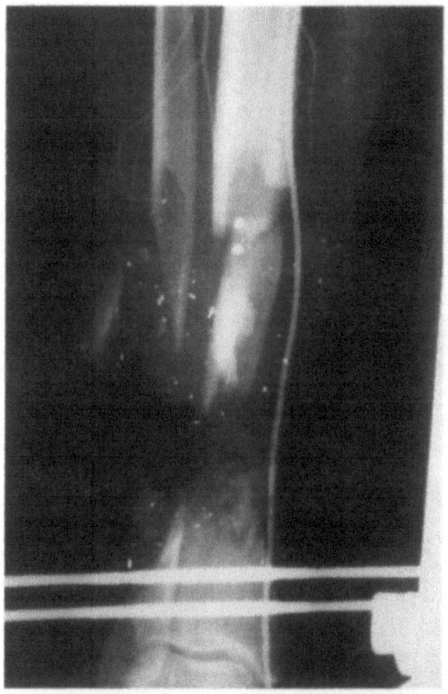

b

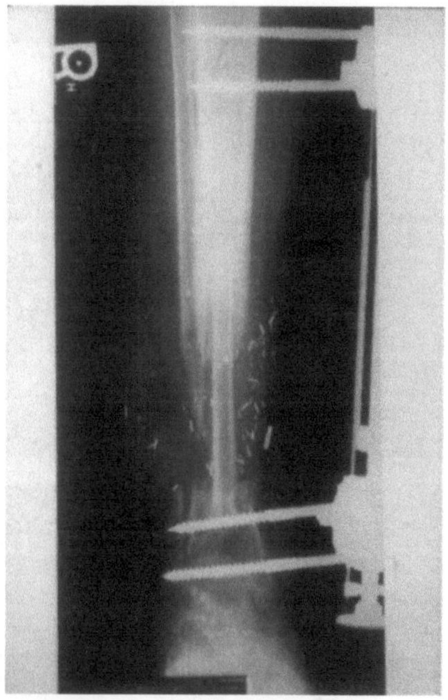

c

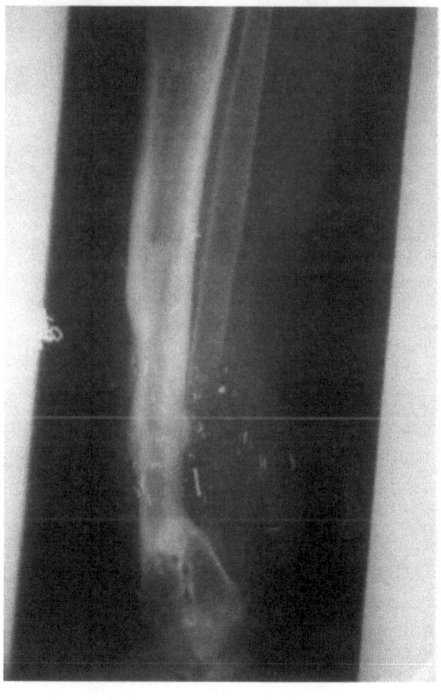

d

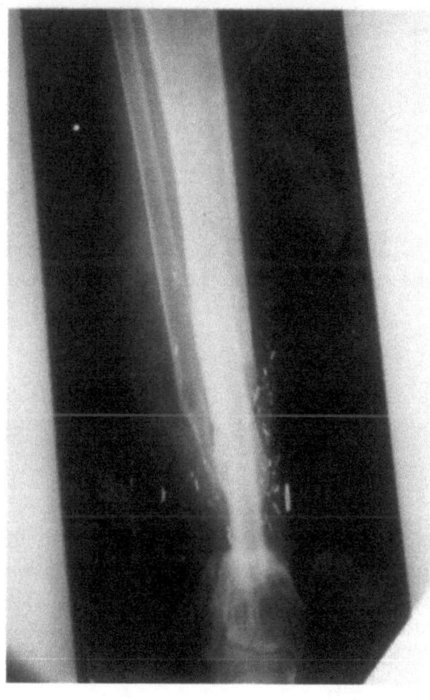

e

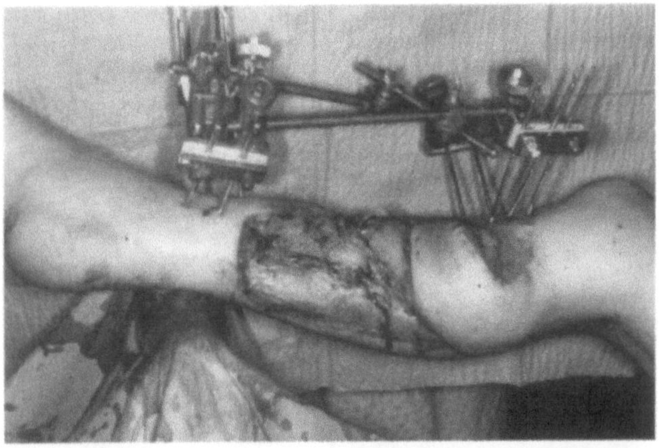
a

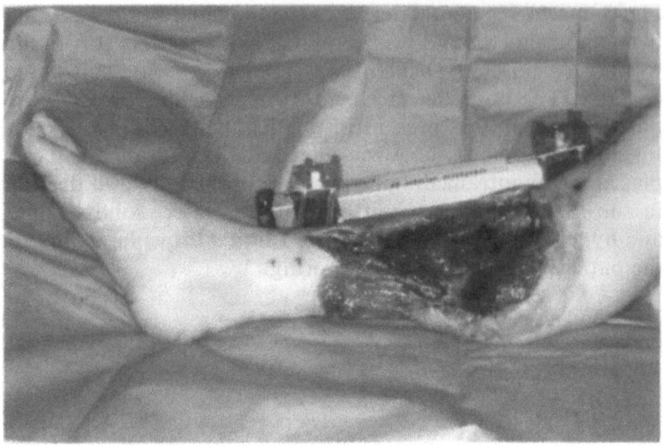
b

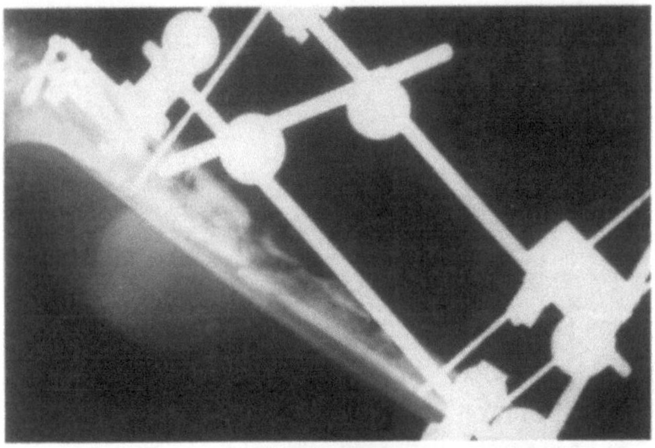
c

Fig. 3-5. a. This 32-year-old patient was referred after failure of a gastrocnemius-soleus pedicle flap. This flap was meant to cover an anterior tibial wound that resulted from a motorcycle accident. There was a gram-negative infection involving both bone and soft tissue. **b.** The pedicle flap was replaced in its original position and the area was meticulously debrided. The external fixator was also replaced to allow easier access to the posterior tibial vessels. (After osteomyelitis, it is wise to follow debridement with muscle transplantation and achieve a closed wound that shows no evidence of infection for several months before proceeding with bone transplantation or grafting.) **c.** The severely infected bone of the midtibia was not salvageable because it was intensely purulent.

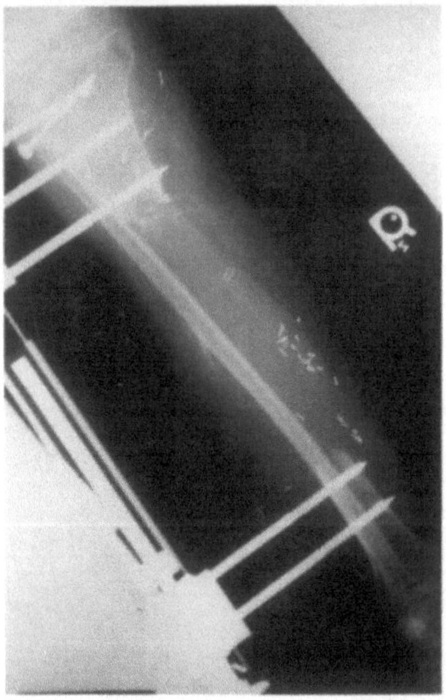
d

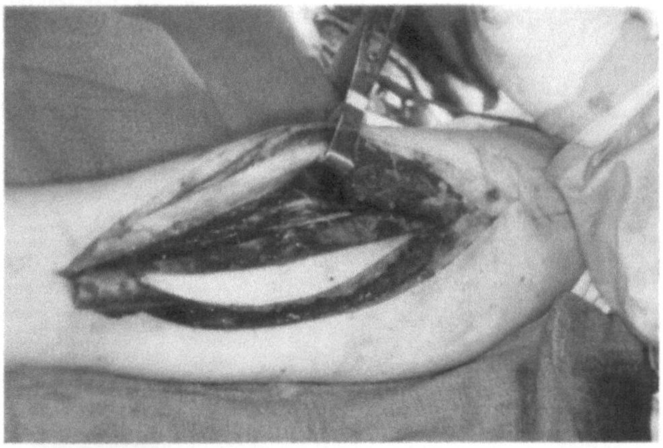
e

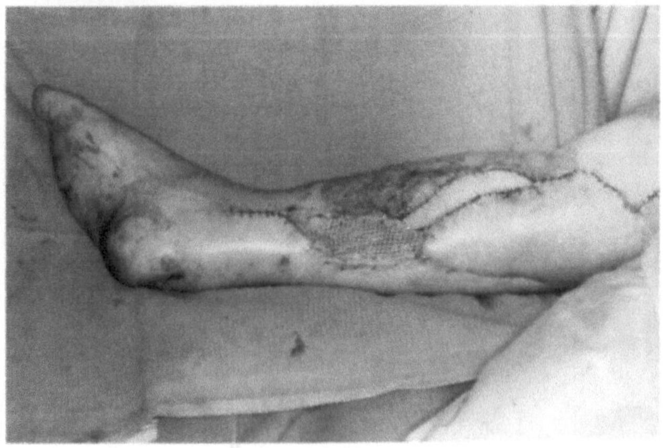
f

Fig. 3-5. d. Following debridement of the grossly infected bone, a large segmental tibial defect remained. **e.** The fibula transplant was harvested and it included an island of skin. **f.** The island of skin was used to confirm vascularity in the transplant.

Fig. 3-5. g. The vascularized fibula transplant was placed in the defect. After 14 months, the transplant had hypertrophied and the patient was initiated on partial weight bearing in a cast brace. At 17 months, he was fully weight bearing. **h.** Excellent soft-tissue cover and solidly healed bone were ultimately achieved.

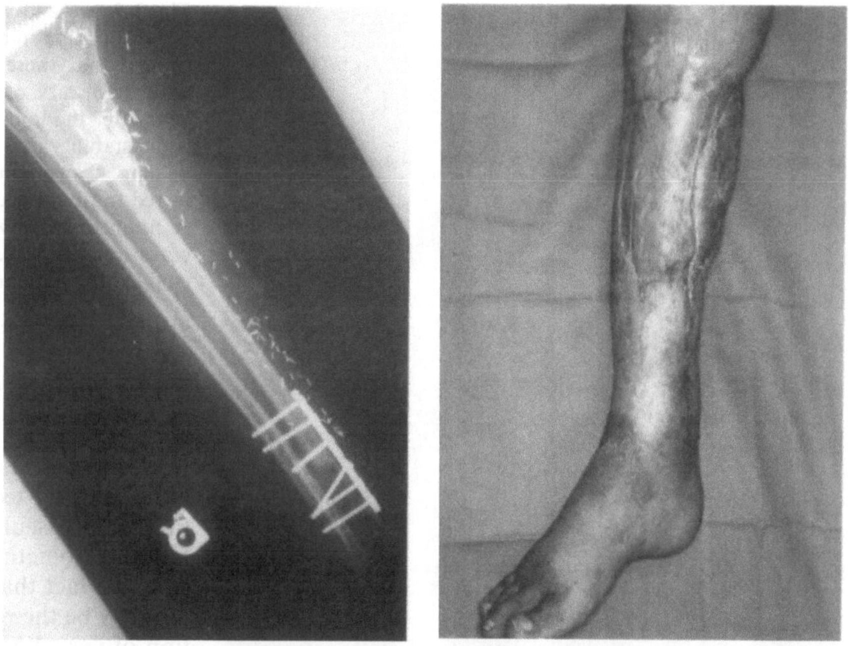

g h

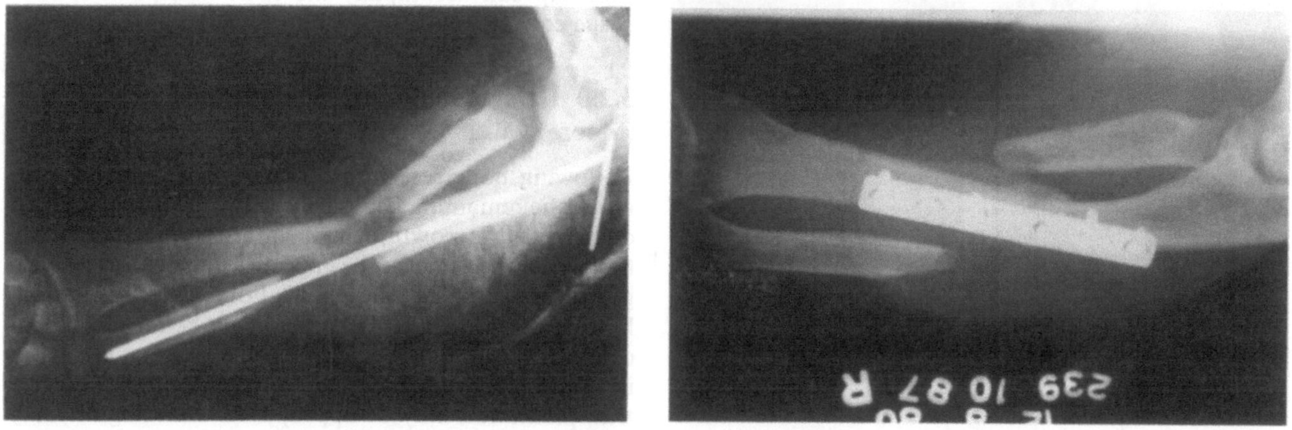

a b

Fig. 3-6. a. This forearm injured in a blast had a 5-cm defect in the ulna and extensive damage to the forearm muscles. It was unlikely that these muscles would provide any pronation or supination. **b.** A one-bone forearm was the best solution in this patient.

3.2.2.2 Extensive Bone Defect: One Intact Bone

A *tibial defect with an intact fibula* holds the possibility of regaining osseous integrity through the fibula. The techniques of proximal and distal tibiofibular synostosis (Fig. 1-13c) and vascular pedicle grafting using the ipsilateral fibula should be considered (Chacha et al. 1981, Maurer and Dillin 1987). These options may be preferable to vascularized fibula transplantation, especially if the site has been previously infected; in my experience, there is a high incidence of postoperative infection when vascularized bone grafting is done in such a previously infected area. If there has been previous osteomyelitis and the fibula is intact, then vascularized fibula transplantation is less desirable. In the absence of previous infection, however, vascularized fibula transplantation supplemented with cancellous bone grafting will usually effect rapid bone healing. In such situations, vascularized bone grafting, allografting, or tibiofibular synostosis may be appropriate, depending on the bone graft bed (Sec. 3.2.2.1).

In the *forearm*, the fibula can successfully replace the radius or ulna with the advantage of restoring pronation and supination. If passive pronation and supination or the muscles that produce these movements are absent, vascularized fibula transplantation is contraindicated and a one-bone forearm is preferable (Castle 1974) (Fig. 3-6). If the defect is in the distal radius, proximal ulna, or both bones, a one-bone forearm is not possible and vascularized bone transplantation may then be indicated (Dell et al. 1984).

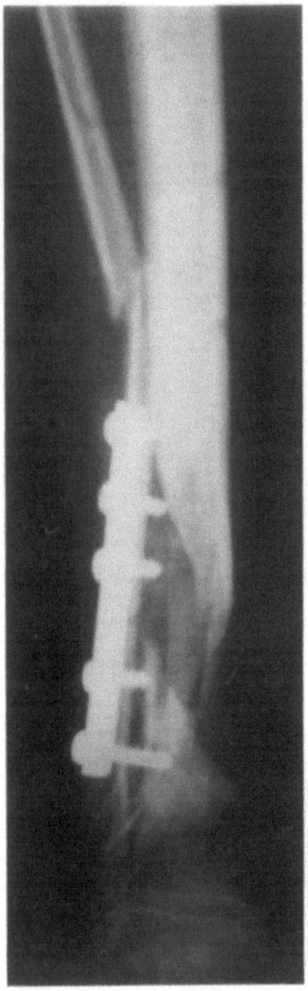
a
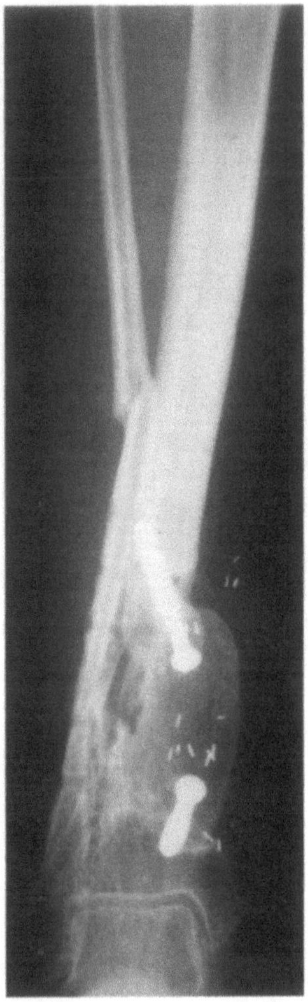
b

Fig. 3-7. a. A 40-year-old woman sustained severe injuries to her distal tibia in an automobile accident. Some stability was present, but there was severe soft-tissue injury, a bone gap with deformity of the fibula, and no evidence of healing a year after the injury despite bone grafting. Because there was some stability and the primary objective was to achieve bone healing, transplantation of vascularized iliac crest was preferred to fibula because of its higher cancellous bone content. A cutaneous flap was included to remedy the poor soft-tissue cover anteriorly. **b.** Two years later, solid healing of the graft enabled the patient to be fully weight bearing without aids.

3.2.2.3 Short Bone Defects With or Without Soft-Tissue Cover

For bone defects shorter than 4–5 cm, nonvascularized bone grafting techniques should usually be attempted first, with vascularized bone grafting being reserved for failures. Sometimes, bone healing does not occur despite the fact that the defect is relatively small. Nonunion may be the result of poor vascularity, and the addition of vascularized cancellous bone (vascularized iliac crest) may solve this problem (Fig. 3-7). A cutaneous skin flap can accompany the bone transplant if soft-tissue cover is poor (Fig. 3-8).

3.2.3 Defects Following Tumor Removal

(Moore et al. 1983)

Following bone resection for benign or malignant tumors, the remaining bed is generally of reasonably good quality, and ingrowth of vasculature from surrounding tissues and healing can be expected. In such cases, allografts are usually successful. Following irradiation, however, vascularized bone may be a better option because of the poor vascularity of the soft tissues. After irradiation or with extensive defects, vascularized fibula transplantation may be appropriate. An allograft may

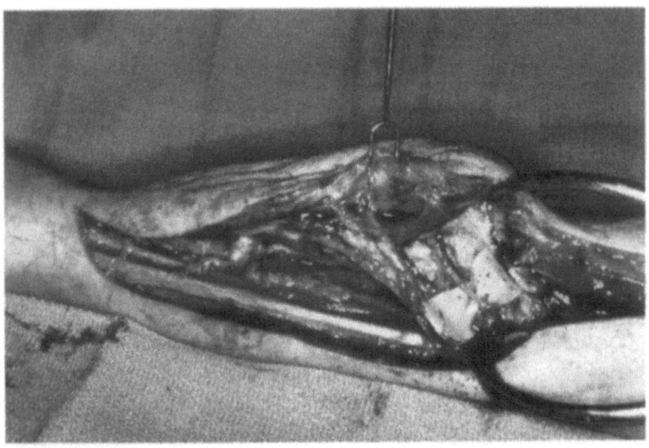
a
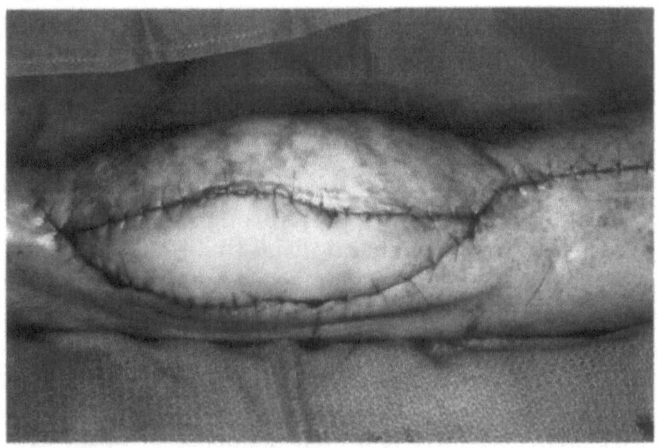
b

Fig. 3-8. (see also Fig. 3–12) **a.** This patient had a persistent tibial nonunion despite multiple bone grafting attempts. A latissimus dorsi muscle flap had been used to provide soft-tissue cover. The recipient vessels are shown and are the same ones that were used for the previous latissimus dorsi transplant. (After approximately 6 months, these vessels can be reused with little danger to the transplant – by then, the transplant can be expected to have established a second blood supply from the tissue bed.) **b.** The wound was covered and the vascularized bone used to bridge the nonunion site.

be combined with a vascularized bone graft from either the fibula or iliac crest. Currently, it is not clear whether the addition of vascularized bone lowers the nonunion rate or the fatigue failure rate after allograft procedures.

3.2.4 Spine Defects

Vascularized fibula transplantation for vertebral stability is promising. The strength of the fibula makes it attractive for this use. Its size allows easy fitting into the vertebra, and the intercostal or lumbar vessel can be used for vascular supply. Still, the long-term results of this application are yet to be seen (Fig. 3-9).

3.2.5 Avascular Necrosis of the Hip

Long-term results of vascularized fibula transplantation for avascular necrosis of the hip have not yet been published. Until such information is forthcoming, this application must be considered experimental.

3.2.6 Acetabular and Proximal Femur Reconstruction

Dissection of the iliac crest based on the deep circumflex iliac artery as an "island graft" will allow rotation of this vascularized bone, which can then be used to reconstruct the proximal femur or acetabulum (Leung and Chow 1984).

3.3 Choice of Transplant

Two vascularized bone transplants are used for extremity reconstruction: the fibula and the iliac crest (Chen and Yan 1983). Their important characteristics are compared in Table 3-1. The fibula is strong, straight, and long, and is therefore ideal for reconstructing major long bones. The donor site is generally benign. In skeletally immature individuals, a distal tibiofibular synostosis must be performed to prevent ankle valgus deformity. The iliac crest is curved, but has a large cancellous component, which is an advantage in promoting early osseous healing.

With these features in mind, the choice of transplant may be considered as follows.

Table 3-1. Comparison of the fibula and iliac crest transplants.

	Fibula transplant	Iliac crest transplant
Donor Site (Fig. 3-10)	Appearance excellent; tibiofibular synostosis required distally	Appearance good; hernia potential
Ease of dissection	Easy (1 hour)	Moderate to difficult (3 hours)
Bone length	5–25 cm (straight)	5–15 cm (surface curved if more than 8 cm is taken)
Pedicle	3–5 cm long with an external diameter of 1.5-3 mm	5–7 cm long with an external diameter of 1.5-3 mm
Bone type	Strong cortex; poorly cancellous	Weak cortex; primarily cancellous
Skin component	Small island of skin can accompany bone (frequently used as a vascular marker; utility for skin cover less well established [Yoshimura et al. 1983])	Large island of skin can accompany bone

Fibula

Used for most vascularized bone reconstruction in the extremities (Figs. 3-3 and 3-4)

For long bone replacement where bone strength is important and structural integrity needs to be restored

Iliac Crest

Used where some stability is present but osseous healing is needed (e.g., tibial nonunions that have repeatedly failed to heal by other methods) (Fig. 3-7)

Used where a curved surface is needed, e.g., for an elbow fusion (Fig. 3-2) – the iliac crest can be curved by a controlled "greenstick" fracture of the outer table, allowing bending of the bone to the appropriate shape

Used for osteocutaneous transplantation where both bone and soft-tissue cover are needed (Gordon et al. 1985, Taylor et al. 1979) (Fig. 3-2)

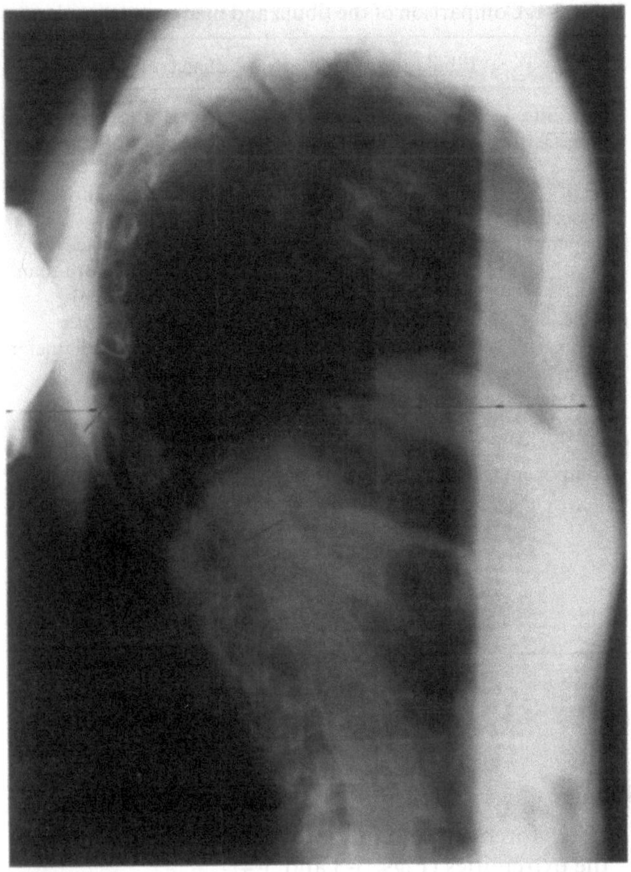
a

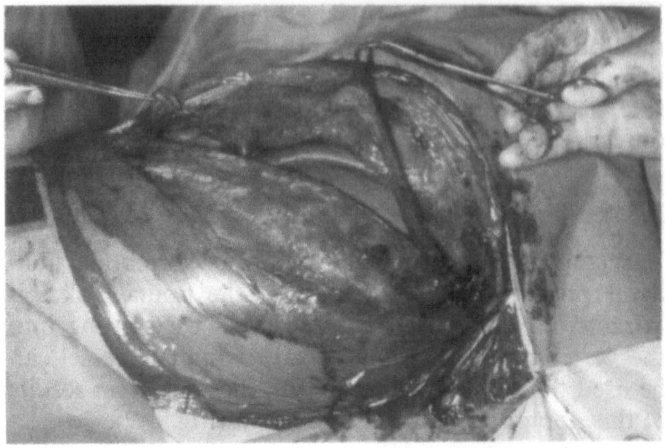
b

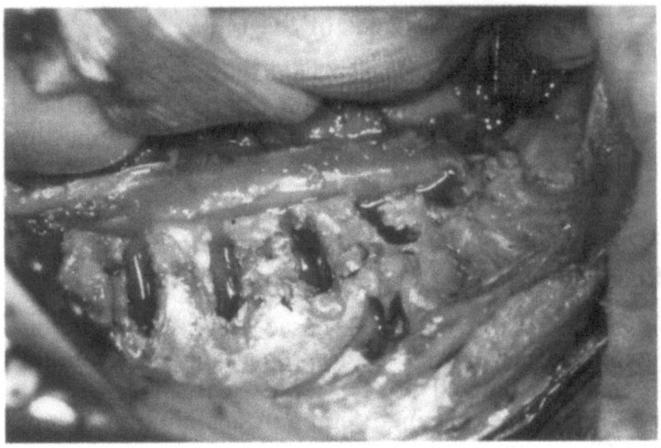
c

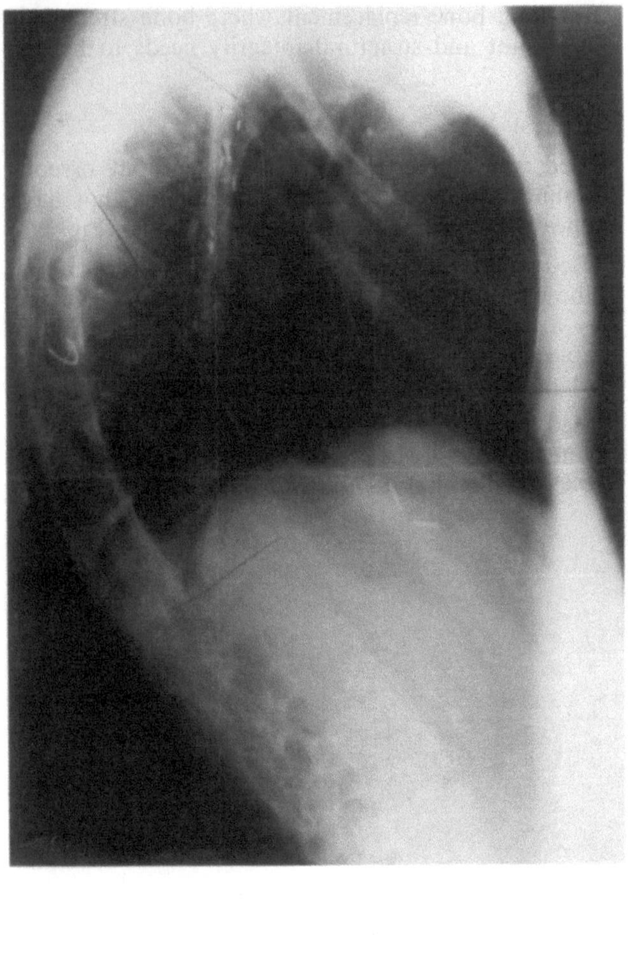
d

Fig. 3-9. (see also Fig. 3-11) **a.** This 13-year-old boy developed severe, progressive kyphosis following the resection of an astrocytoma from the thoracic spine. Following a laminectomy he developed instability with increasing kyphoscoliosis. The kyphosis measured 70°. As a first stage, a posterior fusion in situ with conventional iliac crest bone graft was performed. Bone grafting anteriorly was needed to provide strong support and achieve early healing in order to arrest the progress of the kyphosis. A vascularized fibula transplant was planned. **b.** The second stage was performed four weeks later. The thorax was entered through removal of T7, and the intercostal artery was dissected from this interspace for use as the recipient artery (*held up by clamp*). The hemiazygos vein was used as the recipient vein. **c.** The fibula transplant is seen in place, spanning the interval from T4 to T12. Twenty degrees of correction was obtained at the time of insertion of the fibula graft. **d.** Nine months later, the patient was asymptomatic but continued to wear a brace part time. The fibula graft healed at both ends, had hypertrophied, and can be seen here spanning the region of kyphosis, which has remained stable. (The spinal surgery was performed by John M. Gray, M.D.)

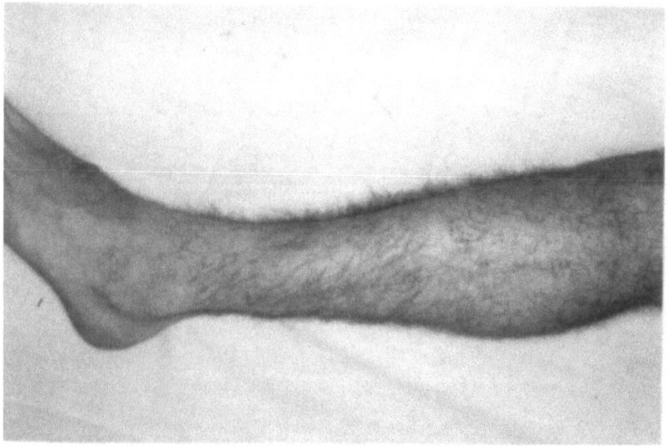

a

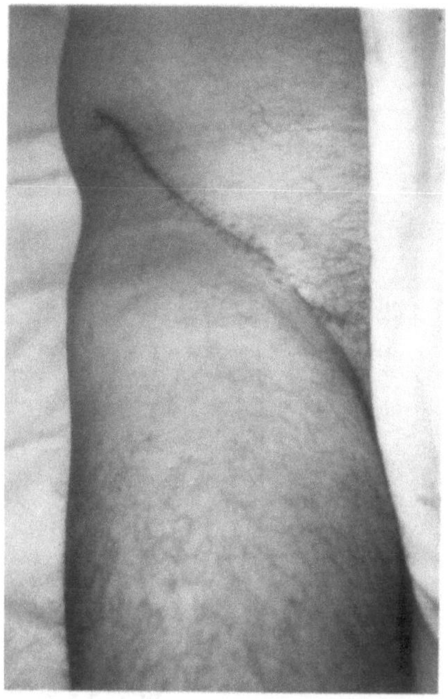

b

Fig. 3-10. a. The donor site following fibula transplantation is usually inconspicuous, and leg function is normal. **b.** The donor site following osteocutaneous groin transplantation is shown. Hernia formation is a potential complication (Sec. 3.5.2h). There are no functional problems in the extremity, but an area of numbness in the anterior thigh usually exists.

Table 3-2. Vascularized bone transplantation for traumatic bone defects of the lower extremity – indications.

Size of bone defect (cm)	Quality of graft bed	Graft indication
<4–5	favorable	nonvascularized bone
	unfavorable*	vascularized bone (iliac crest)
>4–5 (one intact bone)	favorable	allograft, vascularized fibula, or both
	unfavorable	
	no prior infection	vascularized fibula
	prior infection	proximal and distal tibiofibular synostosis
>4–5 (no intact bone)	favorable	allograft, vascularized fibula, or both
	unfavorable	vascularized bone

* is fibrotic, irradiated, or has poor soft-tissue cover

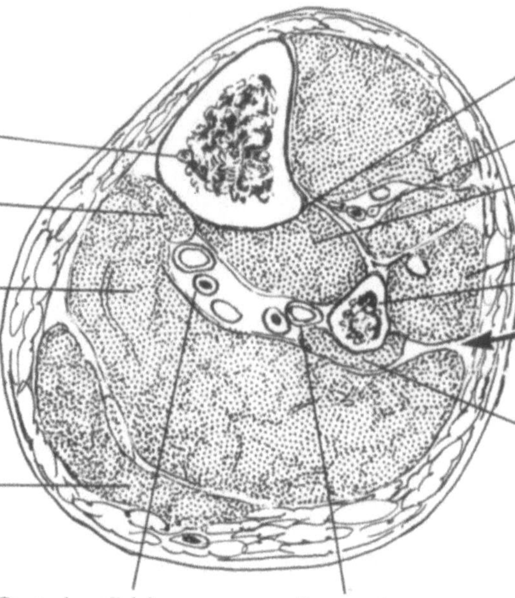

Plate 3-I. Cross section of the leg.

3.4 Vascularized Fibula Transplantation

(Chen and Yan 1983, Gilbert 1981, Taylor 1983, Taylor et al. 1975, Weiland et al. 1983, Wood 1986)

3.4.1 Anatomy (Plates 3-I and 3-II)

The *fibula* is a long, relatively straight and slender bone. It consists of an expanded head proximally, a body, and the lateral malleolus distally. The proximal end lends attachment for the fibular collateral ligament of the knee and biceps femoris tendon, and the lateral malleolus forms the lateral aspect of the ankle. Provided that the head of the fibula is retained for knee stability and the distal fourth is retained for ankle stability, the body can be removed without affecting knee or ankle function. In children, however, a synostosis must be performed distally (Fig. 3-1) to prevent ankle instability.

The *medial surface of the fibular body* gives rise to the anterior muscles of the leg, the interosseous membrane (from the interosseous border), and, posterior to this membrane, the tibialis posterior muscle. The *posterior surface* gives rise to the soleus and flexor hallucis longus, while the *lateral surface* gives rise to the peroneus longus in its proximal two thirds and peroneus brevis in its distal two thirds.

The fibula receives its *periosteal vascular supply* from the surrounding muscles, which are themselves supplied by multiple branches of the peroneal artery. The nutrient artery provides the *endosteal supply* and is also a branch of the peroneal artery. The *peroneal artery* is the largest branch of the posterior tibial artery. Near the ankle, it is connected to the posterior tibial artery by a horizontal communicating branch, and by a perforating branch to the anterior tibial artery. It arises 2–3 cm below the lower border of the popliteus and passes laterally to the fibula. Here, it lies within the substance of the flexor hallucis longus or between this muscle and the tibialis posterior in the posterior compartment of the leg. It travels just posterior to the interosseous membrane and has paired venae comitantes. The *nutrient artery* enters the fibula on the medial surface just posterior to the medial crest; this is in the middle third of the bone. It also gives off branches to surrounding muscles, but there are no other major branches in the middle two fourths of the bone. The peroneal vessels lie near the posterior tibial neurovascular bundle, separated by the tibialis posterior. No nerve accompanies the peroneal vascular bundle.

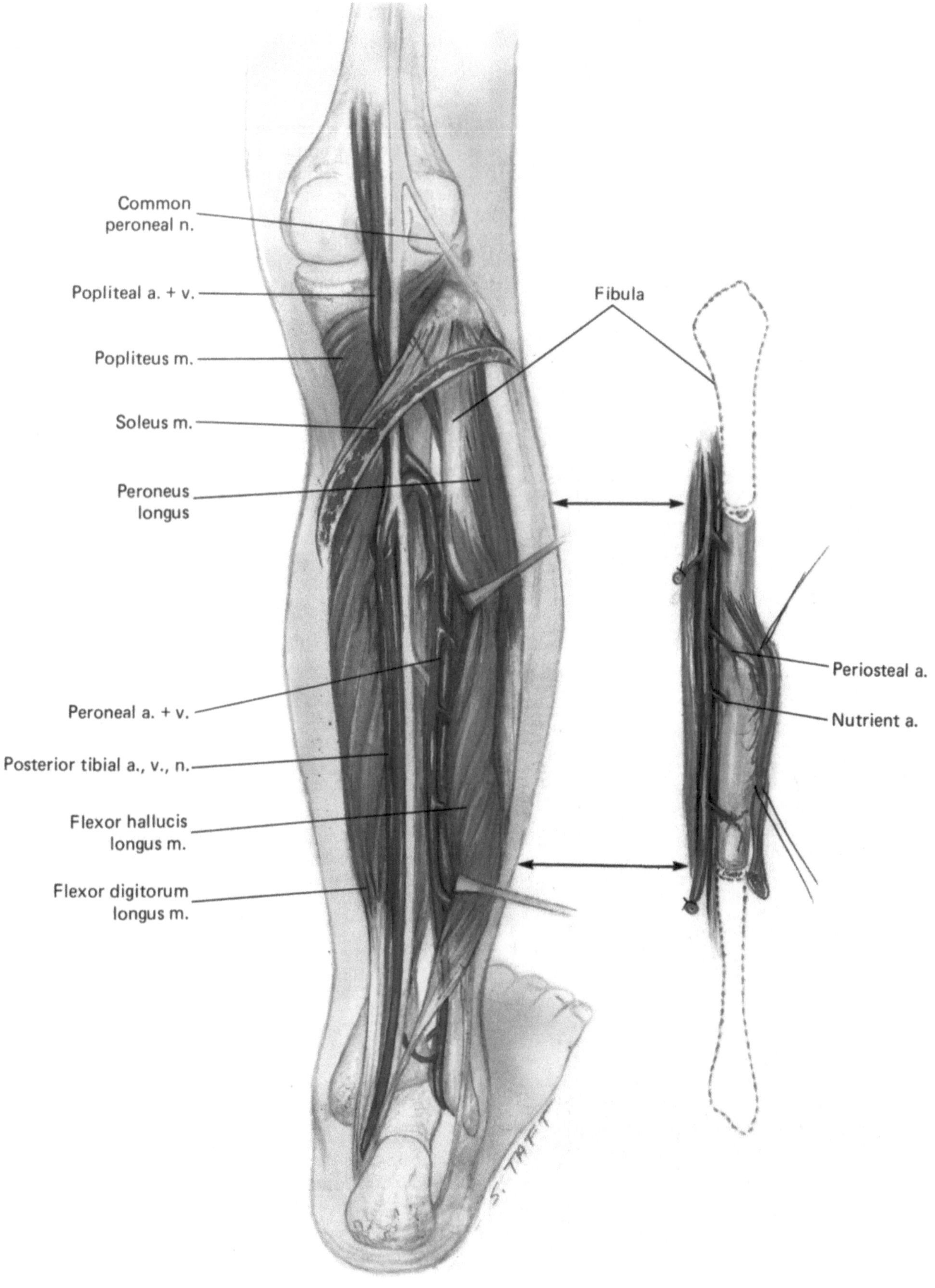

Plate 3-II. Anatomy of the vascularized fibula transplant.

3.4.2 Surgical Technique
(Fig. 3-11; see also Fig. 3-9)

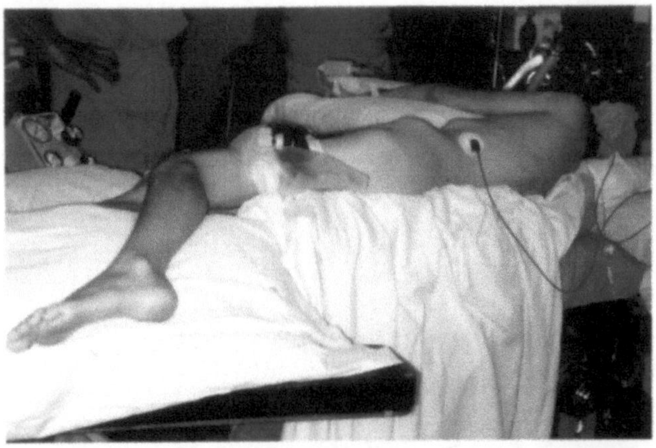
a

a. The leg is positioned on a well-padded arm board which extends from the operating room table. Even with the patient supine, internal rotation of the hip allows the leg to rest with the fibula uppermost.

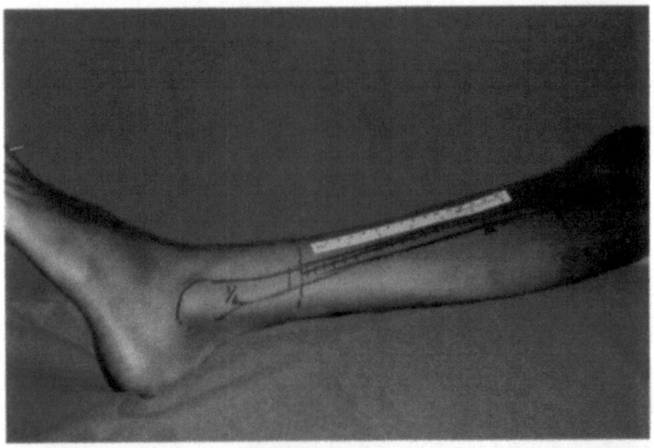
b

b. The surface markings of the fibula can be seen. The distal fourth of the fibula is retained to prevent ankle instability, especially in children. The site where the peroneal nerve crosses over the neck of the fibula is noted. The length of fibula required is measured.

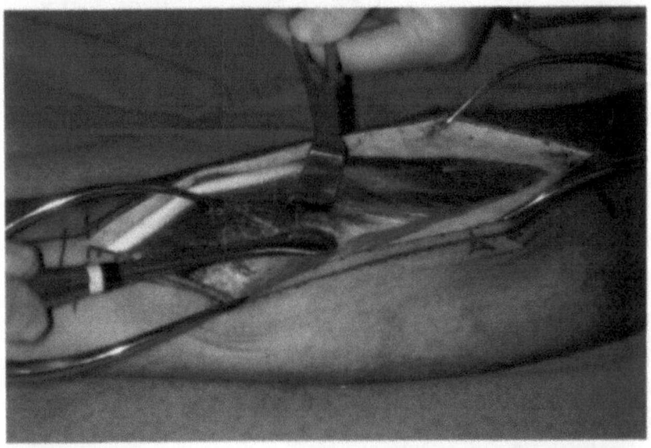
c

c. Under tourniquet control, the incision is made down to deep fascia, which is incised over the subcutaneous border of the fibula. The interval between the peroneal and soleus muscles is separated. A periosteal elevator is used to lightly remove the muscle origin from the superficial surface of the fibula. The periosteum is not removed.

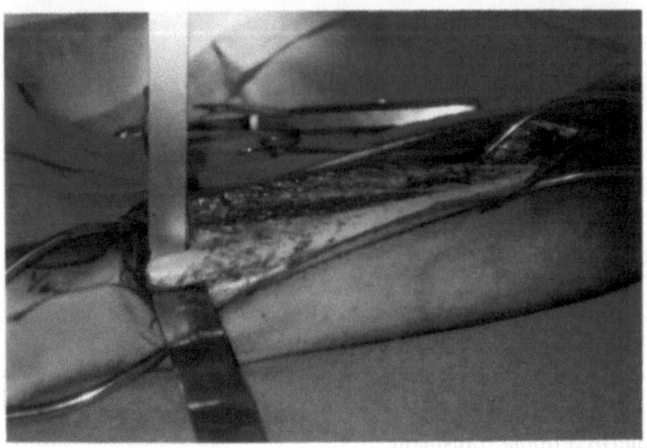
d

d. Using an oscillating saw, the distal osteotomy is made, with care taken to protect the peroneal vessels on the deep surface of the bone.

e. With the muscle carefully retracted, the distal half of the interosseous membrane is divided.

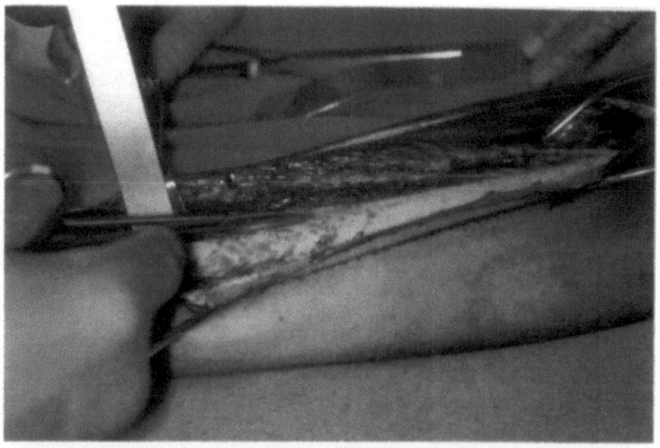

e

f. The proximal osteotomy is made.

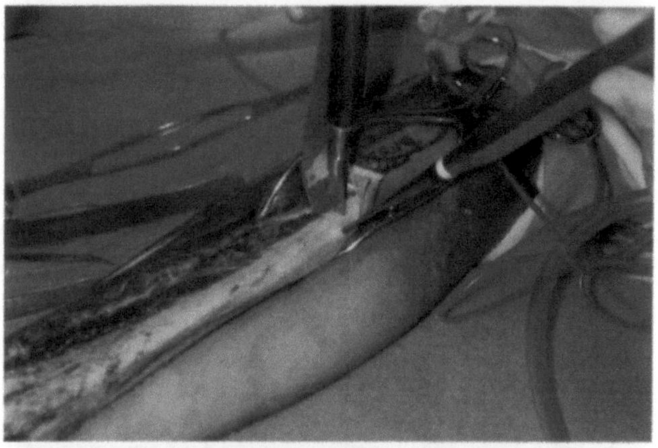

f

g. The fibula can now be rotated externally, bringing the interosseous membrane and the deep surface into view. The rest of the interosseous membrane is divided from the anterior aspect. Proximally, the peroneal vessels can be seen as they approach the fibula, so dissection in this region must be done cautiously. Distally, the fibula can now be grasped with a towel clip and carefully elevated, exposing the peroneal vessels lying deep to the bone in the posterior compartment.

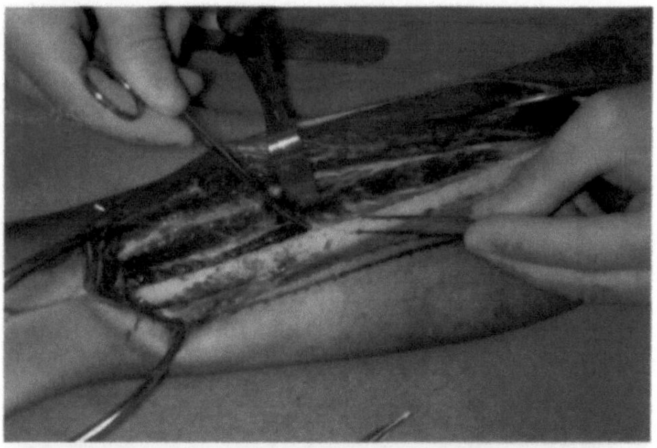

g

h. These vessels are ligated distally. (They can be dissected for further length if a "flow-through" fibula transplant is planned.)

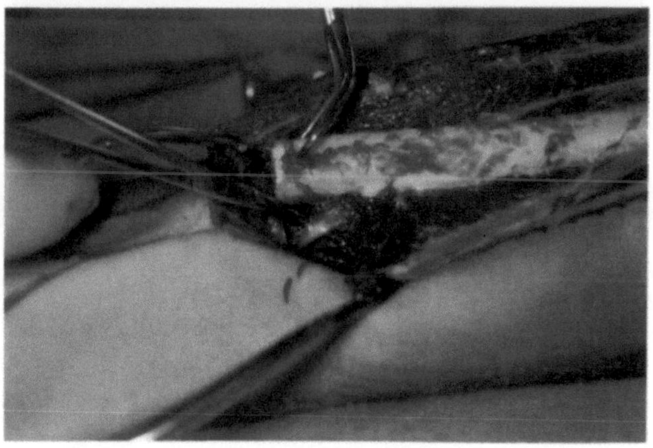

h

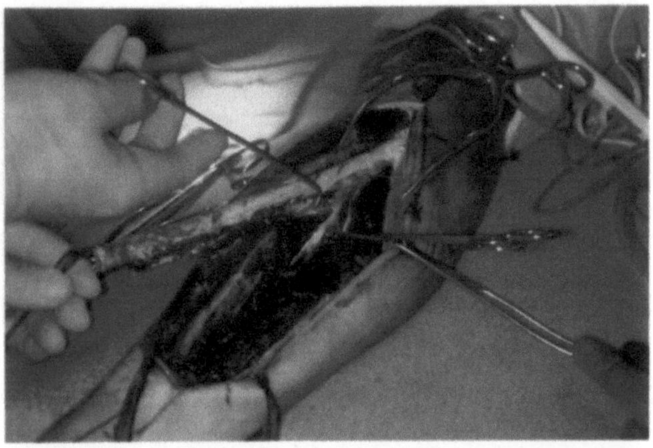

i

i. The fibula is now elevated, dividing deep muscle attachments but ensuring both that the peroneal vessels remain with the bone and that no communications between the vessels and bone are interrupted. (Note the proximity of the posterior tibial nerve.)

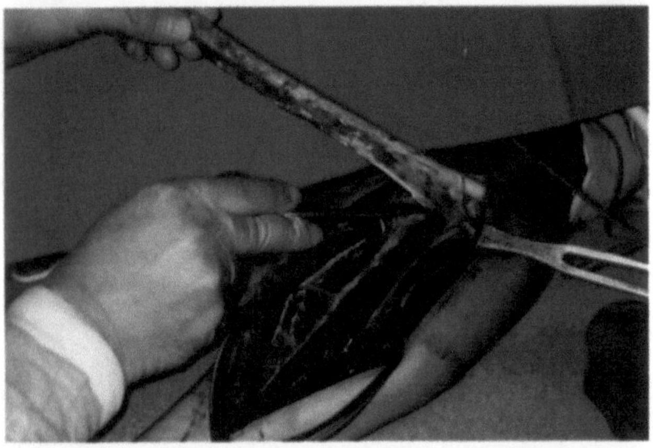

j

j. Proximally, the division between the peroneal vessels and the posterior tibial vessels can be identified. This division is the limit of the proximal dissection of the peroneal vessels, which are shown here. Once the recipient site has been prepared, the vascular pedicle is divided. Greater pedicle length can be obtained if less proximal fibula is required. The nutrient vessel enters the middle third of the bone, which dictates the limit of pedicle length available proximally.

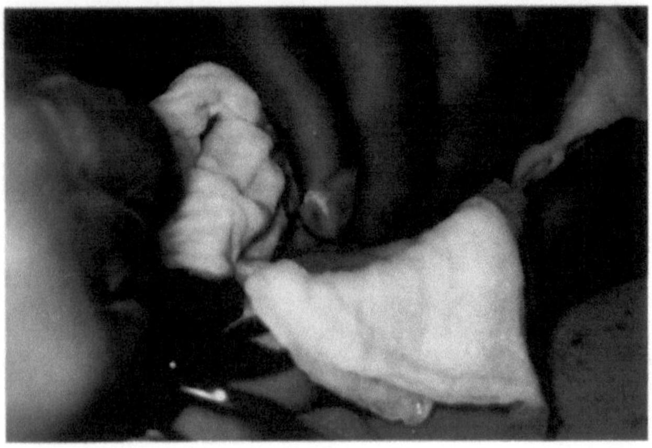

k

k. Good bleeding from the distal medullary cavity and periosteum confirms good circulation.

1. One fourth of the fibula remains. A screw is used to accomplish the distal tibiofibular synostosis.

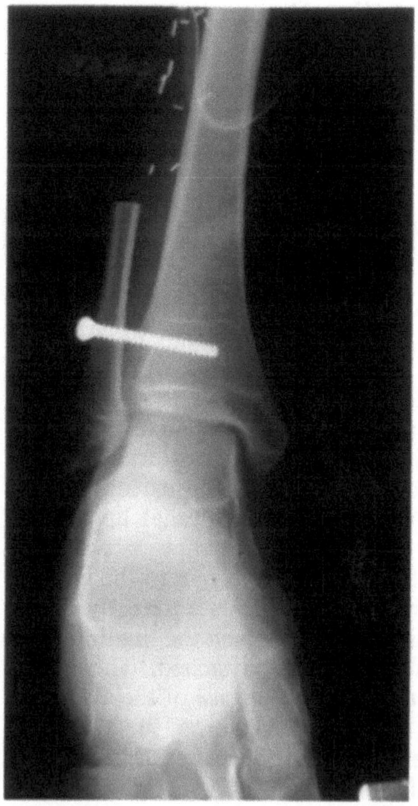

1

3.5 Vascularized Iliac Crest Transplantation

(Huang et al. 1980, Taylor et al. 1979, Taylor 1983, Weiland et al. 1979, Wood 1986)

3.5.1 Anatomy (Plate 3-III)

The *ilium* consists of two parts: a *body* and an *ala*. The body forms two fifths of the acetabulum. The ala is the fan-shaped, expanded portion having an inner and outer surface bounded by the *crest*. The crest is concave in its anterior part, forming the iliac fossa, but is convex behind. The crest has an overhanging external lip to which the fascia lata, external oblique muscle in its anterior half, and tensor fasciae latae muscle are attached. Attached to the internal lip are the iliac fascia and the transversus abdominis muscle. The intermediate line of the crest gives origin to the internal oblique muscle. The iliac crest ends anteriorly in the anterior superior iliac spine, to which the inguinal ligament and sartorius muscle are attached. The iliacus muscle is attached to the pelvic surface of the ala, while the gluteal muscles attach to the external surface.

Between the anterior superior iliac spine and the pubic tubercle is the inferior margin of the external oblique muscle aponeurosis, which is known as the *inguinal ligament*. The *inguinal canal*, which is about 4 cm long, lies above and parallel to the inguinal ligament. The deep inguinal ring lies above the midpoint of the inguinal ligament, while the superficial ring lies above and lateral to the pubic tubercle.

The *external iliac artery* passes under the midpoint of the inguinal ligament, and then becomes the femoral artery. The external iliac artery is crossed by the genital branch of the genitofemoral nerve and the deep circumflex iliac vein. The ductus deferens in the male and the round ligament in the female curve across its medial side. The external iliac vein lies to its medial side. The external iliac artery has two branches. The *inferior epigastric artery* emanates from its medial side just above the inguinal ligament and travels toward the umbilicus. Just lateral to the origin of this artery is the deep inguinal ring with the ductus deferens or round ligament.

The *deep circumflex iliac artery* emanates from the lateral aspect of the external iliac artery slightly distal to the inferior epigastric artery. It passes obliquely toward the anterior superior iliac spine between the transversalis fascia and the iliac fascia. It pierces the transversalis fascia and transversus abdominis to lie between the transversus abdominis and internal oblique muscles. It then passes laterally along the inside of the iliac fossa 1–2 cm from the crest. An ascending branch, frequently of considerable size, originates 1–2 cm medial to the anterior superior iliac spine. The musculocutaneous perforators travel from the deep circumflex iliac vessel to supply the overlying skin along this axis. They emerge from the external oblique muscle adjacent to the upper border of the iliac crest. The largest perforator, which is usually the continuation of the deep circumflex iliac artery, is 6–8 cm beyond the anterior superior iliac spine (Taylor et al. 1979).

Strips of the three muscles of the abdominal wall and the iliacus muscle are retained with the graft to preserve the blood supply to the bone and skin. The deep circumflex iliac vessels provide a pedicle about 6–8 cm long before entering the ilium. Its external diameter is generally 1.5-2.0 mm. The position of the deep circumflex iliac vein varies somewhat, but it can usually be located at a point 2–3 cm lateral to the external iliac artery where the artery and vein converge.

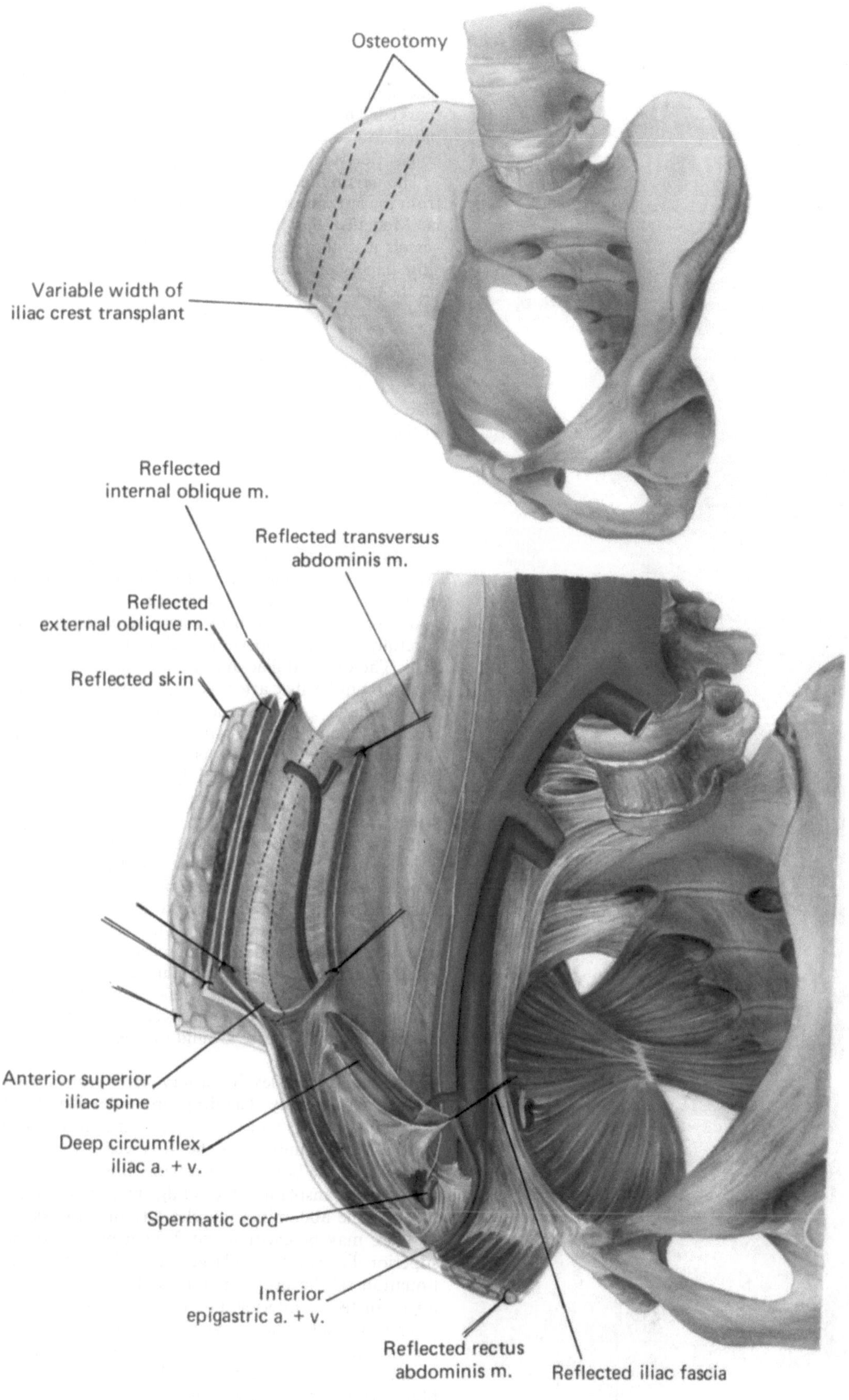

Plate 3-III. Anatomy of the vascularized iliac crest transplant.

3.5.2 Surgical Technique
(Fig. 3-12; see also Fig. 3-8)

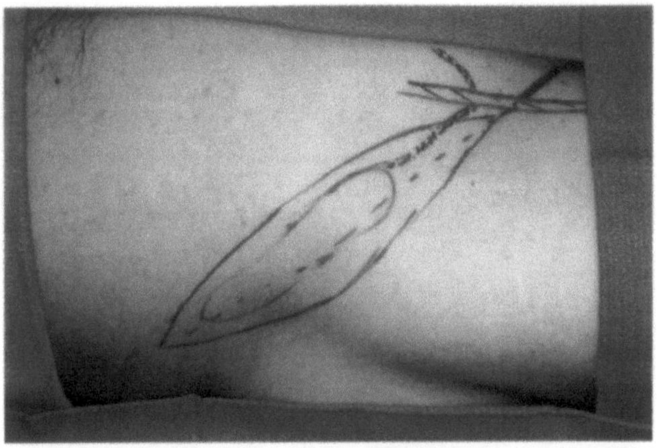

a

a. Surface landmarks are shown here – the anterior superior iliac spine and iliac crest as well as the inguinal ligament are marked. The external iliac and femoral arteries and the anticipated course of the deep circumflex iliac artery and inferior epigastric artery are also shown.

The axis of the cutaneous flap lies along a line extending from the anterior superior iliac spine to the angle of the scapula. Medially, this line is extended toward the external iliac vessels just above and parallel to the inguinal ligament. The skin flap is outlined above and below this axis, depending on the needs of the recipient site.

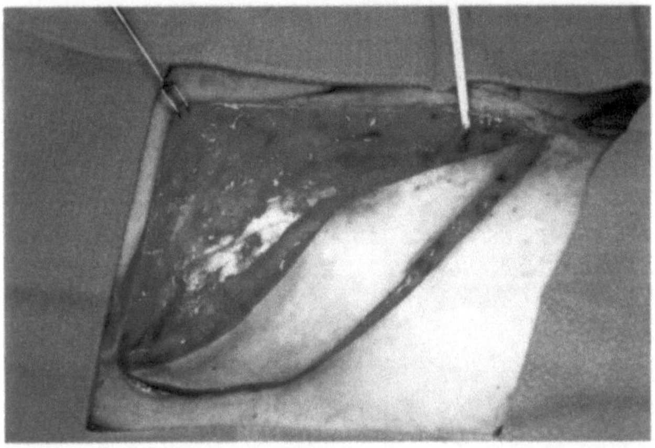

b

b. The upper skin incision is made down to deep fascia. The external oblique muscle is incised a few centimeters from the iliac crest, and the skin margin is sutured to avoid shearing of the cutaneous vessels.

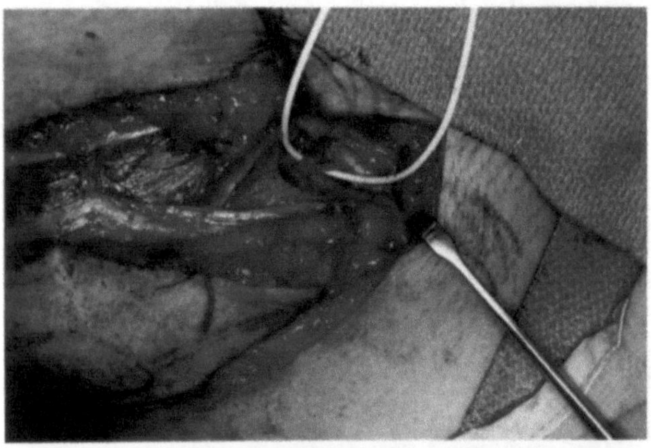

c

c. i. Medially, the superficial inferior epigastric vein may be encountered and may be useful for venous drainage of the cutaneous portion of the transplant.

ii. The *spermatic cord or round ligament* is identified and carefully retracted superiorly and medially.

iii. The external iliac artery and vein are palpated, and the deep circumflex iliac artery is identified and its origin dissected (unfortunately, the vascular anatomy of this region is quite variable [Alpert et al. 1984]). The *deep circumflex iliac artery* emanates from the lateral aspect of the external iliac artery just proximal to the inguinal ligament, generally within 1 cm of it; in the same region, the inferior epigastric artery emanates from it medially.

iv. The *deep circumflex iliac vein* runs with the artery, but 2–3 cm from the external iliac vessels, the artery and vein diverge as they approach the parent vessel. The vein then passes either superficial or deep to the external iliac artery.

v. The transversalis fascia is divided and the internal oblique and transversus abdominis muscles are separated from the inguinal ligament. The deep circumflex iliac artery (*in the vessel loop*) passes through the transversalis fascia and transversus abdominis muscle to lie between this muscle and the internal oblique in its course around the inside of the iliac crest.

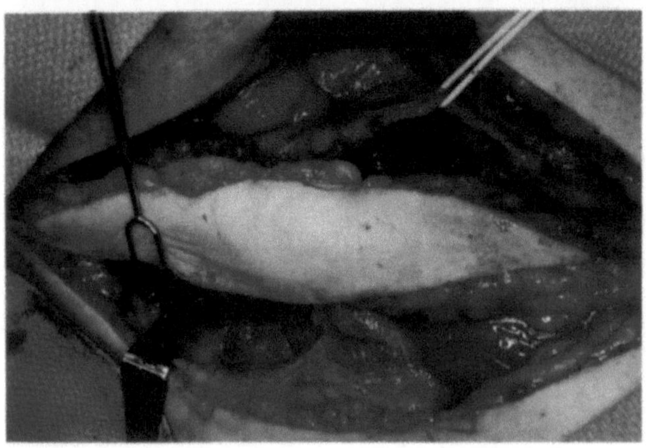

d

d. The deep circumflex iliac artery (*in the vessel loop*) is carefully dissected laterally. The deep circumflex iliac vessels supply the ilium along its inner border near the crest, and the course of the vessels must now be followed to make sure that branches to the bone and overlying muscle and skin are kept with the transplant. Ascending muscular branches pass through the abdominal muscles and into the skin. The first of these may be encountered 2–3 cm medial to the anterior superior iliac spine. The largest ascending branch is the continuation of the deep circumflex iliac vessel, found 6-8 cm posterior to the anterior superior iliac spine.

The internal oblique and transversus abdominis muscles are incised 2–3 cm above the iliac crest, raising this width of muscle along the course of the iliac crest transplant. By blunt dissection, the iliacus muscle is separated from the iliac fossa, leaving periosteum intact.

e. The lower incision of the flap is now made and the outer surface of the bone is dissected. The attachments of the glutei and tensor fasciae latae are dissected from the outer surface of the bone, leaving periosteum intact.

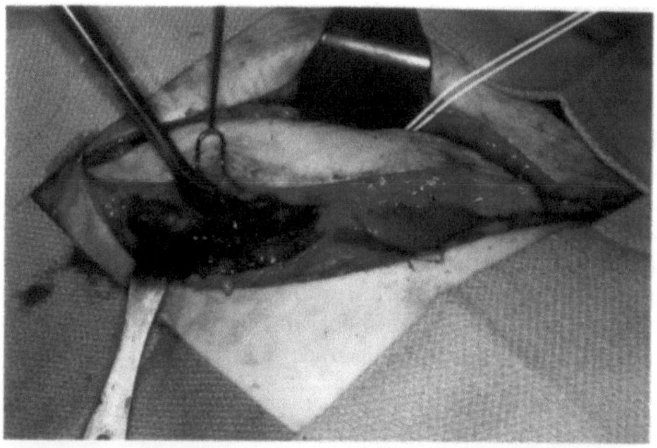

e

f. An oscillating saw is used to make the osteotomies after measuring the width of iliac crest desired. Osteotomies of the outer and inner tables are completed. A straight segment 6–8 cm in length can be obtained. For longer segments of bone that are straight, an osteotomy of the outer table is necessary.

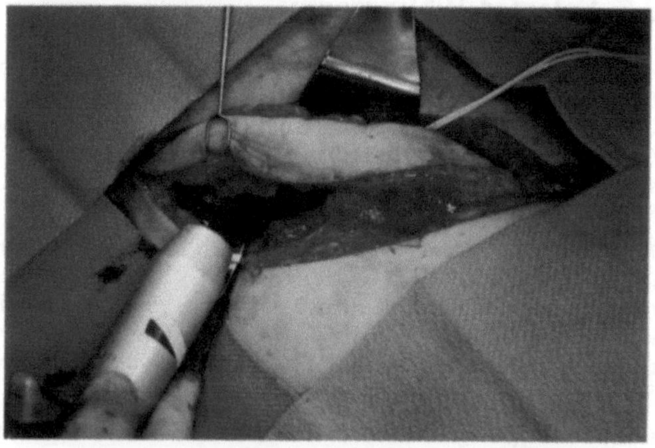

f

g. The inguinal ligament and sartorius are incised medial to the anterior superior iliac spine. This incision leaves the composite transplant fully dissected, based only on the supplying vessels. Good bleeding from the cut surface of the bone and muscle and good color of the skin confirm good vascularity to all parts of the flap. If the cutaneous portion is not required, ascending branches are divided, and the bone with the surrounding cuff of muscle alone is used.

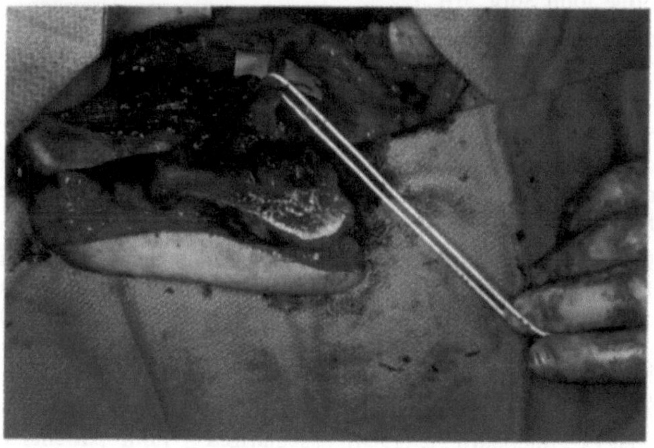

g

h. *Secure closure* of the donor site and lower abdominal muscles is essential to prevent hernia formation. The iliacus fascia and muscle are sutured to the transversalis fascia and muscle. The internal and external obliques are sutured to the glutei and fascia lata. The inguinal ligament is attached laterally and the inguinal canal is repaired if necessary. During closure, flexion of the hip and knee is helpful in reducing tension on the donor site. (See Fig. 3-10b.)

3.6 Postoperative Care

Monitoring the vascularity of buried vascularized bone transplants is difficult. Implanted temperature probes can be used (Chapter 8). An island of skin, which is sometimes carried with a fibula transplant and usually accompanies vascularized iliac crest transplants, enables vascular monitoring. A technetium bone scan will provide some information about the vascularity of the transplant if it is obtained within the first 3–5 days after transplantation. Because the scan is done only once and is expensive, it is not of practical use in assessing the patency of the anastomoses.

The postoperative protocol is similar to that used for muscle or cutaneous transplants; dextran is given (30 cc/hour for 3–5 days), followed by aspirin (325 mg daily for 2 weeks). After constant elevation for a period of 2 weeks, postoperative care of the extremity depends on the stability of the bone fixation. Initially, a splint is applied in the operating room and the dressing is changed frequently during the first 2 weeks. Cast support is generally begun at about day 14, when the swelling has subsided.

3.7 Selected Bibliography

Alpert BS, Parry SW, Buncke HJ, Gordon L (1984) The free groin flap. In Buncke HJ, Furnas DW (eds): Symposium on Clinical Frontiers in Reconstructive Microsurgery, vol. 24. St. Louis, Mosby, pp 71–84

The variability of the vascular anatomy of this region is discussed.

Berggren A, Weiland AJ, Dorfman H (1982) The effect of prolonged ischemia time on osteocyte and osteoblast survival in composite bone grafts revascularized by microvascular anastomoses. Plast Reconstr Surg 69:290

This work underscores the rationale for using vascularized bone transplantation. Bone transplantation with microsurgical anastomosis was performed after 1.5-48 hours of ischemia. Marrow and cortical bone were viable on histologic examination with ischemia times of under 4 hours, while viability was variable with ischemia times of 4–26 hours.

Castle ME (1974) One-bone forearm. J Bone Joint Surg 56A:1223

The criteria for the technique of creating a one-bone forearm are discussed.

Chacha PB, Ahmed M, Daruwalla JS (1981) Vascular pedicle graft of the ipsilateral fibula for non-union of the tibia with a large defect. J Bone Joint Surg 63B:244

An experimental study in Macaca monkeys and clinical experience with 11 patients outline the use of the ipsilateral fibula for treating tibial defects. Various prior methods are described, and the surgical technique of ipsilateral vascular pedicle grafting of the fibula is detailed.

Chen ZW, Yan W (1983) The study and clinical application of the osteocutaneous flap of the fibula. J Microsurg 4:11

The osteocutaneous fibula transplant is described, emphasizing its advantages over the iliac crest and rib transplants for extremity reconstruction.

Dell PC, Burchardt H, Glowczewskie FP Jr (1985) A roentgenographic, biomechanical, and histological evaluation of vascularized and non-vascularized segmental fibular canine autografts. J Bone Joint Surg 67A:105

The authors describe the differences between vascularized and nonvascularized bone grafts. They suggest that vascularized bone grafting may be the superior method for poor graft beds and abnormal bone.

Dell PC, Sheppard JE (1984) Vascularized bone grafts in the treatment of infected forearm nonunions. J Hand Surg 9A:653

Four patients with infected nonunion of the forearm bones underwent wide resection to control infection, followed by vascularized fibula transplantation. All healed, but one required additional cancellous bone grafting.

Gilbert A (1981) Free vascularized bone grafts. Intern Surg 66:27

A brief discussion of the surgical technique for rib, fibula, and iliac crest vascularized transfer is presented. The lateral approach to the fibula between the soleus and peroneal muscles is described.

Gordon L, Buncke HJ, Alpert BS, et al (1985) Free vascularized osteocutaneous transplants from the groin for delayed primary closure in the management of loss of soft tissue and bone in the hand and wrist. J Bone Joint Surg 67A:958

The use of an osteocutaneous transplant consisting of bone (for the metacarpal and carpal loss) and skin (to provide soft-tissue cover) is described in two patients with massive injury to the dorsum of the hand.

Gordon L, Weulker N, Jergesen H (1986) Vascularized fibular grafting for the treatment of congenital pseudarthrosis of the tibia. Orthopedics 9:825

Use of the fibula in treating this difficult problem is promising and appears to be superior to nonvascularized bone grafting techniques. Surgical technique and preliminary results in six patients are described.

Huang GK, Liu ZZ, Shen YL, et al (1980) Microvascular free transfer of iliac bone based on the deep circumflex iliac vessels. J Microsurg 2:113

Details of the anatomy (including the variability of the deep circumflex vessels) of this transplant as well as the surgical technique are described.

Jupiter JB, Bour CJ, May JW (1987) The reconstruction of defects in the femoral shaft with vascularized transfers of fibula bone. J Bone Joint Surg 69A:365

In seven patients, defects of the femur were reconstructed by vascularized fibula transplantation. Primary skeletal healing occurred in five, while two patients required subsequent bone grafting at the proximal osteosynthesis site. Details of the technique and results are presented.

Leung PC, Chow YYN (1984) Reconstruction of proximal femoral defects with a vascular-pedicled graft. J Bone Joint Surg 66B:32

The iliac crest graft based on the deep circumflex iliac artery is described for reconstructing the proximal femur.

Mankin HJ, Doppelt S, Tomford W (1983) Clinical experience with allograft implantation: The first ten years. Clin Orthop 174:69

Details of the clinical use of allografts, mostly for patients who had undergone tumor resection, are presented. The infection rate was 13.2%; the allograft fracture rate was 16.5%, often with prolonged difficulty in healing after fracture.

Maurer R, Dillin L (1987) Multistaged surgical management of posttraumatic segmental tibial bone loss. Clin Orthop 216:93

The technique of and clinical experience with proximal and distal tibiofibular synostosis are described.

Moore JR, Weiland AJ, Daniel RK (1983) Use of free vascularized bone grafts in the treatment of bone tumors. Clin Orthop 175:37

Immediate vascularized fibula transplantation was used in seven cases of locally aggressive bone tumors and in three cases of congenital pseudarthrosis of the tibia. Early healing and hypertrophy without recurrence of tumor was achieved in all but one patient.

Ostrup LT, Fredrickson JM (1974) Distant transfer of a free living bone graft by microvascular anastomoses. Plast Reconstr Surg 54:274

The fates of vascularized and nonvascularized bone grafts are discussed. This important early experimental work using rib grafts served as the basis for subsequent microvascular bone transplantation.

Pho RWH, Levack B, Satku K, et al (1985) Free vascularized fibula graft in the treatment of congenital pseudarthrosis of the tibia. J Bone Joint Surg 67B:64

Five patients with a relatively short follow-up are described.

Taylor GI (1983) The current status of free vascularized bone grafts. Clin Plast Surg 10:185

This article outlines the indications for and technique of fibula and iliac crest transplantation. The details of preoperative planning, use of bone models, and surgical technique are analyzed. Case studies are presented and may be helpful to the reader in evaluating potential solutions to similar clinical problems. This article is not a report on a clinical series of bone transplants.

Taylor GI, Miller GDH, Ham FJ (1975) The free vascularized bone graft. A clinical extension of microneurovascular techniques. Plast Reconstr Surg 55:533

This landmark article describes the first vascularized fibula transplant with emphasis on anatomy, nutrient supply, and physiologic basis. The posterior surgical approach (described by Henry) through the popliteal fossa is employed. (This approach is no longer used; the far simpler, lateral approach for harvesting the fibula is now favored.)

Taylor GI, Townsend P, Corlett R (1979) Superiority of the deep circumflex iliac vessels as the supply for free groin flaps. Plast Reconstr Surg 64:745

The surgical technique and clinical uses of the osteocutaneous groin flap based on the deep circumflex iliac vessel are described in detail.

Weiland AJ, Daniel RK (1979) Microvascular anastomoses for bone grafts in the treatment of massive defects in bone. J Bone Joint Surg 61:98

The techniques of and early experience with bone grafting are described. Use of the external fixator for stabilizing vascular bone transplants and the addition of cancellous bone at the osteosynthesis sites are mentioned.

Weiland AJ, Kleinert HE, Kutz JE, et al (1979) Free vascularized bone grafts in surgery of the upper extremity. J Hand Surg 4:129

The alternatives to and basis of vascularized fibula transplantation as well as the vascular anatomy of the fibula are outlined. A table that compares the characteristics of the rib, iliac crest, and fibula is also included. Five clinical cases involving the upper extremity (two involving tumors, three involving trauma) are presented. The surgical techniques of iliac crest osteocutaneous and fibula transplantation are briefly described; the Henry approach to the fibula, which has now been replaced by the simpler, lateral approach, is used.

Weiland AJ, Moore JR, Daniel RK (1983) Vascularized bone autografts. Experience with 41 cases. Clin Orthop 174:87

Details of the anatomy and surgical technique are clearly outlined and the results in 41 patients are analyzed. Indications are discussed.

Weiland AJ, Moore JR, Tolo VT (1987) Vascularized fibular grafts in the treatment of congenital pseudarthrosis. Presented at the Eighth Combined Meeting of the Orthopaedic Association of the English-Speaking World, Washington, DC, May 5

Twenty cases of congenital pseudarthrosis were treated with vascularized fibula transplantation. At the time of follow-up, which ranged from 1.5-9 years, union had been achieved in 15. Fractures below the fibular graft occurred in two patients, both of whom healed with conventional bone grafting techniques. Five patients experienced nonunion; this persisted in four patients despite bone grafting, and amputation was performed in the fifth. Residual anterior bowing and valgus angulation were present in half of the patients and was the most common problem.

Wood MB (1986) Free vascularized bone transfers for nonunions, segmental gaps, and following tumor resection. Orthopedics 9:810

The rationale, indications, and choice of donor bone for this procedure are reviewed. The results of a series of 49 cases that had a union rate of 82% are presented.

Yoshimura M, Shimamura K, Yoshinobu I (1983) Free vascularized fibular transplant. A new method for monitoring circulation of the grafted fibula. J Bone Joint Surg 65A:1295

A cutaneous "buoy" taken with the fibula transplant is described for monitoring vascularity. A larger skin flap can be used for combination defects involving bone and soft tissue. Anatomy and surgical technique are described in detail.

4 Toe Transplantation for Hand Reconstruction

4.1 Overview

Many techniques are available to reconstruct an absent or deformed thumb or finger. For numerous problems in the hand, transplantation of all or part of a toe has benefits over such other available methods as thumb lengthening, osteoplastic reconstruction, and pollicization. Toe transplantation provides digital pulp and nail support along with sensation and motion in the digit (Lister et al. 1983, Poppen et al. 1983). The obvious disadvantage of this procedure is the loss of all or part of a toe from the foot. The anticipated benefits for the hand as well as the potential problems for the foot, which must be clearly understood by both the patient and surgeon, will be considered in this chapter.

In order to successfully fashion thumbs and fingers from toes, the anatomic and functional differences between them must be well understood. Toes are structurally very similar to fingers, if one considers their basic anatomy. One important difference, however, is that the great toe does not rotate in utero as does the thumb. Because anatomy and function are directly related, any difference in anatomy between toes and fingers reflects the specialized and unique functions for which they are adapted.

The *great toe* is approximately 20% larger than the thumb, but a slow process of atrophy occurs following transplantation. This atrophy is perhaps a result of the decreased amount of callus and lighter "duty" of the thumb compared with the great toe. In time, then, the great toe becomes a cosmetically and functionally outstanding replacement for the absent thumb.

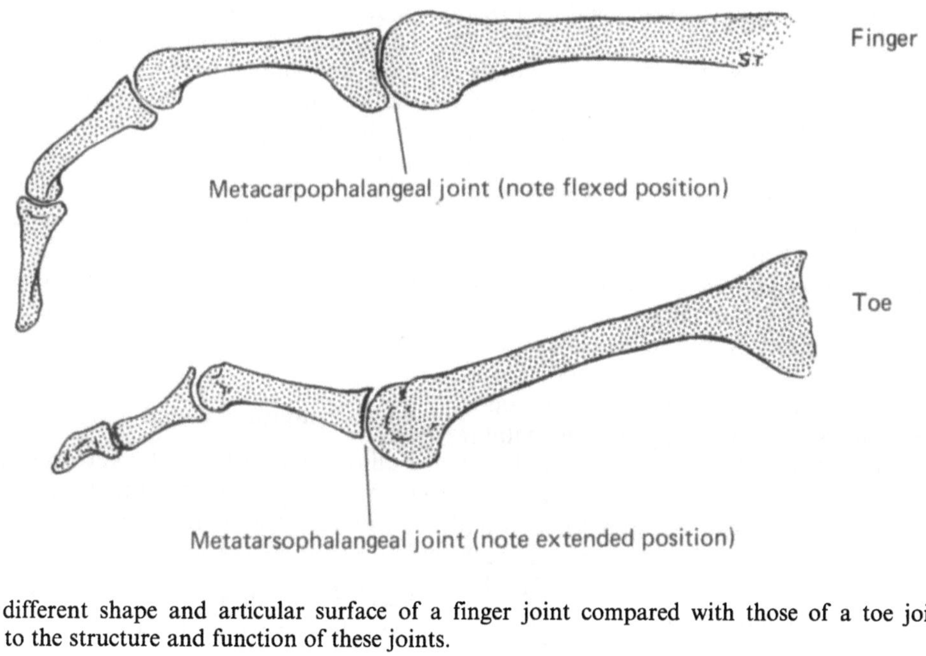

Plate 4-I. Note the different shape and articular surface of a finger joint compared with those of a toe joint. The joint capsules are adapted to the structure and function of these joints.

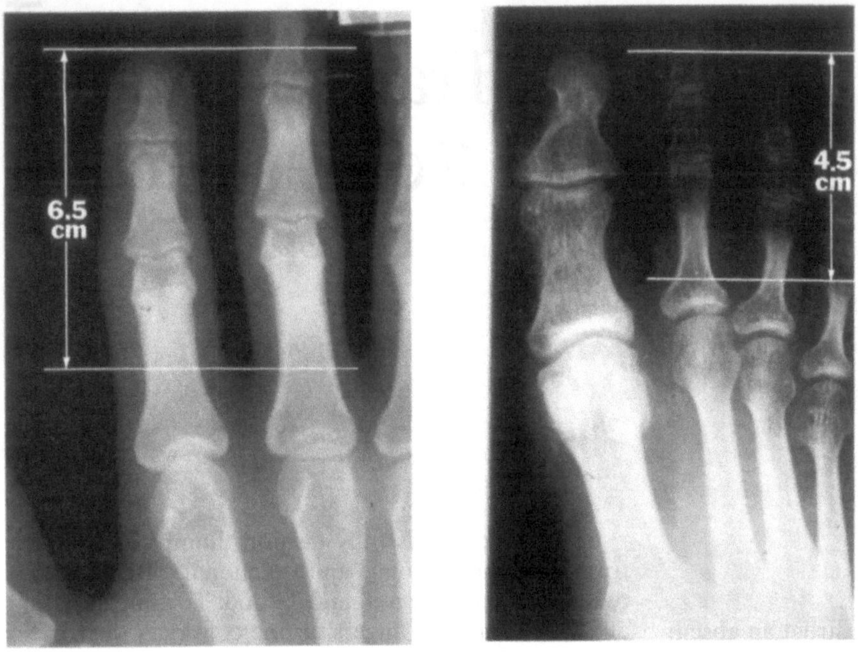

a b

Fig. 4-1. a. The distance from the end of the finger to the base of the web space is 6.5 cm. **b.** The distance from the end of the toe to the base of the web space is 4.5 cm.

The *second toe* has a smaller nail than does a finger, the distal phalanx is somewhat bulbous, and the *interphalangeal joints* are flexed to a greater extent than the interphalangeal joints of a finger. Temporary pinning of the distal phalanx following second-toe transplantation may partially correct the flexed attitude of the distal part of the transplanted second toe. Also, the *metatarsophalangeal joint* is a hyperextension joint, in contrast with the metacarpophalangeal joint, which flexes readily. For this reason, when a second toe is used to replace a finger, the functional outcome will be far superior if the metacarpophalangeal joint is intact in the hand and the transplant is attached distal to it (Sec. 4.3.1.2) (Plate 4-I).

Compared with the fingers, the toes have smaller phalanges, and the *web spaces* are closer to the distal end (Fig. 4-1). To achieve appropriate finger length, the length of toe required is measured from the toe's distal end, and because of the position of the web space, skin grafting or flap cover is frequently necessary for the proximal part of the transplant. Also, the fatty tissue of the web space is often bulbous, so this area may subsequently need careful debulking.

Several transplant options from the foot are possible for the reconstruction of hand defects. These consist of the *great toe*, the *second toe* distal to the metatarsophalangeal joint, the second toe along with the metatarsophalangeal joint and part of the metatarsal, and parts of one or more toes. In reconstructing a thumb, the soft tissues of the great toe can be used to surround an iliac crest graft by the so-called "*wrap-around*" technique (Morrison et al. 1980) (Figs. 4-6 and 4-21). For specific defects of the hand, the *metatarsophalangeal joint* (Figs. 4-19 and 4-24), *proximal interphalangeal joint* (Fig. 4-25) (Kuo et al. 1984, Mathes et al. 1980, O'Brien et al. 1984, Tsai et al. 1982), other *parts of the toes* such as the pulp or distal phalanx, soft tissues, or other combinations of soft tissue and bone can be transplanted (Foucher et al. 1980) (Fig. 4-23).

4.2 Indications

4.2.1 Trauma

The most common indication for toe-to-hand transplantation is traumatic loss of the thumb or fingers. A *careful history* is essential because the details of the injury are often helpful. The zone of injury, which may be considerably more proximal than the site of amputation, determines both the site of vascular repair and the length of vessel that must be taken with the toe. In the case of burns, superficial veins are often absent and the surgeon should plan to use a vena comitans as a recipient vein.

Primary toe transplantation immediately after a traumatic injury is unwise. At that point, the patient cannot fully appreciate the magnitude of his or her loss and is not in a state of mind to consider the problems stemming from loss of a toe.

4.2.2 Tumors

Following resection of aggressive tumors, toe transplantation may restore function once the likelihood of the patient's survival has been established.

4.2.3 Congenital Defects (Gilbert 1982, May et al. 1981, Michon et al. 1984)

Although technically demanding, thumb and finger reconstruction for congenital defects using toe transplantation can be rewarding. Continued growth in the transplanted toe can be expected (Mathes et al. 1980; Nunley et al. 1987, Sec. 5.7). Pollicization is indicated when four fingers are present, and especially for *longitudinal deficiencies* such as radial club hand. When two or three digits are present, the pollicization of one leaves only one or two fingers for opposition, and toe transplantation may be considered (Fig. 4-10). For longitudinal deficiencies, however, recipient structures may be rudimentary or absent, which is why dissection should always begin in the hand to confirm their presence. With *transverse congenital deformities* such as constriction bands, the recipient structures are generally near the site of amputation, making transplantation easier (Fig. 4-16).

4.3 Choice of Transplant

4.3.1 Recipient Site Considerations

4.3.1.1 Thumb Reconstruction

The purpose of toe-to-thumb transplantation is to provide an opposable thumb for *large and small object grasp.* Many patients have the capability of grasping small objects with even a very short thumb. The greatest benefit of toe transplantation, however, lies in restoring the ability to grasp large objects. The individual needs of the patient should be carefully evaluated. Often, a hand therapist who tests many specific occupational functions can be very helpful. A prosthetic thumb can sometimes aid in evaluating the prognosis and assess whether surgery will be beneficial. Computerized mapping of the abnormal hand wherein a thumb or finger of variable dimensions is "added" can give the patient a good idea of the anticipated appearance.

The thumb can be reconstructed with the great toe, the second toe, or by the wrap-around technique, and the advantages and disadvantages of each must be considered within the context of amputation level (Fig. 4-2). Amputations that are *distal to the interphalangeal joint* of the thumb are best treated with lengthening procedures or first-web-space deepening if indeed any surgery is necessary. The great toe will often be too bulbous if placed in this location, while a second toe will be too narrow.

A great toe transplant is indicated for amputations occurring in the region of the *midmetacarpal to the interphalangeal joint* (Fig. 4-5). It is important that the reconstructed thumb not be too long, so the bone of the toe should be resected back to the appropriate level.

There remains much controversy regarding what the best transplant would be for amputations distal to the midportion of the metacarpal that have some intact thenar muscle function where either a *great toe, a second toe, or the wrap-around* technique can be used. From the perspective of thumb function, the *great toe* provides a broader pulp with stronger pinch and grasp than does a second toe. In addition, the great toe and thumb are more similar in terms of size. The great toe is slightly angled toward the fibular side at the interphalangeal joint and its initial size is greater compared with the thumb. Nevertheless, the ultimate functional and cosmetic results are generally excellent. The *second toe* is an acceptable replacement for the thumb, but the pulp surface is narrow, the interphalangeal joint is flexed, and the appearance is not as good as that following the great-toe or wrap-around procedure (Fig. 4-7). The benefits of using the second toe primarily relate to considerations at the donor site (Sec. 4.3.2).

The *wrap-around technique* (Doi et al. 1985, Morrison et al. 1980) results in a thumb that has excellent appearance and is narrower than the great toe (Fig. 4-6), but there are two disadvantages. An iliac crest bone graft is used to provide the osseous structure of the new thumb, and bone resorption occasionally follows this procedure. The other disadvantage is that movement at the interphalangeal joint is not possible; this is particularly important if the amputation is proximal to the metacarpophalangeal joint (Fig. 4-5). The technique can be modified to include the distal phalanx of the great toe, with less likelihood of bone resorption. A normal carpometacarpal joint is therefore essential if this technique is used. The procedure should not be used in children because growth potential is absent.

Amputations *proximal to the midportion of the metacarpal* will result in a thumb that is too short if the great toe is removed at the metatarsophalangeal joint level. It is my opinion that the great toe should not be removed proximal to this level in order to avoid subsequent gait problems relating to push-off and balance. Indeed, the sesamoid bones at the head of the first metatarsal should be left intact on the plantar surface to circumvent such problems (Plate 4-II).

With these factors in mind, amputations of the thumb that are *proximal to the midportion of the metacarpal* should be reconstructed with the second toe. The second ray may be removed, including the metatarsophalangeal joint and part of the second metatarsal, but specific plans for coverage on both sides of the metatarsal must be made (Fig. 4-9). Often, split-thickness skin grafting will be adequate, but in some cases a preliminary skin flap improves the ultimate result of the transplant.

Thumb reconstruction is considerably more of a problem when none of the metacarpal remains (Gordon, Rosen et al. 1984). In many such amputations, pollicization of the index finger is the best choice. If multiple digits have been injured, a toe transplant may be the best alternative. The metatarsal base can be placed on the *trapezium*, with the eventual formation of a "pseudojoint" over time (Fig. 4-8). Toes have also been placed on the *distal radius* in unusual cases of adactyly (Furnas and Achauer 1983, Meals and Lesavoy 1983, Zhong-Jig and Chen 1984). When considering the length of toe needed, the method of osteosynthesis must be planned at the same time because some methods call for overlapping and others are performed end-to-end (Sec. 4.4). It must be realized that amputations proximal to the metacarpophalangeal joint may

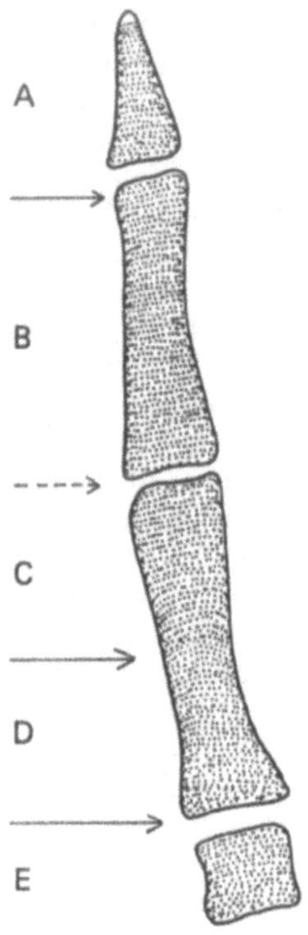

Fig. 4-2. The options for toe-to-thumb transplantation depend on the level of amputation. A – No surgery is indicated (occasionally, web deepening or thumb lengthening). B – Great-toe vs. second-toe vs. wrap-around procedure (Sec. 4.3.1.1). C – Great-toe vs. second-toe vs. wrap-around procedure (may need opposition transfer). D – Second-toe (needs opposition transfer) vs. pollicization. E – Pollicization vs. second-toe (rarely).

not have sufficient musculature remaining, and an opposition tendon or muscle transfer may be needed to provide active movement of the transplant. Usually, a hand tendon is available (e.g., the extensor indicis proprius or flexor digitorum superficialis) or the abductor digiti minimi can be used (Huber transfer). Occasionally, this is not possible and a functional microvascular transplant should be considered (Gordon, Rosen et al. 1984) (Fig. 4-8).

If the thumb has been amputated at the *metacarpophalangeal joint*, then the proximal phalanx of the toe, including the proximal articular surface, can be placed on the articular surface of the distal metacarpal of the thumb. Such a composite joint is reconstructed by removing the joint capsule of the toe circumferentially and suturing it to the soft tissues around the neck of the metacarpal (Wilson et al. 1984).

4.3.1.2 Finger Reconstruction

Second-toe transplantation to replace an amputated finger is indicated when there is inadequate opposition for the thumb, such as in *congenital adactyly* (Fig. 4-16) or *where all the digits have been traumatically amputated* (Fig. 4-14). Toes transplanted *proximal to the metacarpophalangeal joint* will have considerably less total active motion than those distal to this joint (Gordon et al. 1985) because the metatarsophalangeal joint of the second ray is a hyperextension joint (Plate 4-I). If the *metacarpophalangeal joint is intact* and the toe transplant is performed distal to it, movement in the finger is likely to be adequate. If only *one finger is present* and is stiff or insensate and has limited pinch function with the thumb, the addition of a toe may provide considerably stronger pinch and a broader surface for large object grasp (Fig. 4-11).

When *one or two fingers* have been amputated, the indications for replacement with a toe transplant are less clear. Indeed, when a single digit has been amputated, toe transplantation should only be performed in rare situations, and must be regarded primarily as a cosmetic operation that will restore the arcade of the digits. Ray amputation of the index or small fingers or ray transfer for central finger loss, however, will provide an excellent functional as well as cosmetic result (Fig. 5-10). In patients who use their hands for five-fingered activities such as playing a musical instrument or using a keyboard, replacement of one or two fingers may be appropriate in rare circumstances (Fig. 4-13).

Generally, the most ulnarward digits should be reconstructed to give the best large and small object grasp. In patients with *adactyly*, two toes from the same foot have been used to provide an opposable surface that is quite broad (Lister et al. 1983). This procedure produces a substantial defect in the foot, the long-term results of which have not yet been clearly delineated. For the present, I feel that this donor site defect is too great for this procedure to be used routinely.

Adactyly may also be treated by transplanting a second toe from each foot either simultaneously or in sequential operations to provide two digits for opposition. These digits are placed next to each other on the long and ring, or ring and small finger rays to provide a good surface for pinch (Gordon et al. 1985).

4.3.1.3 Thumb and Finger Reconstruction

When neither *thumb nor fingers* are present, a great toe from one foot and a second toe from the other may be used to reconstruct a thumb and a single finger for opposition (Gordon et al. 1985) (Fig. 4-17). Hands with no thumb or fingers may be reconstructed by other treatment combinations, such as great-toe transplantation combined with a prosthesis (Fig. 4-18), or second-toe transplantation combined with thumb lengthening (Fig. 4-15).

4.3.2 Donor Site Considerations

Removal of the *great toe* produces a moderate cosmetic defect in the foot (Fig. 4-3). Function continues to be good and careful gait analysis has not revealed any substantial short- or long-term problems (Lipton et al.

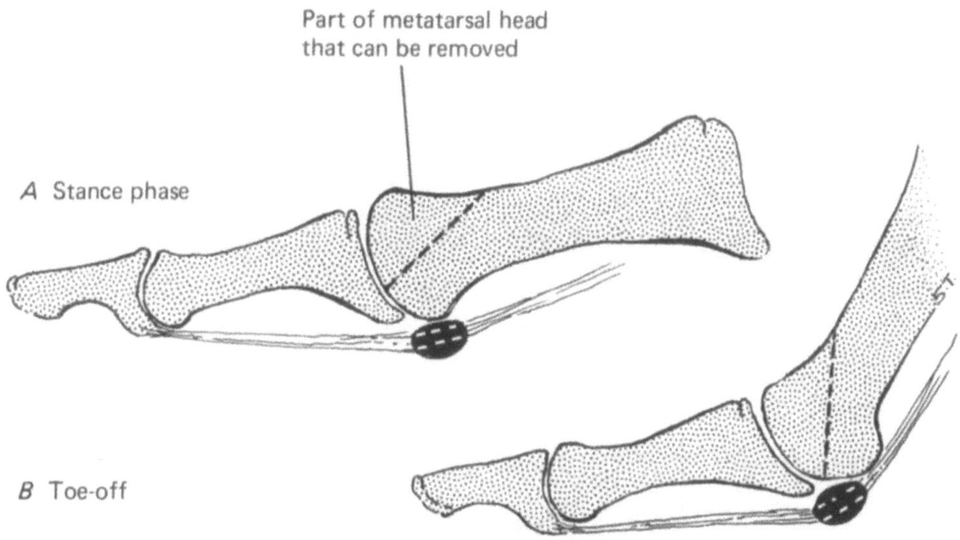

Plate 4-II. The first metatarsal head and sesamoid bones should not be removed when the great toe is transplanted. A portion of the dorsal surface of the first metatarsal may be removed without affecting the weight-bearing surface. The plantar surface of the first metatarsal head and the sesamoid bones are important in stance (*A*) and at toe-off in the gait cycle (***B***).

1987, Poppen et al. 1981). Weight bearing is shifted somewhat toward the lateral side of the foot. The first metatarsal head and sesamoid bones should be left intact for balance and push-off (Plate 4-II) (Frykman et al. 1986). Cultural preferences in addition to cosmetic and functional considerations may produce objections to using the great toe. Such an objection may be encountered in oriental patients who wear slippers much of the time, or in patients who, for religious or cultural reasons, cannot accept the loss of the great toe.

Removal of the *second toe*, in contrast, produces minimal functional or cosmetic deficit in the foot (Fig. 4-3) (Frykman et al. 1986). If the second toe is used, most of the second ray to the base of the metatarsal is removed, and the third ray is moved next to the first ray, reconstructing a new intermetatarsal ligament. This technique allows primary skin closure. The deficit in the foot will then be imperceptible to the casual observer unless the toes are counted. For this reason, the second toe is my choice in higher-risk patients, such as those with a history of vascular disease, diabetes, or microvascular thrombosis (Fig. 4-7). I also advocate second-toe transplantation for reconstructing congenital defects in order to limit the possibility of abnormal foot growth and gait problems in the young child.

The donor site following a *wrap-around procedure* is considered by some to be better than that after amputation of the great toe. Skin grafting and a cross-toe flap are needed to reconstruct the toe, which ends up shorter, scarred, and lacking a nail. The appearance is often poor, healing is slow, and complications are not infrequent. Some surgeons therefore favor amputation of the remainder of the great toe when this technique is used.

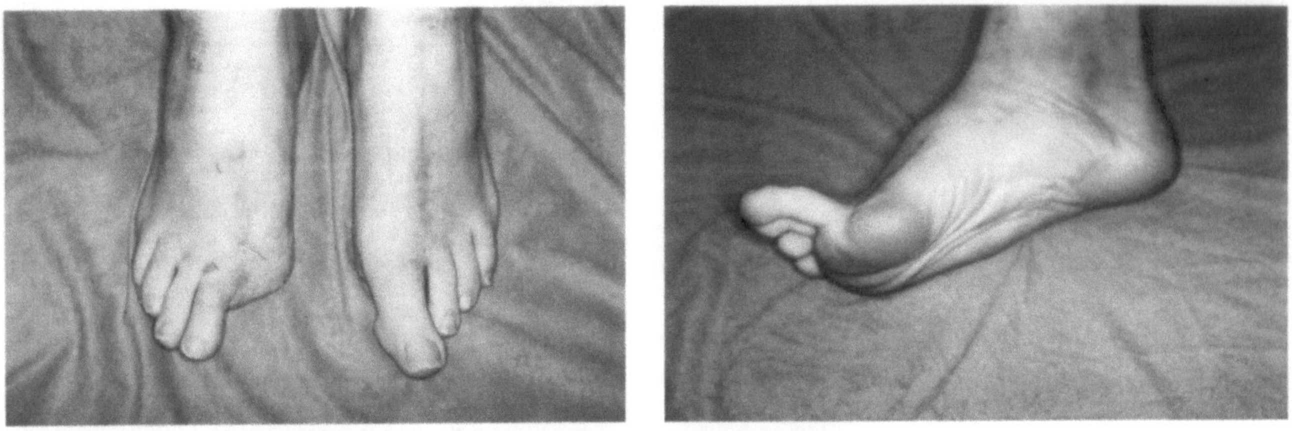

a b

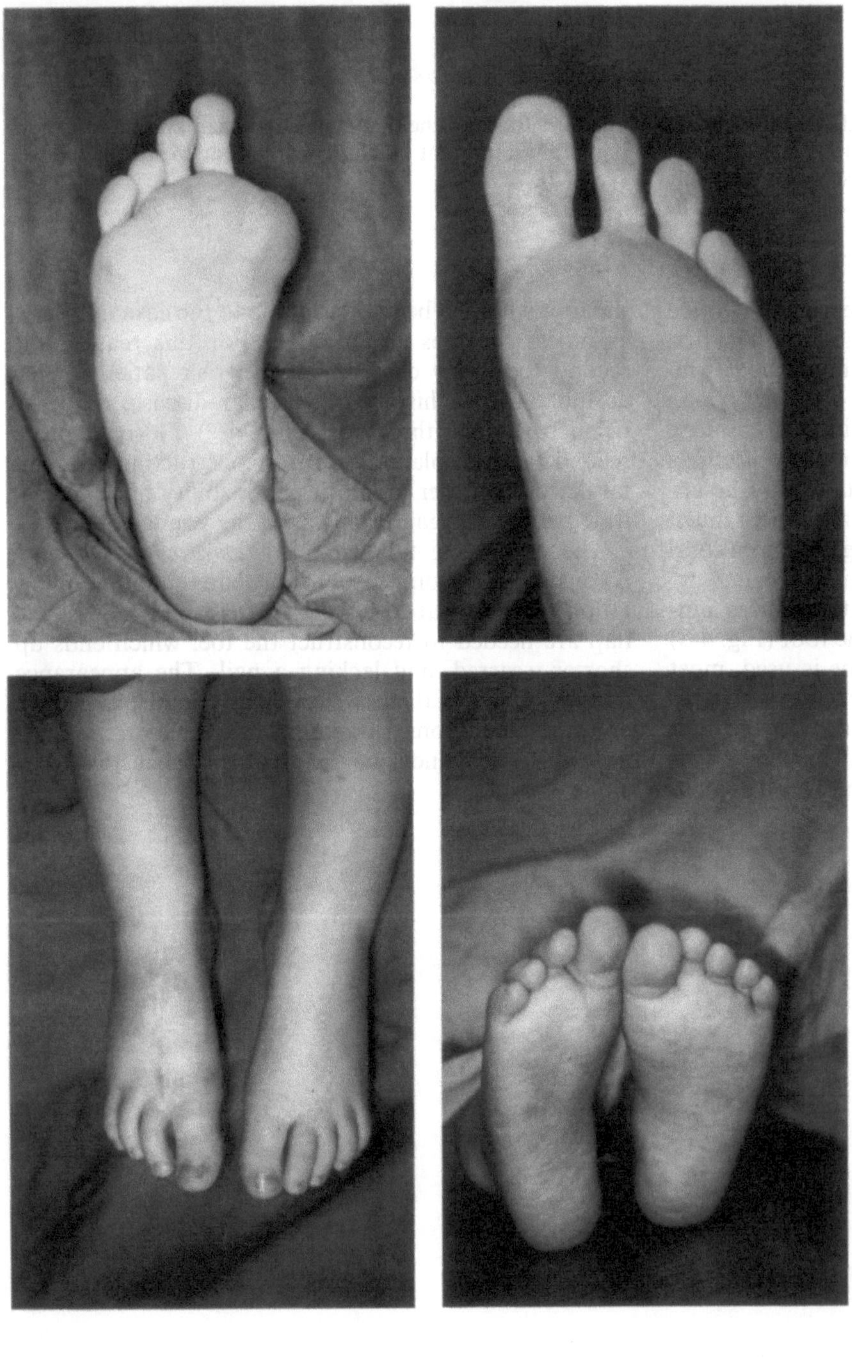

c d e f

Fig. 4-3. a. The donor sites following transplantation of a great toe and second toe are shown from the dorsal aspect. **b** and **c.** A great-toe transplant seen from the plantar surface. Retention of the sesamoid bone and maintaining the length of the first metatarsal is important for weight bearing; this is evidenced by the callus formation under the metatarsal head, which continues to be used for weight bearing and balance. **d.** A second-toe transplant seen from the plantar surface. **e** and **f.** A second-toe transplant in a 22-month-old child.

4.4 Preoperative Planning

4.4.1 Arterial System

An *arteriogram of the hand* is essential in posttraumatic cases to establish which vessels are available and confirm the vascular supply to the remaining digits. The supply to the remaining digits should not be disturbed. Dominant radial supply or independent radial and ulnar supply is not infrequent (Coleman and Anson 1961, Sec. 2.9; Jones and O'Brien 1985) (Fig. 2-1). In congenital cases, the vessels are extremely small and arteriography is more difficult. It has not been my practice to perform arteriography in small children.

Because *the vascular anatomy* in the foot has considerable variability, a lateral projection arteriogram is performed to delineate the dorsal and plantar circulation (Gu et al. 1985, Leung et al. 1983, Wu et al. 1980). Spasm can be a problem in obtaining information about the distal vasculature, so vasodilating agents or a general anesthetic may sometimes be indicated when doing the arteriogram. The position of the first dorsal metatarsal artery, i.e., dorsal or plantar, may be seen on an oblique arteriogram of the foot. Also, if this artery curves under the first metatarsal on the anteroposterior view, a plantar vessel can be anticipated. A detailed knowledge of the vascular anatomy of the first metatarsal artery is the key to the arterial dissection for both second- and great-toe transplantation (Leung et al. 1980, Wu et al. 1980) (Plates 4-III and 4-V; Fig. 1-23c).

4.4.2 Venous System

The veins should be outlined on the *dorsum of the foot* by elevating the tourniquet so that blood pressure is between systolic and diastolic. The veins on the *dorsal aspect of the hand* forming the dorsal venous network drain into the basilic and cephalic veins; these are of large caliber and make excellent recipient vessels. After a burn, or if there has been extensive skin grafting on the dorsal aspect of the hand, these vessels may be absent, in which case the venae comitantes of the radial artery should be used.

4.4.3 Osteosynthesis

Length is a key factor for both appearance and function of the transplanted toe. A reconstructed thumb or finger that is slightly shorter than its contralateral counterpart will generally function well. When planning length, the arcade of the digits must be kept in mind. One should also be aware that the method of bone fixation will affect the ultimate length and should therefore be planned carefully. Bone fixation can be accomplished with (1) the end-to-end technique, using Kirschner wires or interosseous wires (Fig. 5-24), or (2) the overlapping technique, wherein the toe bone is hollowed out and a peg is fashioned on the thumb. This creates a mortise-and-tenon joint with good bone contact, and it is secured with a single oblique Kirschner wire to control rotation.

4.4.4 Skin Flaps

Skin flaps, transplant length, and the position of the vascular pedicle can be planned with a *clay model* (Figs. 4-8, 4-16, and 4-19). For example, if the first web space has poor soft-tissue cover, as large a skin flap as possible should be taken with the toe.

When the ipsilateral toe is used, the skin on the lateral aspect of the great toe and the first toe web space can be included to provide cover or release a contracture of the first web space in the hand. In addition, the arterial pedicle will then be in the correct position to anastomose the dorsalis pedis vessel to the radial artery just before this artery enters between the two heads of the first dorsal interosseous muscle. When fingers are being reconstructed, the webs and position of the vessels should be planned similarly.

The *web space of the toe* lies at the mid-proximal phalanx level of the toes. If the osteotomy site of the toe transplant is more proximal, skin cover proximal to this level will be inadequate and either a split-thickness skin graft or another method of skin cover will be necessary (Fig. 4-1).

Any first *web space contracture* should be released; this can be accomplished with coronal incisions over the thumb amputation stump with flap elevation on the radial and ulnar sides, which should allow for the skin on the ulnar aspect of the amputation stump to drop into the first web space. If this measure is anticipated to be inadequate, a preliminary procedure to provide adequate soft-tissue coverage may be necessary prior to toe-to-thumb transplantation.

In deciding whether to use the *left or right great toe*, one must consider (1) that the ipsilateral toe taken with some skin from the first web space will provide better cover for the first web space of the hand; (2) that the ipsilateral great toe will be angled about 10° toward the index finger at the interphalangeal joint and may compromise large object grasp slightly (May et al. 1978); and (3) the position of the arteries. Transplanting the ipsilateral toe will place the dorsalis pedis vessel close to the radial artery as this artery enters between the two heads of the first dorsal interosseous muscle.

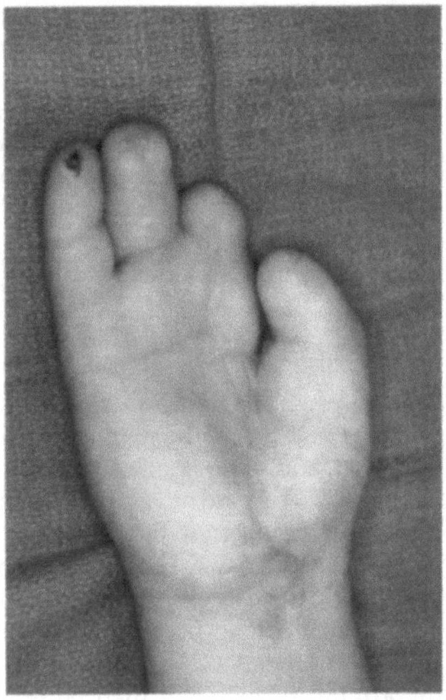

a

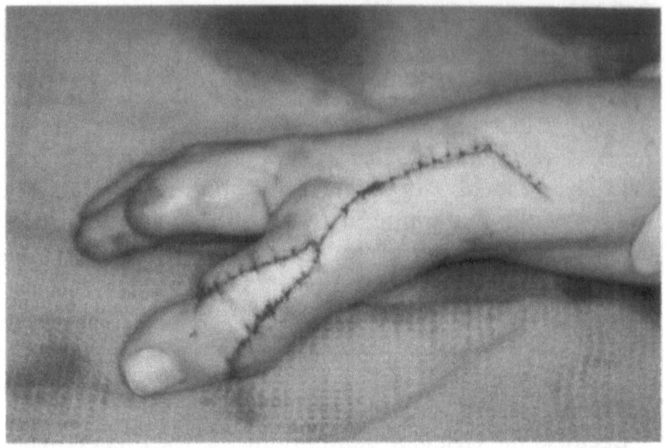

b

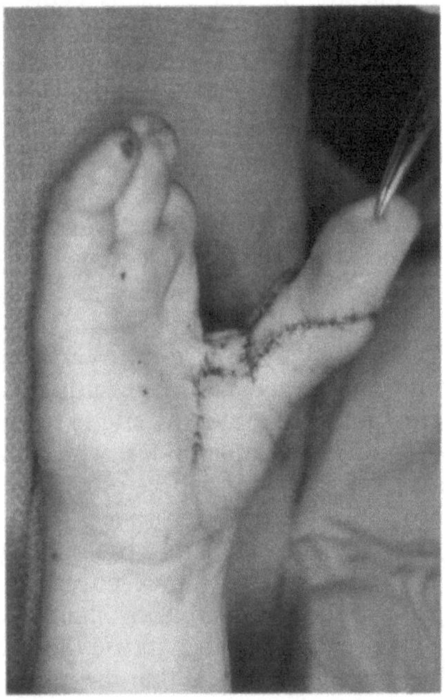

c

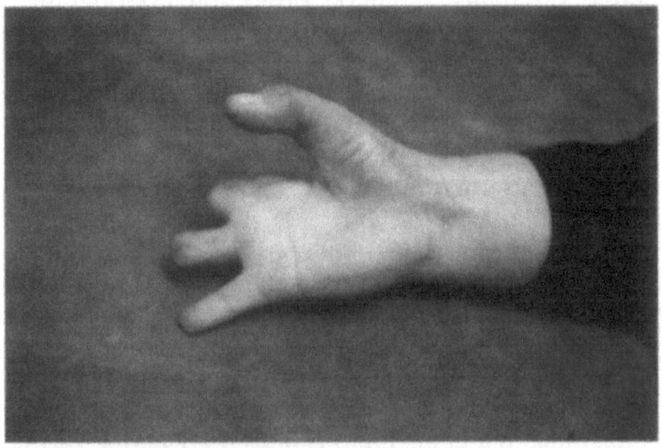

d

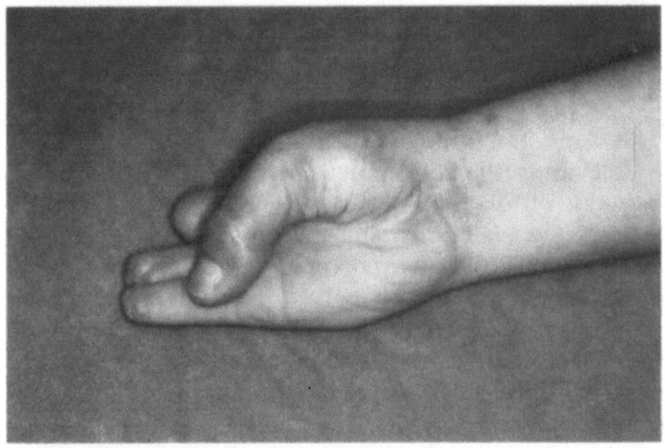

e

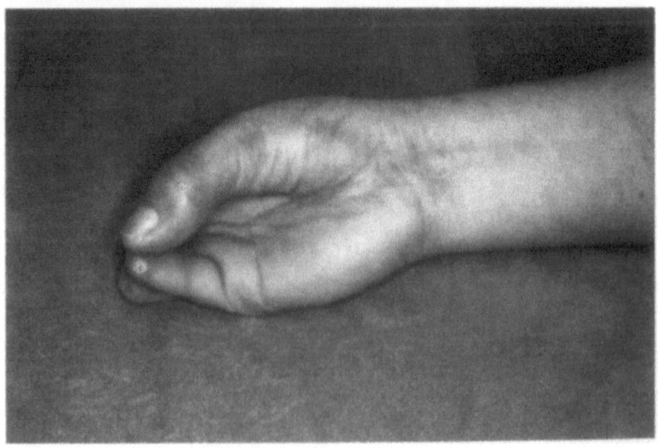

f

Fig. 4-4 a–f. Thumb amputation at the proximal phalangeal level: whole great-toe transplant. a. This patient had been a respiratory therapy student. She lost her thumb and fingers after a radial artery catheter was placed in class (see also Figs. 1-26 and 2-1). She had a first web space contracture, extremely limited mobility of the thumb stump, and virtually no function in the hand. **b** and **c.** By making a sagittal incision over the tip of the thumb stump, the ulnar flap was elevated and used to widen the first web space. The thumb was then planned with flaps to fit appropriately over the end of the bone. With the ulnar artery being the dominant vessel supplying this patient's hand, the arterial anastomosis was performed between the dorsalis pedis vessel and the radial artery proximal to the wrist. **d–f.** The transplant looks very similar to a thumb. The patient is able to pinch against the small finger and has regained both large and small object grasp.

Fig. 4-5a–e. Thumb amputation at the distal metacarpal level: whole great-toe transplant. a. The great toe appears slightly broader than the thumb when the two are seen next to each other. When seen separately, the appearance is good. **b.** Especially if there is no movement in the metacarpophalangeal joint, a functional interphalangeal joint is important. Fifteen to 30° of motion can usually be achieved (Frykman et al. 1986). **c** and **d.** Good dexterity and large object grasp were restored. **e.** Seven-millimeter two-point discrimination (Frykman et al. 1986).

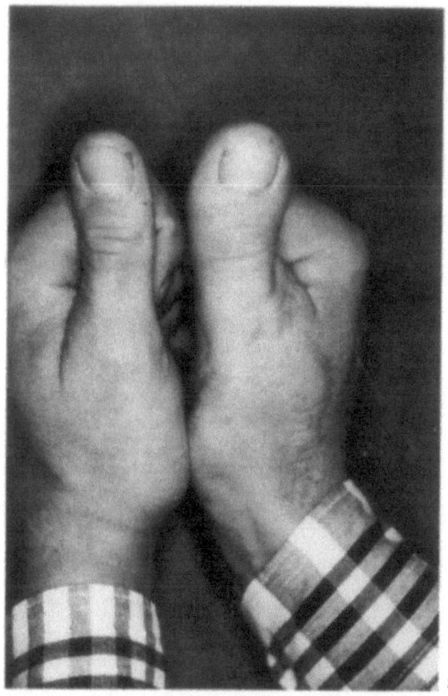

a

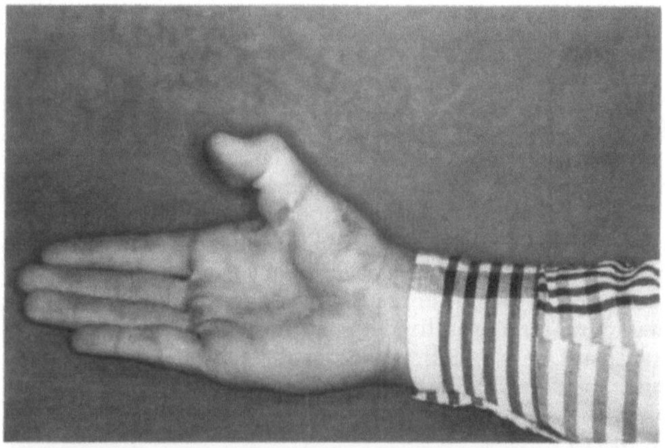

b

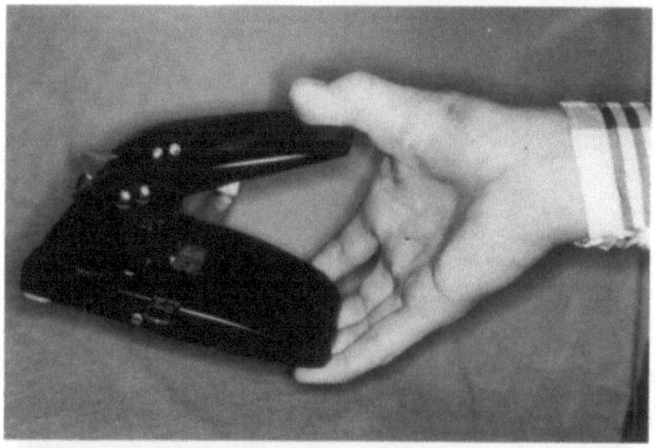

c

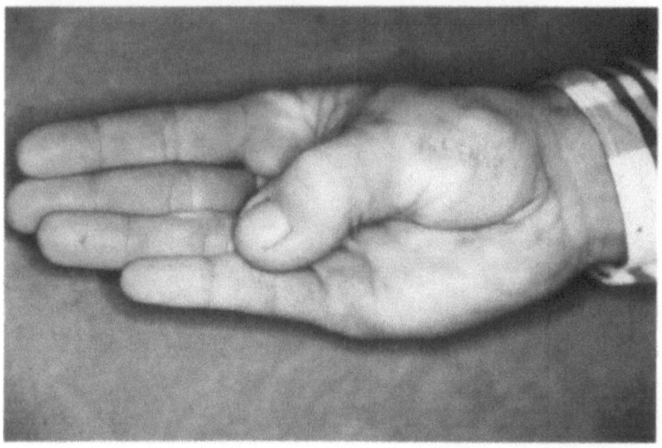

d

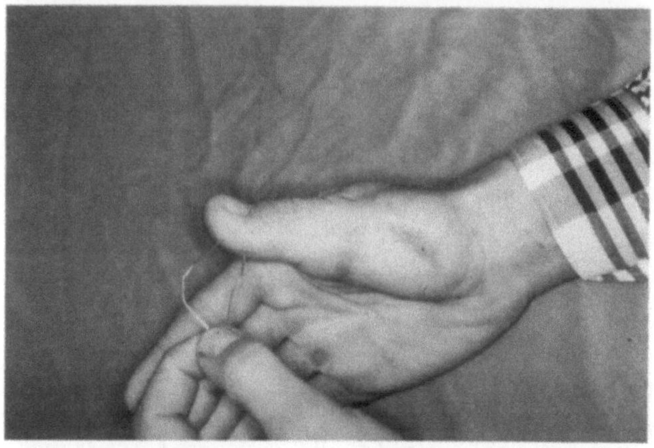

e

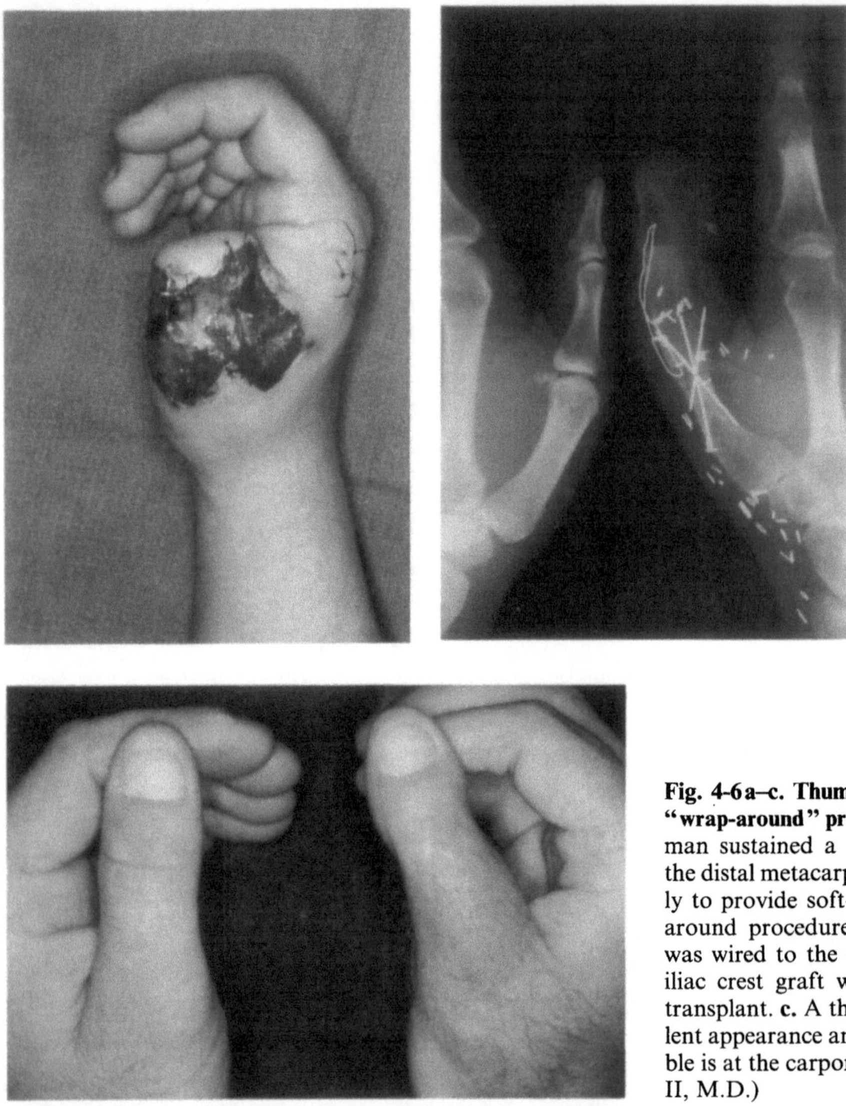

a b

c

Fig. 4-6a–c. Thumb amputation at the distal metacarpal level: "wrap-around" procedure (see also Fig. 4-21). **a.** A 22-year-old man sustained a thumb amputation with a crush injury of the distal metacarpal. A tubed groin flap was used preliminarily to provide soft-tissue cover in anticipation of a toe wrap-around procedure. **b.** An iliac crest corticocancellous graft was wired to the distal metacarpal. The distal aspect of this iliac crest graft was fixed to the distal phalanx of the toe transplant. **c.** A thumb was reconstructed which had an excellent appearance and good function. The only movement possible is at the carpometacarpal joint. (Courtesy of Hill Hastings II, M.D.)

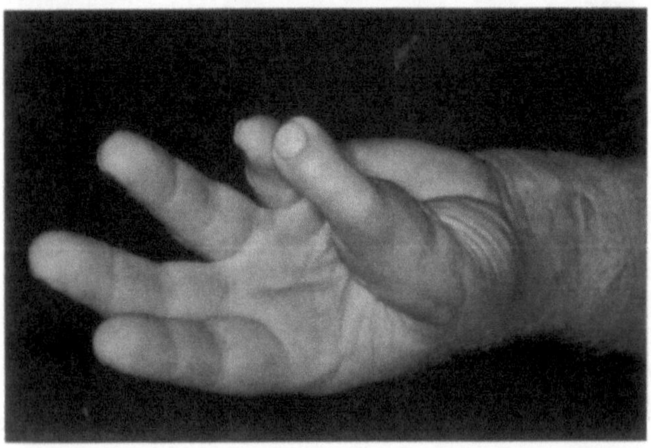

Fig. 4-7. Thumb amputation in a high-risk patient: second toe-to-thumb transplant. This patient has polycythemia. He chose to undergo second-toe transplantation because the appearance of the donor site is better than that of any other transplant; this was an important consideration because I felt he had a slightly greater risk of losing the transplant. This transplant is considerably narrower than a normal thumb or a thumb reconstructed from either a great toe or by the wrap-around procedure. It is flexed at the interphalangeal joint and has the appearance of a toe. Despite the transplant's narrower pulp surface and lesser strength compared with a transplanted great toe, this patient regained adequate function and was satisfied with the result.

Fig. 4-8a–h. Thumb amputation at the trapezium level: second-toe ray transplant including the second metatarsal. a. In an accident involving an auger, this man's thumb was amputated at the trapezium level. There were severe injuries to all of the other fingers, partial amputation of the ring and small fingers, and nerve and tendon damage to the index and long fingers. **b.** A second-toe transplant including the second metatarsal was planned to provide some opposition. Because of severe injuries to the radial aspect of the hand, the index finger had poor sensation on the radial side. This deficit in addition to the injuries to the other digits made pollicization a less desirable alternative. **c.** Following the toe transplant, an *adduction contracture* was present in the first web space, and the thumb had no *active opposition*. A flap was needed in the first web space to release the contracture, and active motor function was required to enable opposition and thumb abduction. A Huber abductor digiti minimi transfer was considered as an active motor, but additional tissue was needed to allow passive motion in the web space. A serratus muscle transplant satisfied both of these requirements simultaneously. The web space was released and the recurrent branch of the median nerve was dissected and divided proximal to the neuroma for repair to the long thoracic nerve fascicles. **d.** One slip of the serratus anterior was used to widen the web space, and a second slip brought subcutaneously to the radial aspect of the thumb provided abduction. **e.** This muscle transplant released the first web space contracture and restored good active abduction and opposition. The muscle is flat and profiles evenly with the surrounding palmar skin. The similarity between the actual reconstruction and the clay model is evident. (*Continued*)

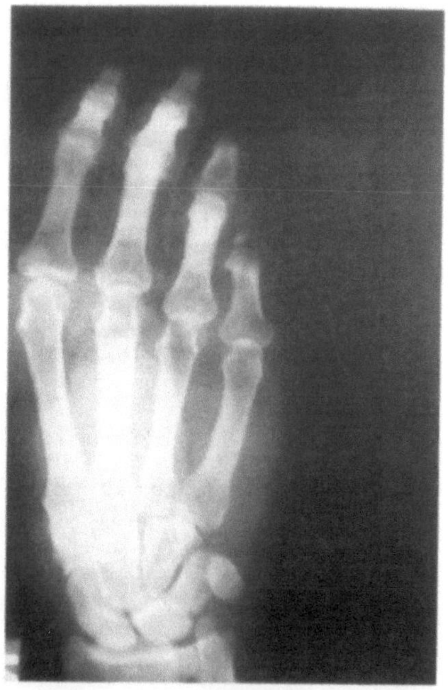

a

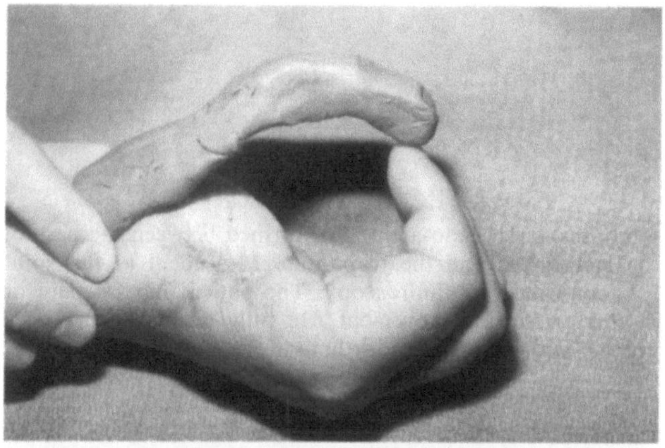

b

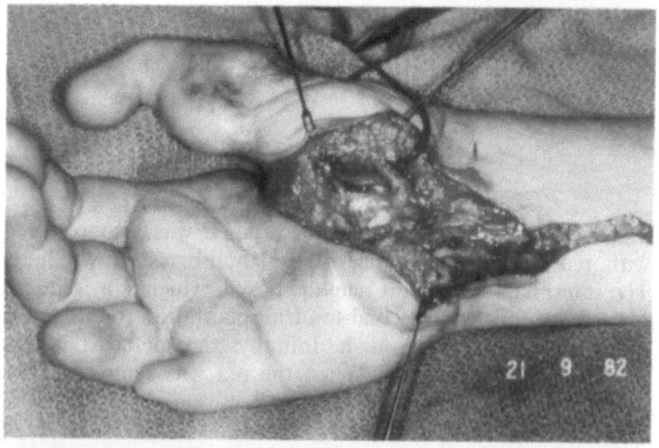

c

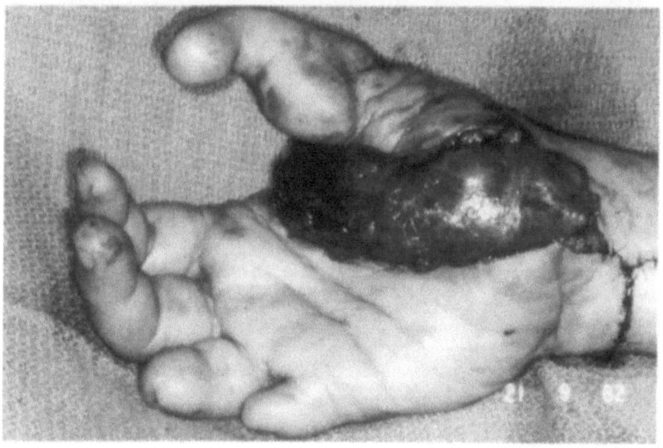

d

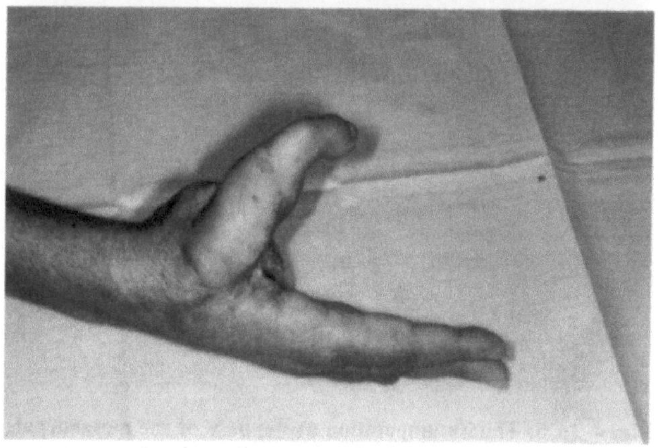

e

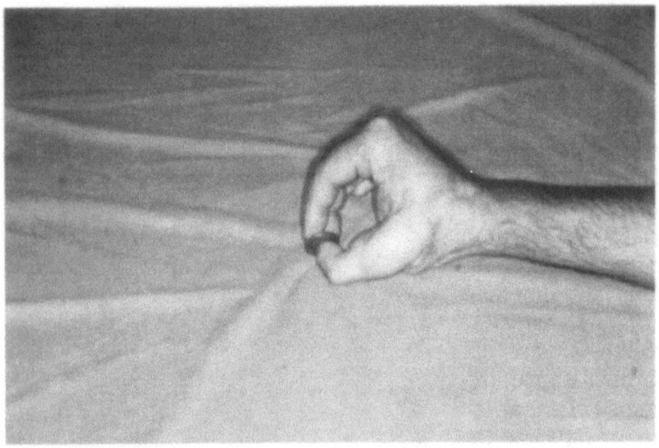
f

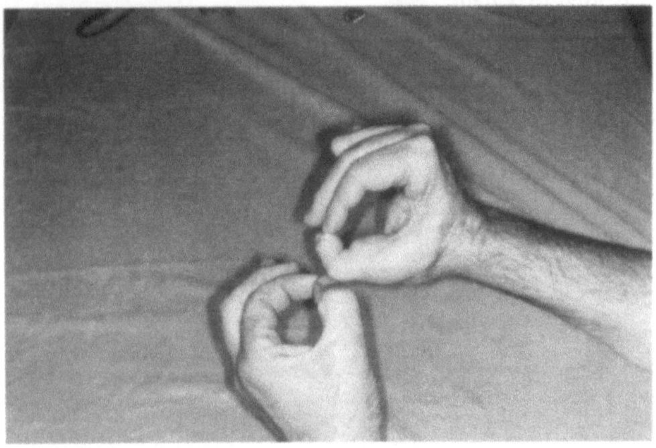
g

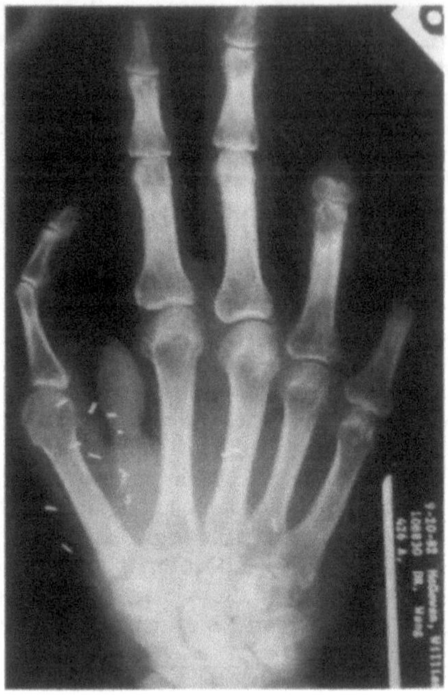
h

Fig. 4-8f, g. Excellent small object pinch was also restored with reasonable appearance of the thumb, as shown here. The interphalangeal joint remains flexed, which is a frequent occurrence following second-toe transplantation to either the finger or thumb position. **h.** Initially, the metacarpal was pinned to the trapezium. When the pin was removed after 4 months, a "pseudo-arthrosis" formed between the base of the metacarpal and the trapezium. Movement at this joint was confirmed by fluoroscopy. The patient has no pain or discomfort during movement. He fully resumed work as a butcher without problems or limitations.

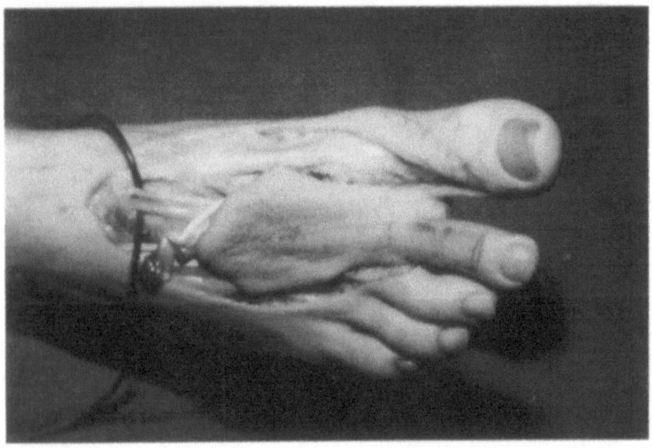
a

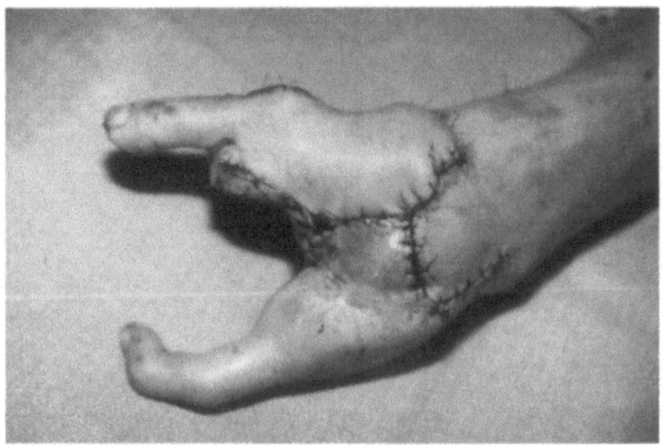
b

Fig. 4-9a, b. Thumb amputation at the base of the metacarpal: second-toe ray transplant with a dorsalis pedis flap. a. When the second-toe ray including the metatarsal is transplanted, the sides of the metatarsal need soft-tissue cover, although the interosseous muscle may cover a part of this area. The cover options are (1) a preliminary cutaneous flap, (2) a split-thickness skin graft on the muscle tissue, (3) a dorsalis pedis flap taken with the toe transplant, and (4) a flap done at the time of the toe transplant. If a dorsalis pedis flap is taken, skin grafting will be required after removing the second-toe ray. This grafting is a disadvantage because it can lead to delayed healing in the foot. Here, a dorsalis pedis flap with the second toe is seen dissected. Proximally, the vessels and extensor tendon have been dissected. **b.** This second-toe transplant was used in the thumb position to provide opposition against a stiff small finger. The flap was well vascularized, but additional skin grafting was required on the palmar surface.

Fig. 4-10a–f. Thumb agenesis: second-toe to thumb transplant. a. This 22-month-old girl had bilateral symmetrical congenital hand deformities, with a rudimentary thumb and two poorly functioning digits. A thumb for opposition was needed. In such a deficiency, it is necessary to first dissect the vessels, nerves, and tendons in the hand to assess whether recipient structures are present and toe transplantation will be worthwhile. **b.** The toe was dissected. The dorsalis pedis vessel, digital nerves, and tendons were ready to be divided at the point affording the appropriate length. **c.** The improvement in the hand was compared with the opposite side. The cosmetic and functional deficit in the foot is minimal (Fig. 4-3). **d.** Large object grasp has been provided. **e.** Good, passive motion and excellent sensation is present in the transplant. Further reconstruction to provide pulp-to-pulp pinch is planned when the child is older. **f.** Solid healing of the transplant to the metacarpal is evident.

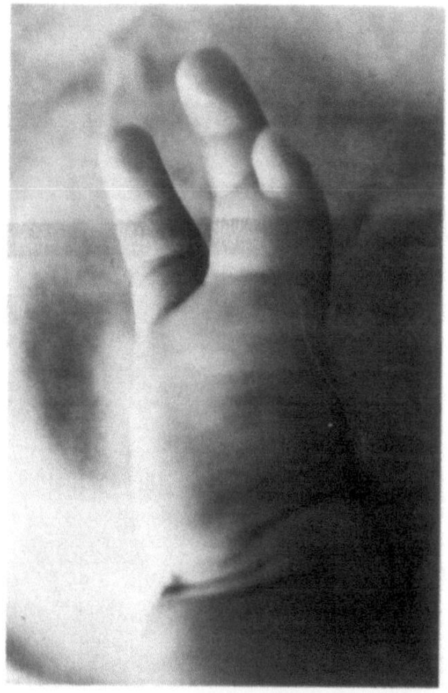

a

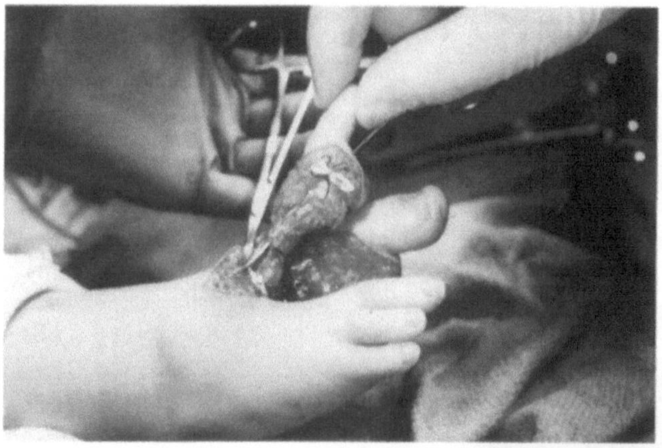

b

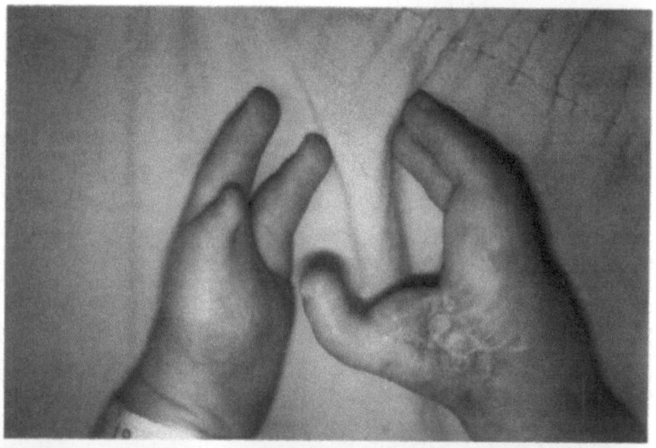

c

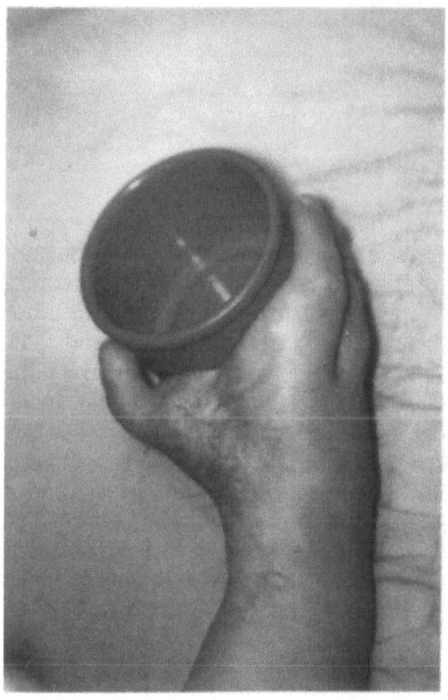

d

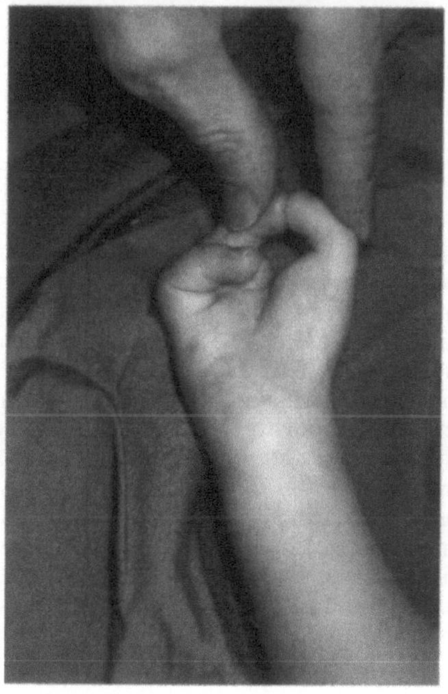

e

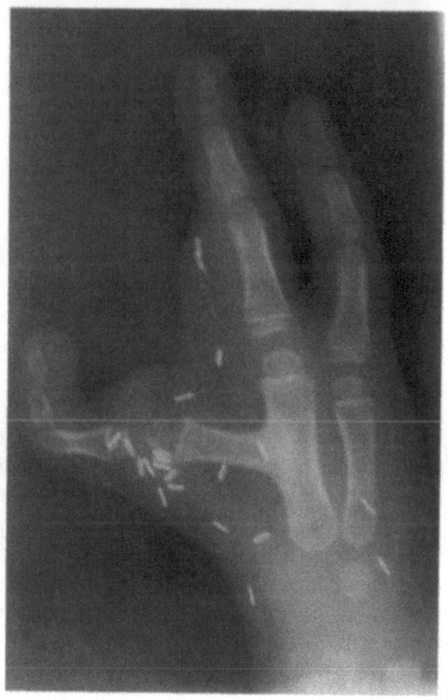

f

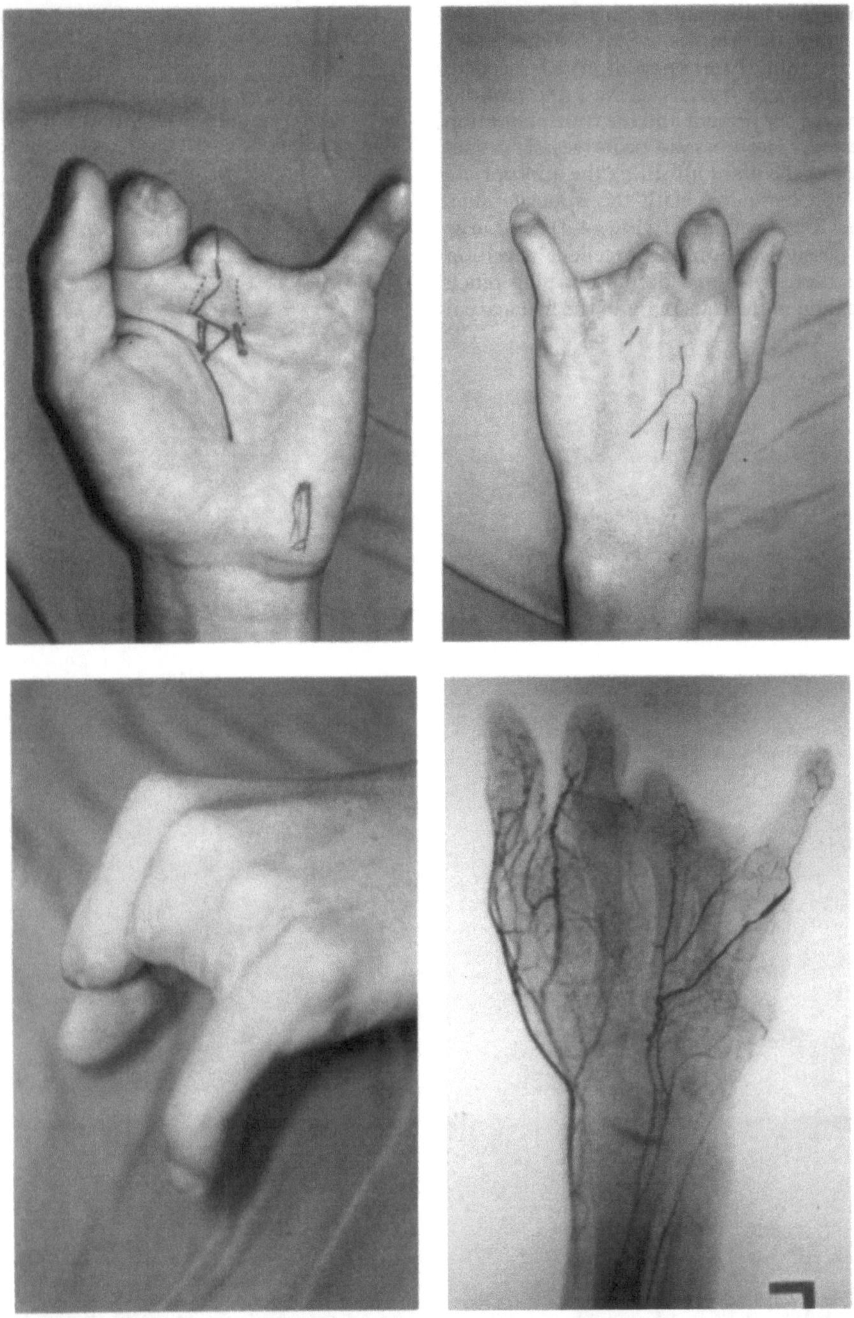

a b c d

Fig. 4-11 a–j. Multiple finger amputation distal to the metacarpophalangeal joint (one finger remaining): second-toe transplant (see also Fig. 4-22). **a.** Following a saw injury, this patient had had one finger replanted which became insensate and stiff. On the palmar surface, a second toe was to be transferred to the long finger position to restore pinch and provide a broader surface for tubular and large object grasp. A longitudinal incision over the tip of the long finger amputation stump opened the digit, permitting easy positioning of the toe transplant and bone fixation. The anticipated position of the digital nerves and position of the common digital vessels heard on Doppler examination were marked out on the hand. **b.** On the dorsal surface, the superficial veins were mapped out. **c.** Good flexion and extension of the metacarpophalangeal joints were present in the fingers. This feature is extremely important for the ultimate functioning of this transplant. **d.** The preoperative arteriogram revealed separate arterial supply to the ulnar and radial parts of the hand (see also Figs. 1-26 and 2-1). It is essential in this situation to use a digital vessel or the radial artery end-to-side. **e.** Dissection of the palmar structures revealed a good digital artery, common digital nerve, and flexor tendons. **f.** On the dorsal side, a long vein was harvested with the toe for anastomosis to the dorsal venous system of the hand. **g–j.** A broad surface has been established for grasp of large objects. The patient uses the transplant for pinch and manipulation of small objects and for key pinch and other activities requiring strength.

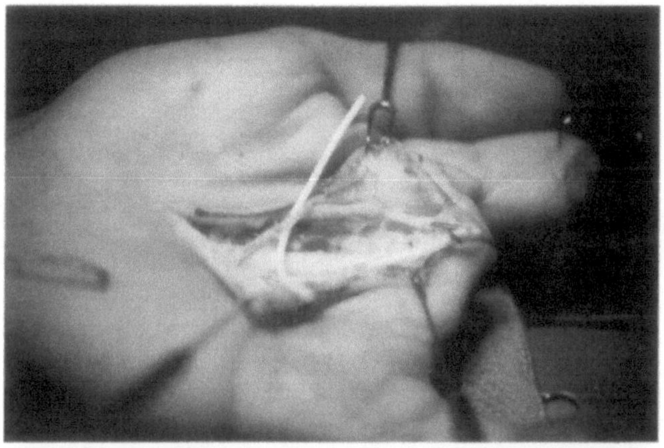
e

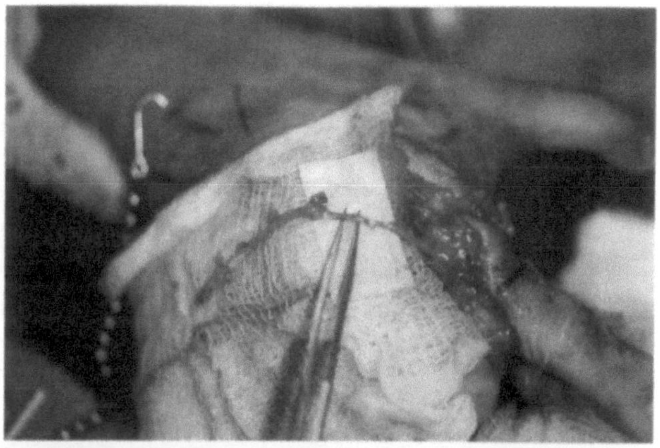
f

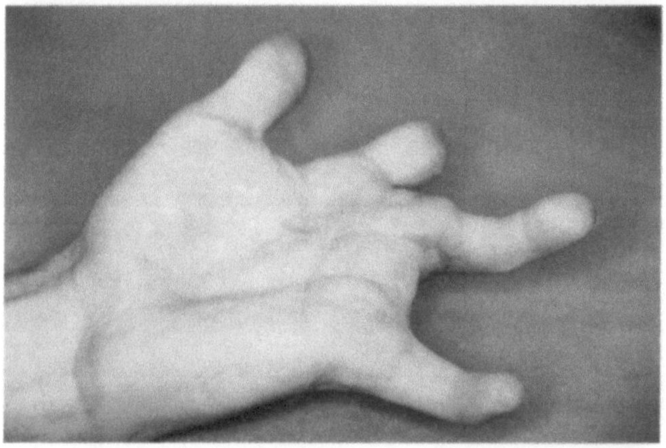
g

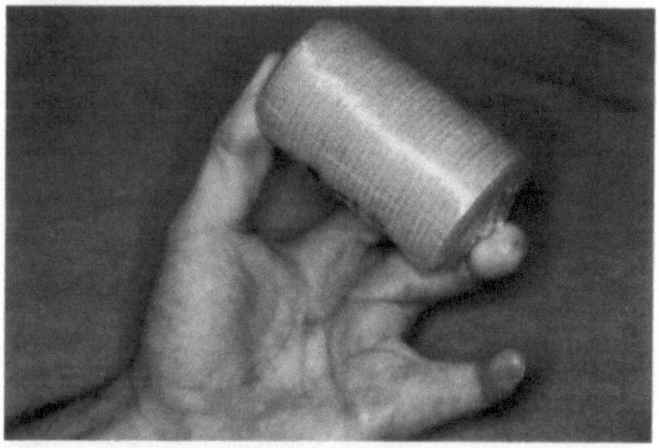
h

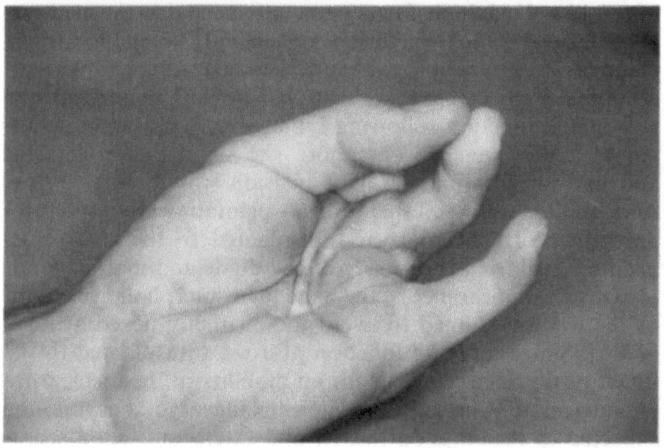
i

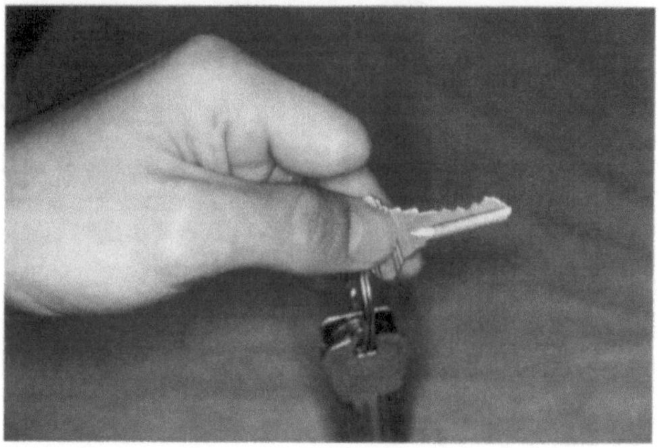
j

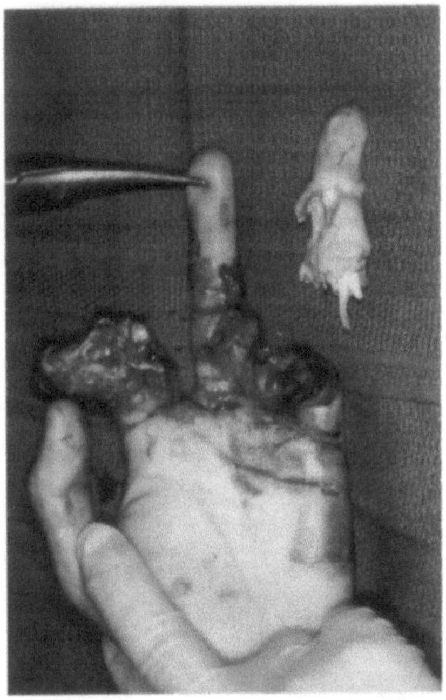
a

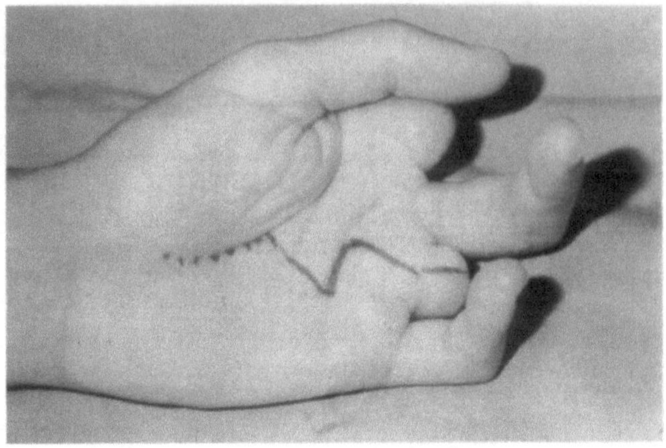
b

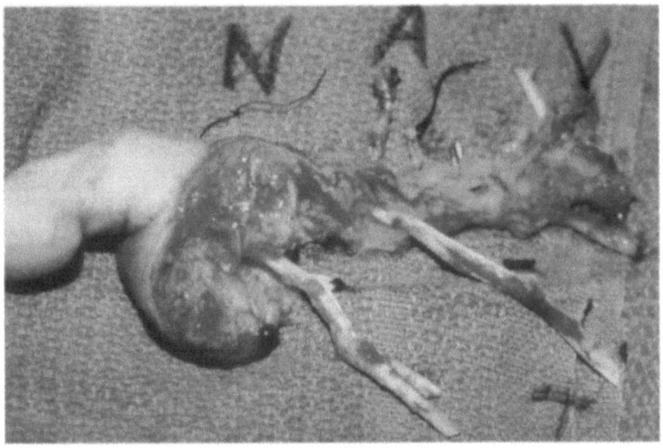
c

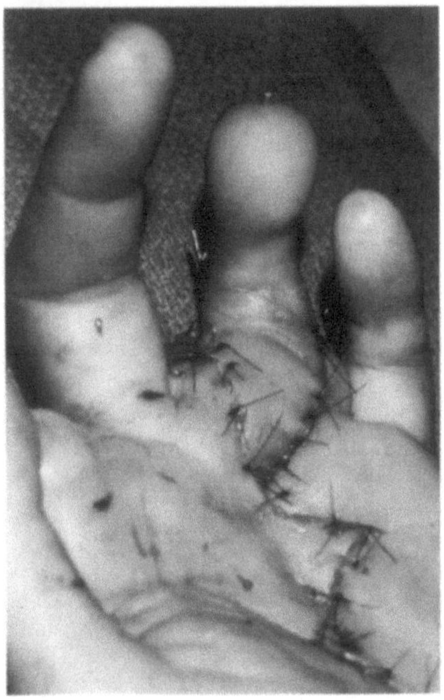
d

Fig. 4-12a–d. Multiple finger amputation distal to the metacarpophalangeal joint (two fingers remaining): second-toe transplant. a. A 30-year-old woman sustained severe injuries to all of her digits in a saw accident. **b.** The long finger regained reasonable function following repair, but sensation was impaired and movement was poor. The small finger was stiff and had limited function. The incision was marked out. **c.** A second toe was harvested for transplantation; the structures are shown. **d.** The toe was transplanted to the ring finger position, restoring the arcade of the digits and markedly improving the appearance of the hand. The interphalangeal joint of the toe was pinned to avoid the distinctly flexed attitude of this joint. (Ultimate function of a toe transplanted to the finger position largely depends on mobility at the metacarpophalangeal joint because the interphalangeal joints cannot be expected to regain good flexion and extension. Good sensation, however, is usually restored.)

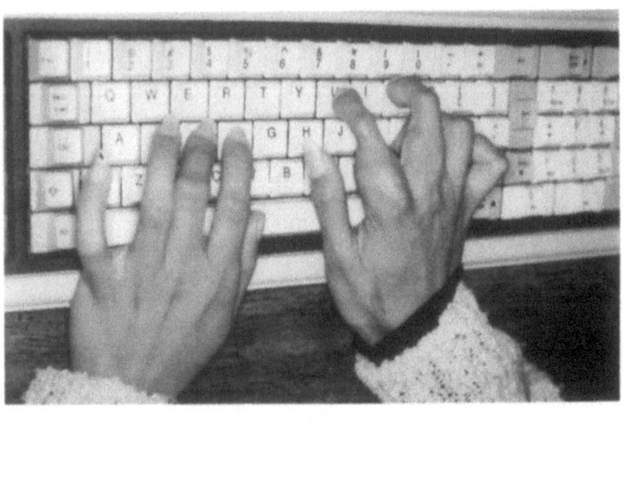

Fig. 4-13. Multiple finger amputation distal to the metacarpophalangeal joint (normal ring and small fingers): double second-toe transplant. This patient sustained an amputation of the index and long fingers and was unable to work as a typist. She was also particularly distressed by the appearance of her hand. Despite the use of a cosmetic prosthesis, she continued to have problems and was unable to work. A double second-toe transplant (one toe from each foot) restored the normal arcade of the digits. Although these digits have the appearance of toes on close scrutiny – being in a flexed position at the interphalangeal joints – the patient indicated that this is never noticed and she is exceedingly pleased with the result. She is once again able to work as a typist. Toe transplantation may be indicated in such unusual circumstances where five-fingered activities and cosmetic considerations are important.

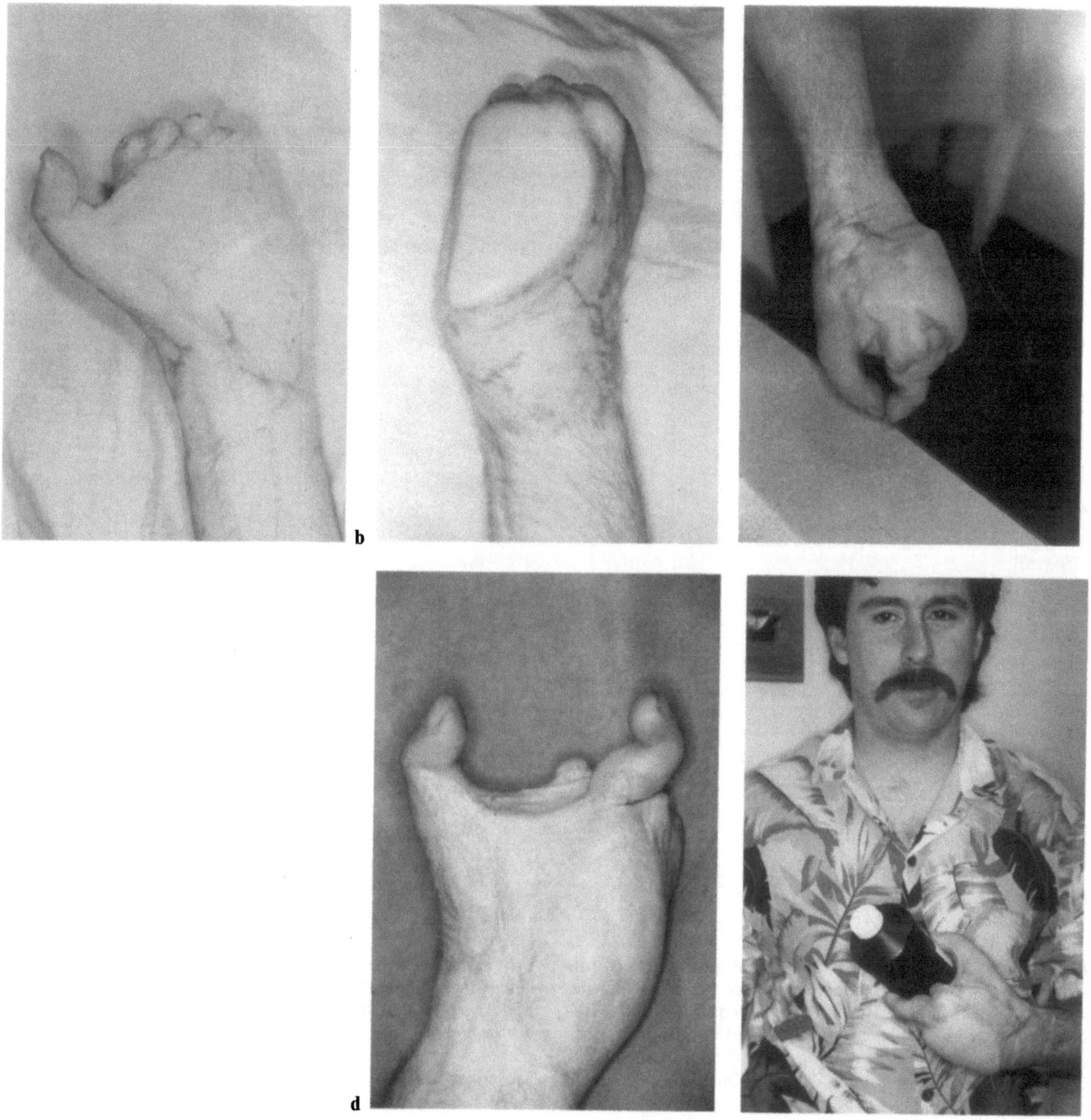

a b c d e

Fig. 4-14a–e. Adactyly with an intact thumb (traumatic): second-toe transplant (see also Fig. 1-8). **a** and **b.** This patient sustained an exceedingly severe crush injury to his hand. A double microvascular muscle transplant provided cover, with the latissimus dorsi used dorsally and the serratus anterior placed on the palmar surface (Fig. 1-8). His thumb had good sensation and some motion, but a mobile digit was needed on the ulnar side to provide pinch. In a preliminary operation, silicone tendon rods were placed under the muscle transplant on the palmar and dorsal sides to provide gliding surfaces for the flexor and extensor tendons of the proposed toe transplant. **c–e.** The patient regained excellent large and small object grasp. There was good movement and sensation in the finger with good end-to-end pinch.

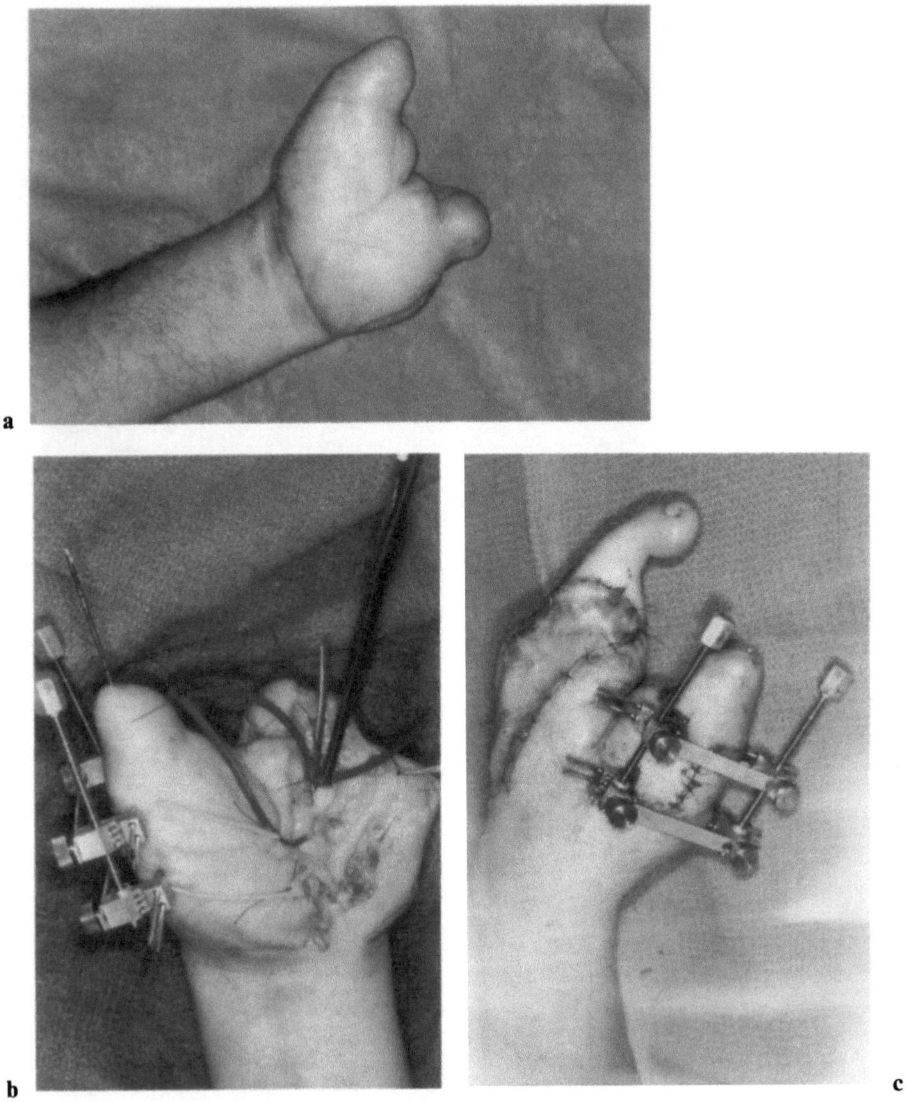

Fig. 4-15a–c. Adactyly with a short thumb remnant (posttraumatic): second-toe transplantation combined with thumb lengthening. a. Reconstruction of this hand required a new digit on the ulnar side as well as adequate thumb length for opposition. The option of double toe transplantation was considered, but because the thenar muscles were still functional and could provide active opposition, thumb lengthening was chosen. **b.** The lengthening apparatus was placed on the thumb metacarpal. The recipient structures were dissected to receive the second-toe transplant. **c.** The second-toe transplant is seen in place. Note that a skin graft was needed to cover the dorsal aspect of the second metatarsal.

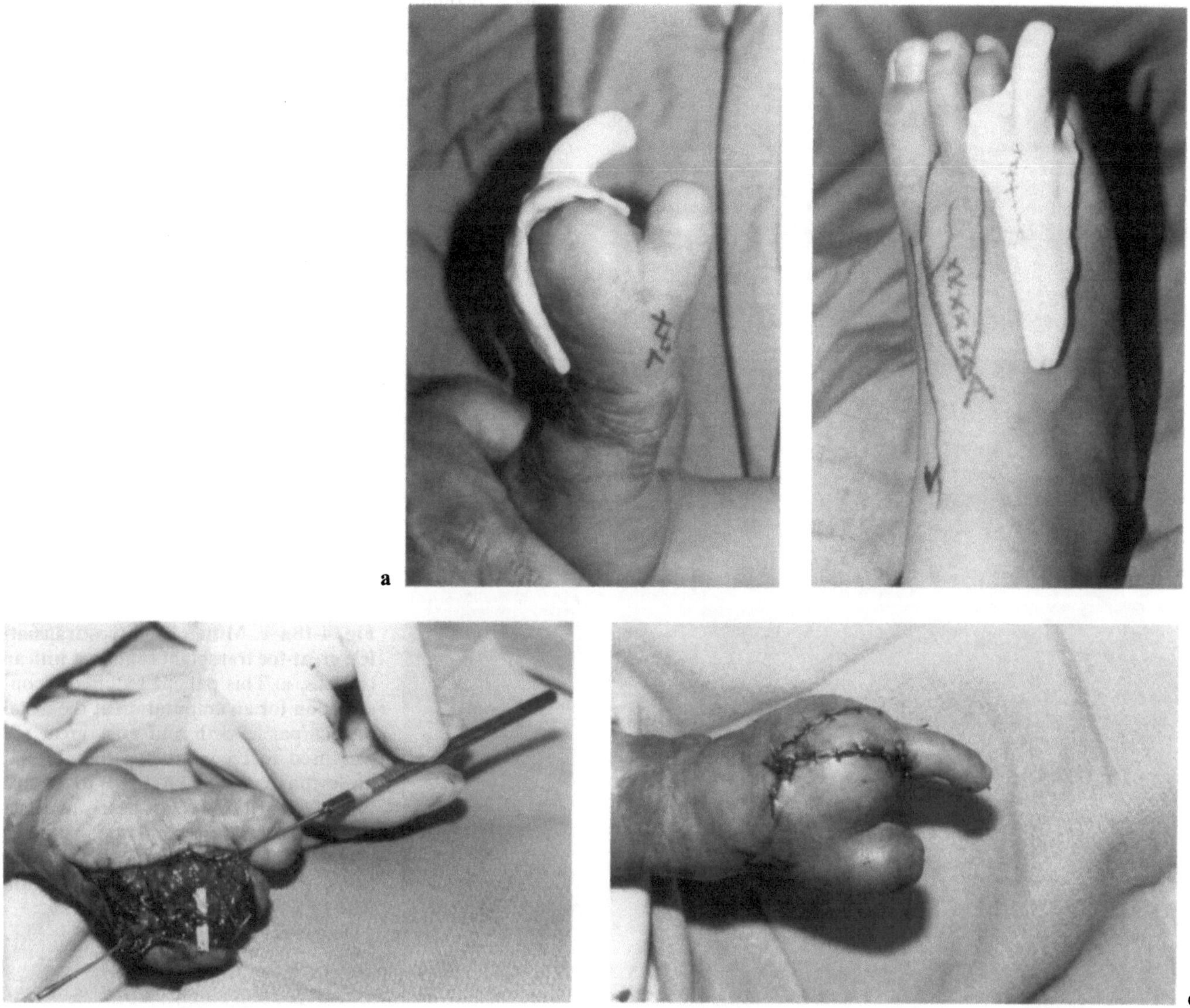

a b c d

Fig. 4-16a–d. Congenital multiple finger loss: transplant of a second toe to the long finger position. a and **b.** Congenital amputation of the fingers left this 3-year-old boy with only a short thumb in his left hand. A second-toe transplant was planned to provide a mobile, opposing digit. A clay model was used to plan the position of the vascular repairs and skin flaps, and the length, position, and rotation of the transplant on the hand. **c.** The vessels and nerves were present near the site of amputation. **d.** The toe in position on the hand resembles the clay model. At the time of foot closure, an extra segment of the second metatarsal was taken. It was anticipated that this bone would be used for later thumb lengthening.

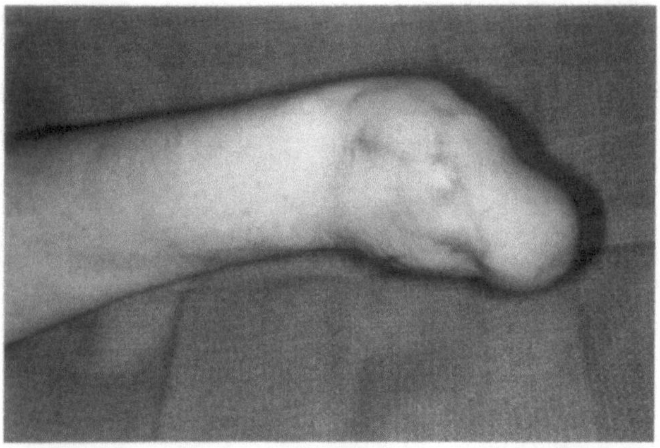
a

Fig. 4-17 a–c. Mitten hand (posttraumatic): great-toe and second-toe transplant. a. This 42-year-old chemist lost all of his fingers and thumb in a laboratory explosion. **b.** A great toe from one foot was used to reconstruct a thumb, and a second toe from the opposite foot was used to fashion an opposable digit; this restored reasonable grasp. **c.** Although there is no strong pulp-to-pulp pinch, pinch is possible between the thumb and index finger if he uses a broad-barrel pen.

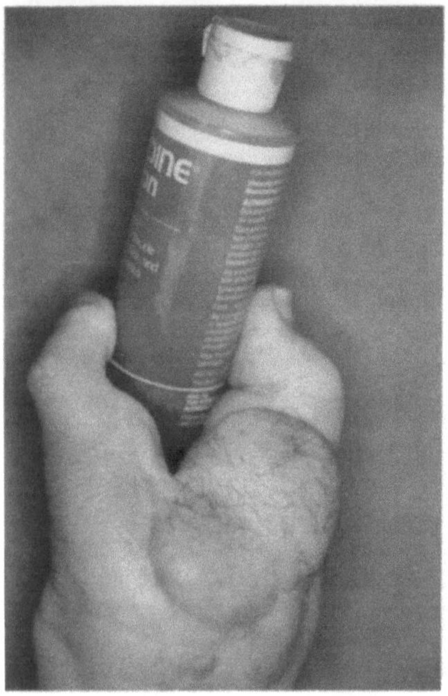
b

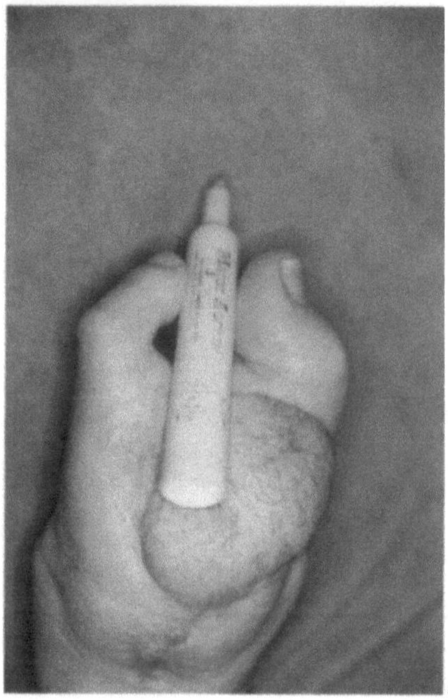
c

Fig. 4-18 a–c. Mitten hand (posttraumatic): great-toe transplant combined with an orthosis. a. This patient required reconstruction for an amputation at the distal metacarpal level. **b** and **c.** A great toe was used to reconstruct a thumb, and an orthosis was then used to enable pinch. An orthosis is not nearly as effective as a sensate second toe, but it is a reasonable alternative in some situations. (Courtesy of Richard J. Smith, MD†)

†Deceased. ▽

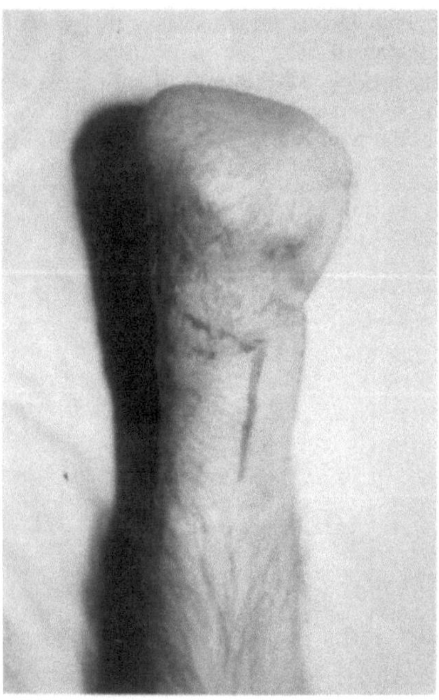
a

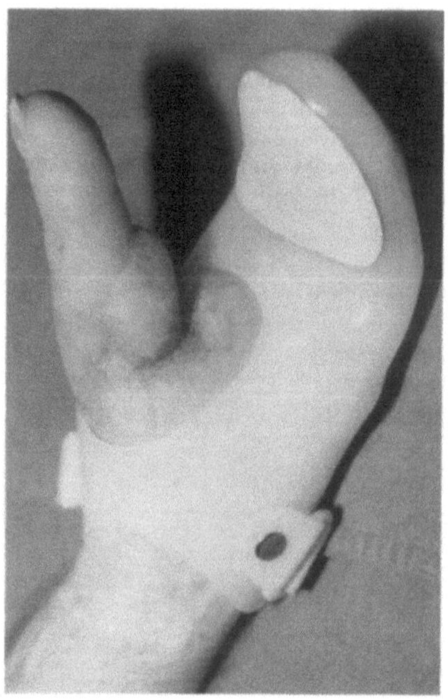
b

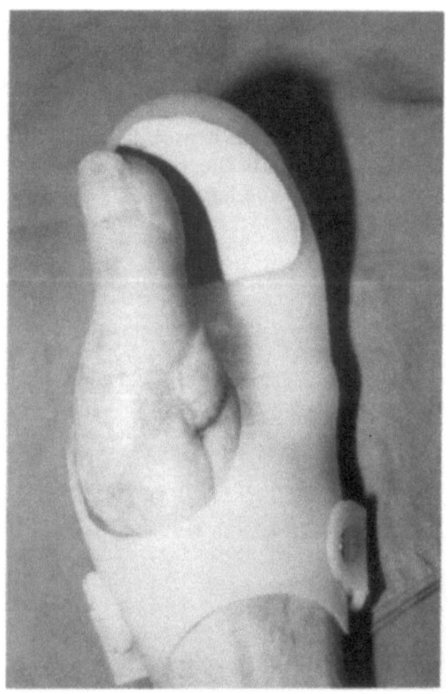
c

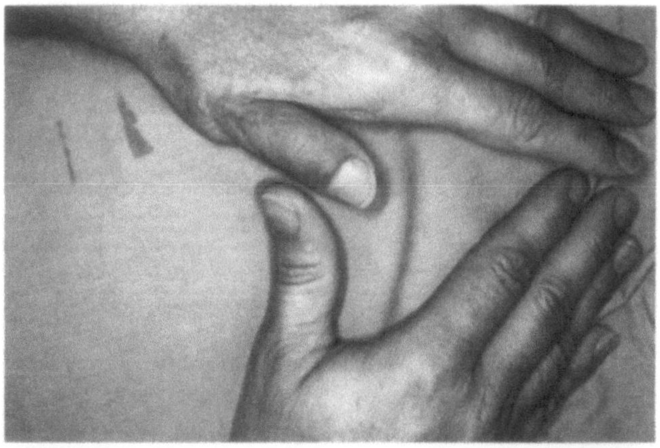
a

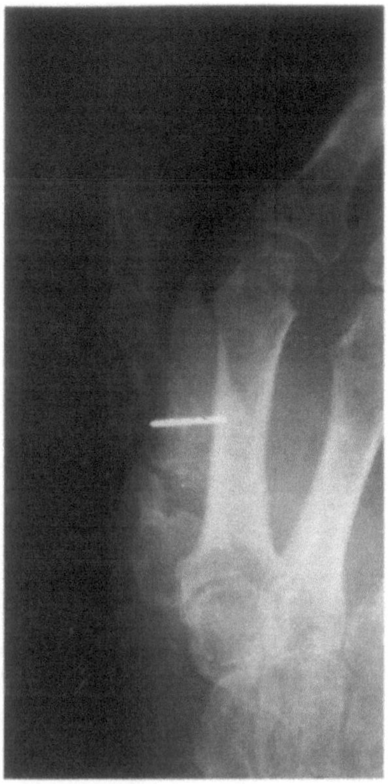
b

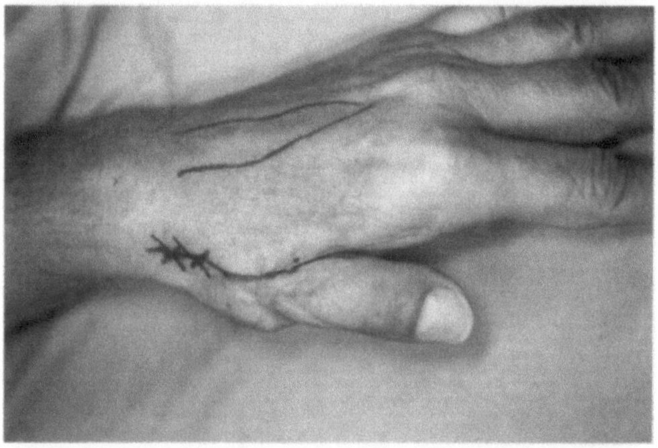
c

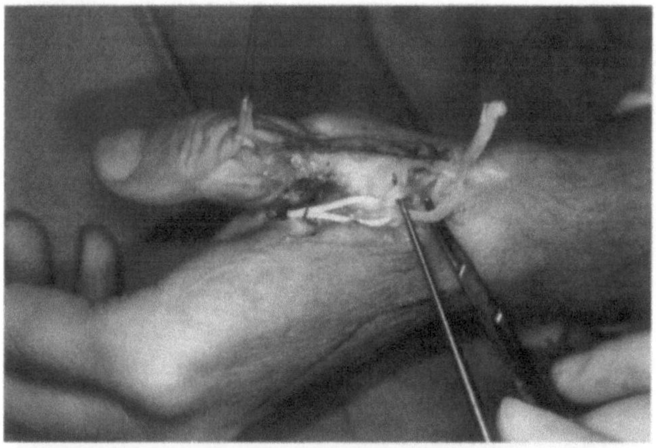
d

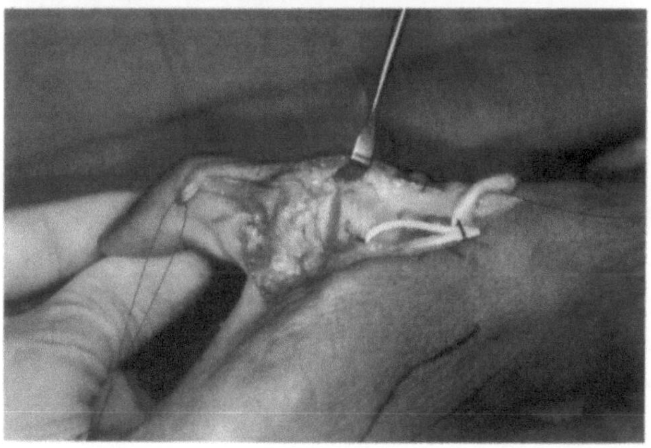
e

Fig. 4-19 a–j. Metacarpal and metacarpophalangeal joint loss in the thumb (posttraumatic): metatarsophalangeal joint of the second toe to the thumb metacarpophalangeal joint (see also Fig. 4-24). **a.** This patient injured his right thumb in a rifle accident. There was a marked web space contracture with no passive movement. The reconstruction option chosen was to graft bone to lengthen the thumb, and release the web space contracture. This release would require a substantial amount of tissue. The bone transplant would have to include a joint because the trapeziometacarpal joint provided the only mobility. **b.** This radiograph shows the damage, which included loss of the metacarpal and metacarpophalangeal joints and marked shortening. **c.** A web space release was planned. The radial artery could be palpated on the dorsal surface of the first metacarpal space. The dorsal veins are seen outlined. **d.** The extensor tendons were dissected proximally and distally, and the radial artery is shown just before it enters between the two heads of the first dorsal interosseous muscle. A large superficial vein is also shown. **e.** The osteotomy prepared the site for the vascularized joint transplant. *Continued*

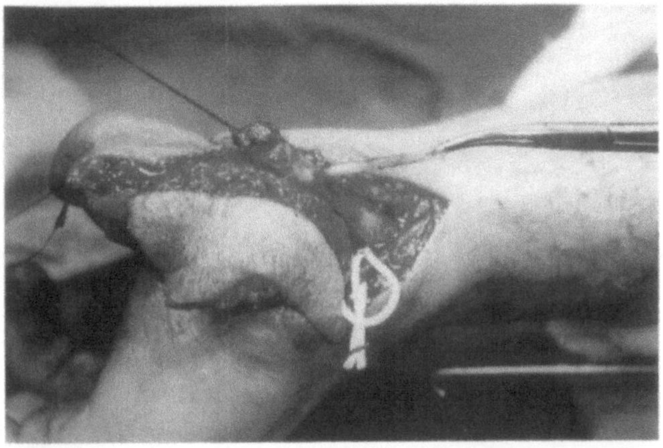
f

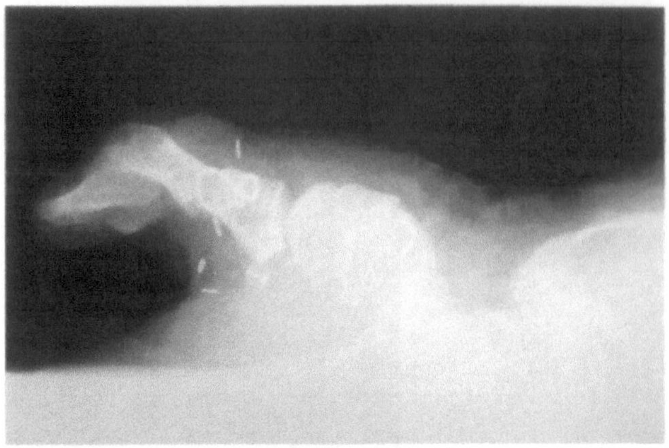
g

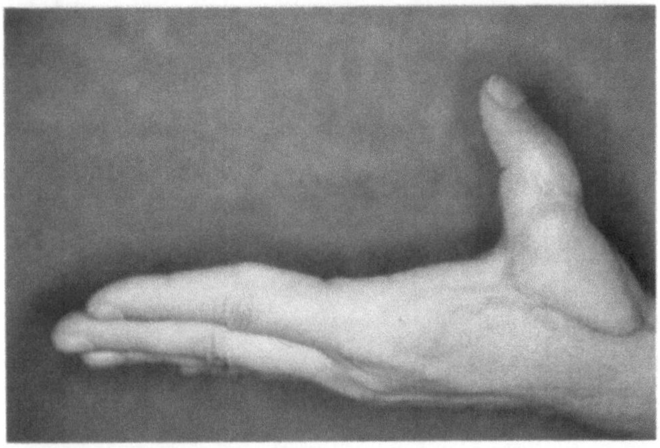
h

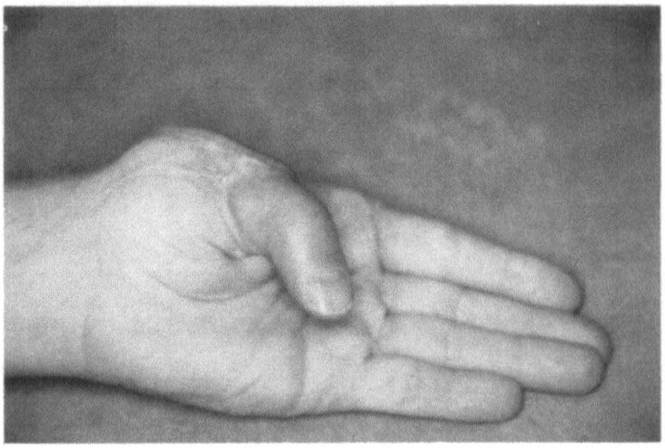
i

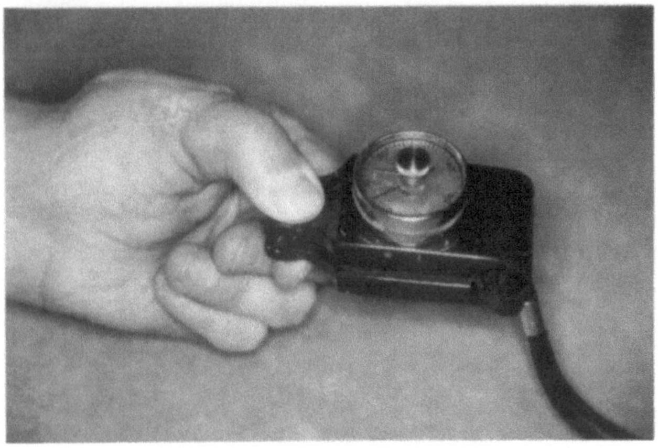
j

Fig. 4-19. f. The joint was wired into place and a weave stitch was used to repair the extensor tendons. Note that the cutaneous flap was carefully planned to provide soft-tissue cover in the first web space for abduction of the thumb. **g.** This radiograph shows the position of the joint transplant and the intraosseous wiring, which provided good fixation both proximally and distally. **h–j.** Good thumb length was restored. The patient is able to abduct well and can flex the thumb to a point 1 cm from the base of the small finger. He has good pinch strength between the thumb and index finger.

4.5 Anatomy (Plate 4-IV)

The great and second toes are hyperextended at the metatarsophalangeal joint, slightly flexed at the proximal interphalangeal joint, and extended at the distal interphalangeal joint (Plate 4-I). The longitudinal arch of the foot ends at the metatarsal head, which bears the weight of the body during gait. This overall structure differs from that of fingers, which have a longitudinally flexed arch that terminates at their end. Both the joint surfaces and joint capsules are adapted to their positions. The web spaces of the foot are located more distally than those of the hand (Fig. 4-1).

The *superficial transverse metatarsal ligaments* reinforce and connect the digital slips of the plantar aponeurosis. The articular capsule of the metatarsophalangeal joint is loose. Dorsally, it is reinforced by fibers from the extensor tendons and is attached closer to the articular border than it is on the plantar side. The *plantar ligament* is analogous to the palmar plate of the fingers. On each side of the joint lies a collateral ligament. The plantar ligament of the great toe is replaced by the sesamoid bones and a strong interconnecting ligament between them. All of the plantar ligaments are connected by *deep transverse metatarsal ligaments* which connect adjacent metatarsal heads and joint capsules.

At ankle level, the *anterior tibial artery* lies between the extensor hallucis longus and extensor digitorum longus tendons. At the ankle it becomes the *dorsalis pedis artery* which passes over the dorsum of the foot to the first intermetatarsal space. Just proximal to this space, it is crossed by the extensor hallucis brevis tendon, and at the base it divides into the *deep plantar artery* (also called the perforating branch), which dives plantarward to the plantar arch, and the *first dorsal metatarsal artery*, which proceeds distally in the first metatarsal space. Distally, this vessel divides into two branches which supply the adjacent sides of the first web space.

The *origin of the first dorsal metatarsal artery is of considerable surgical importance* and can be somewhat variable (Plate 4-V). In about two thirds of patients, the first dorsal metatarsal artery emanates from the dorsalis pedis artery and travels in a relatively dorsal plane (Plate 4-VA and B). This course can be dorsal to the interosseous muscle (Plate 4-VA), within the muscle, or deep to it (Plate 4-VB), but the artery courses dorsal to the deep transverse metatarsal ligament (Plate 4-VA and B). Other configurations are seen in about one third of patients. The first dorsal metatarsal may arise from the dorsalis pedis or deep plantar artery, but the principal vessel to the toes runs deep to the deep transverse metatarsal ligament (Plate 4-VC). Occasionally, the vessels to the great and second toes may arise from the plantar arterial arch (Plate 4–VD) (Egloff 1984, Leung et al. 1983).

The dorsalis pedis artery has paired *venae comitantes.*

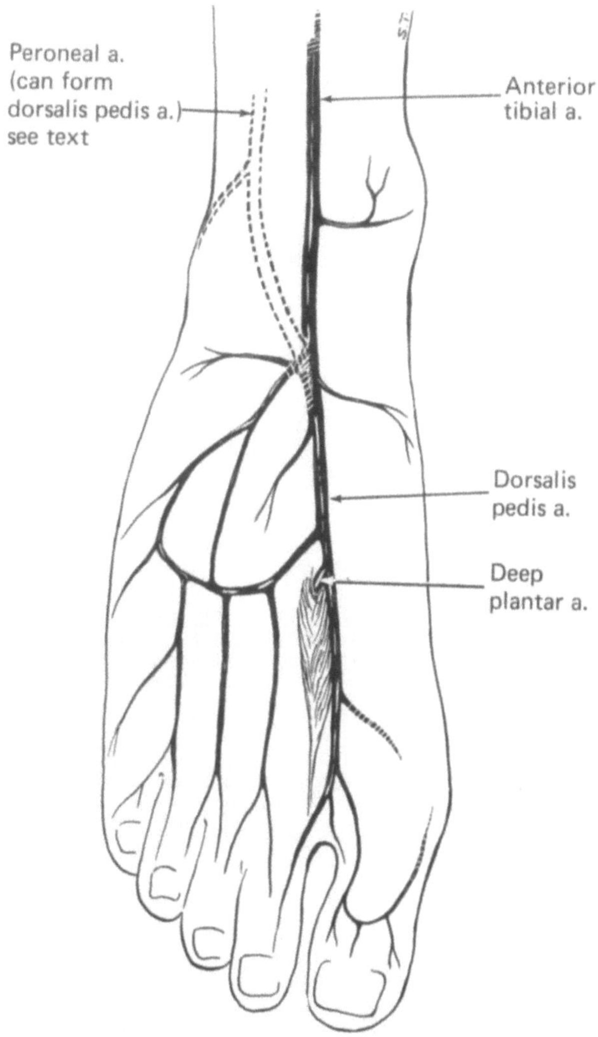

Plate 4-III. The dorsalis pedis artery can arise from the peroneal artery on the lateral aspect of the ankle (see also Fig. 1-23c).

Superficial veins on the dorsum of the foot form a venous arch and drain into the saphenous system.

The *deep peroneal nerve* divides just distal to the ankle into medial and lateral branches. The medial branch passes distally just lateral or medial to the dorsalis pedis artery and divides into two dorsal digital nerves which supply the *adjacent sides of the first web space* (Fig. 2-12c). The *superficial peroneal nerve* pierces the deep fascia proximal to the ankle between the peroneus longus and extensor digitorum longus, and divides into two branches. The medial and intermediate dorsal cutaneous nerves cross the ankle to supply the *dorsum of the foot* (Fig. 2-12b), while the nerve supply to the *plantar surfaces* of the medial 3 1/2 toes arises from the *medial plantar nerve*. The medial plantar nerve gives off the proper digital nerve to the great toe, and three common digital nerves which pass between the divisions of the plantar aponeurosis; these common digital nerves divide into proper digital nerves which pass plantar to the digital arteries along both sides of each toe.

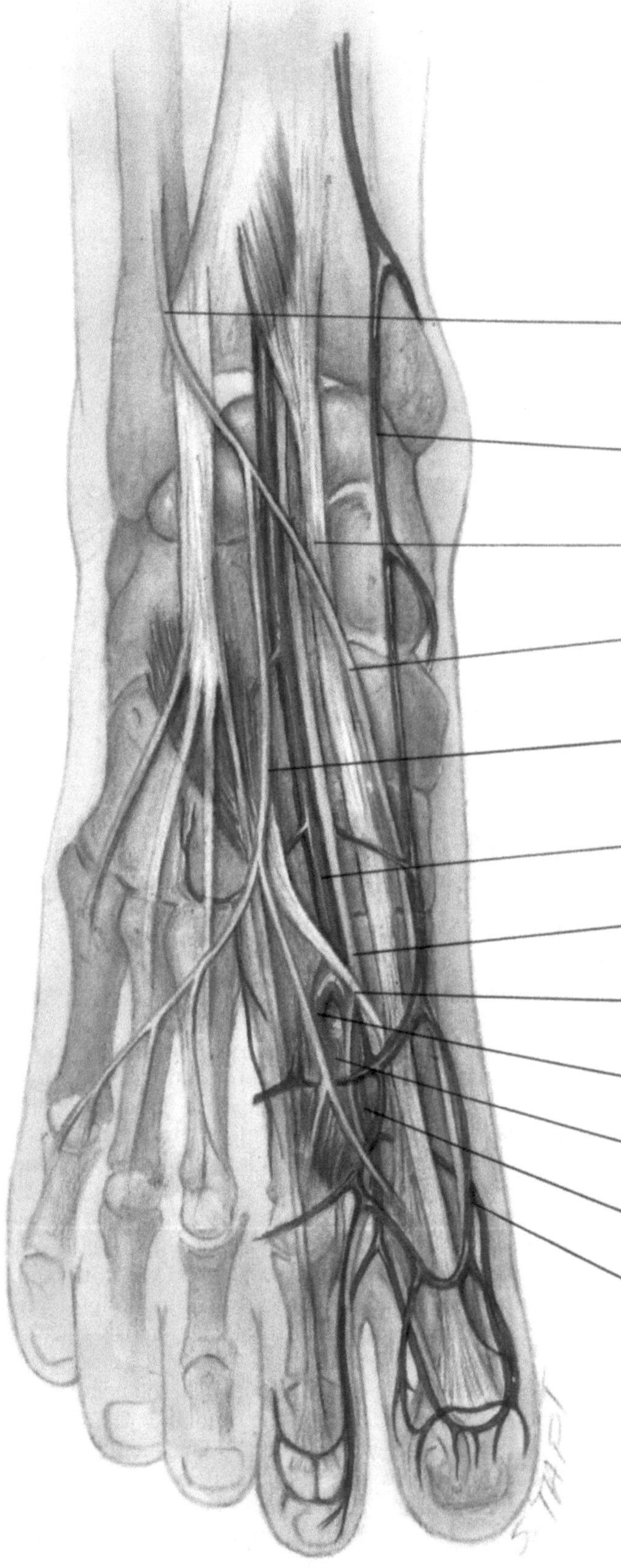

Plate 4-IV. Anatomy of the dorsum of the foot.

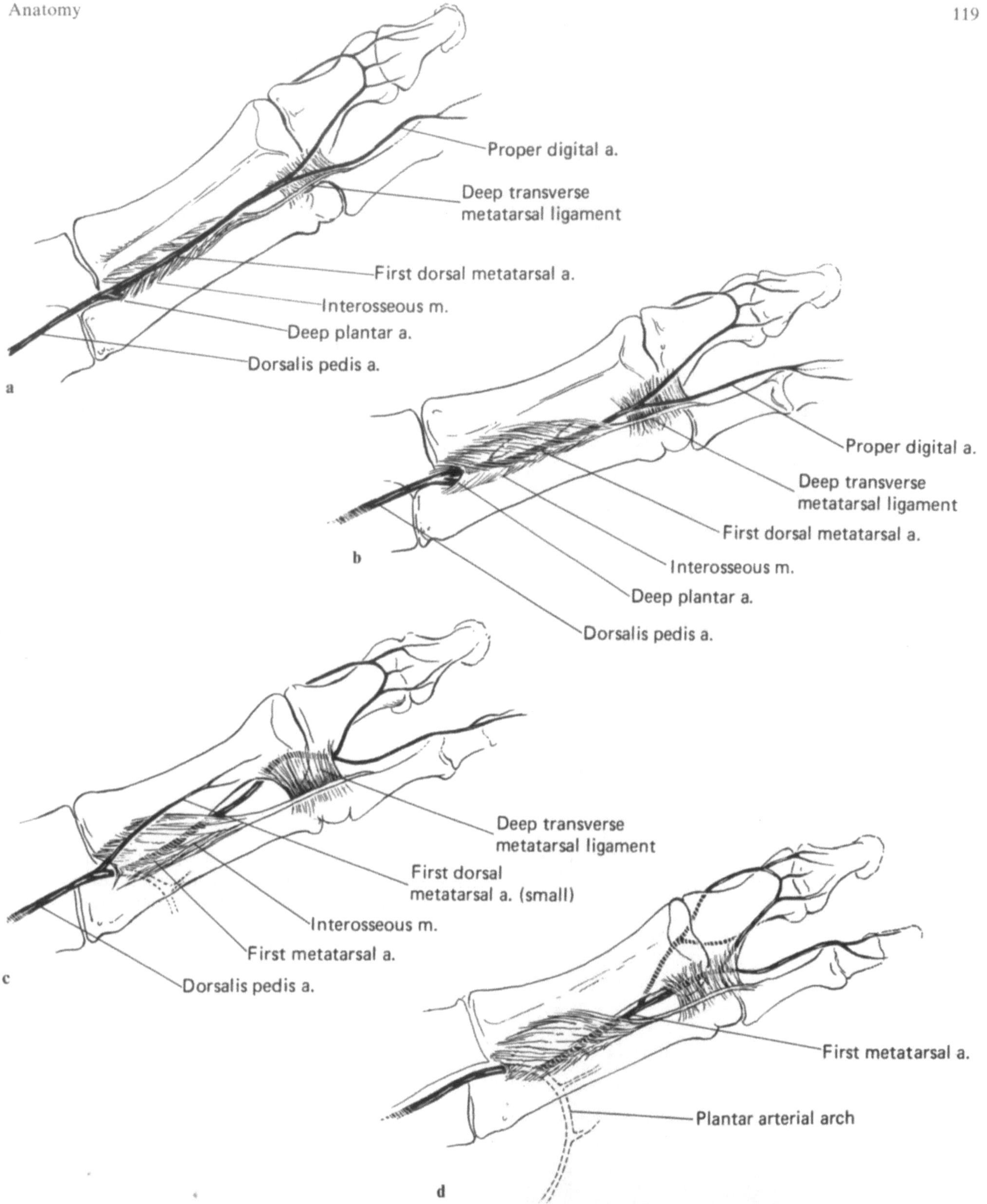

Plate 4-V. a. The dorsalis pedis artery divides into the deep plantar artery and the first dorsal metatarsal artery (FDMA). The FDMA continues superficial to the interosseous muscle and deep transverse metatarsal ligament, and divides into the proper digital arteries supplying the adjacent sides of the first web space. **b.** The FDMA can travel in or deep to the interosseous muscle, but remains superficial to the deep transverse metatarsal ligament. **c.** The FDMA is small and inadequate for supplying the toes. The metatarsal artery originates from the dorsalis pedis artery or the deep plantar artery, and runs deep to the interosseous muscle and deep transverse metatarsal ligament. This artery tends to curve under the first metatarsal bone. **d.** The first metatarsal artery emanates from the plantar arterial arch and runs deep to the interosseous muscle and deep transverse metatarsal ligament. The FDMA is small or absent.

4.6 Surgical Technique

4.6.1 Whole Great Toe Transplantation

(May et al. 1978) (Fig. 4-20)

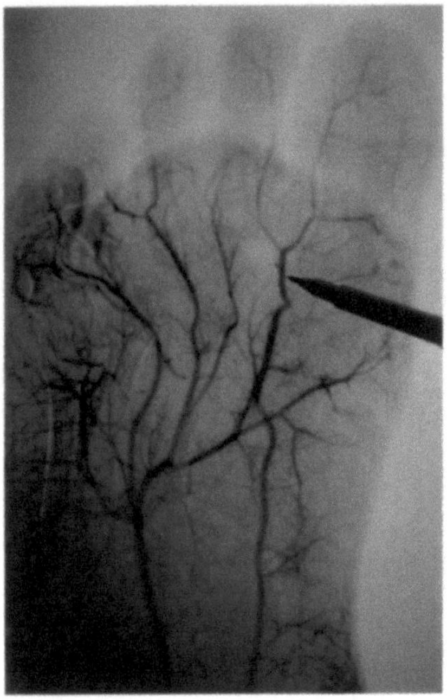

ai

a. i. *The arteriogram* of the foot shows the dorsalis pedis artery and first dorsal metatarsal vessel. The position of this vessel, i.e., whether it is dorsal or plantar, may be seen on an oblique view, but this information is often evident on the anteroposterior film. As noted in Section 4.5, the course and origin of the first dorsal metatarsal artery is variable. If this vessel runs near or curves beneath the first metatarsal in the anteroposterior view, a plantar vessel is likely. In this patient, the dorsalis pedis can be seen diving plantarward as the deep plantar artery to join the plantar arch. As it does so, the first metatarsal artery emanates from the deep plantar artery; a plantar vessel can therefore be expected.

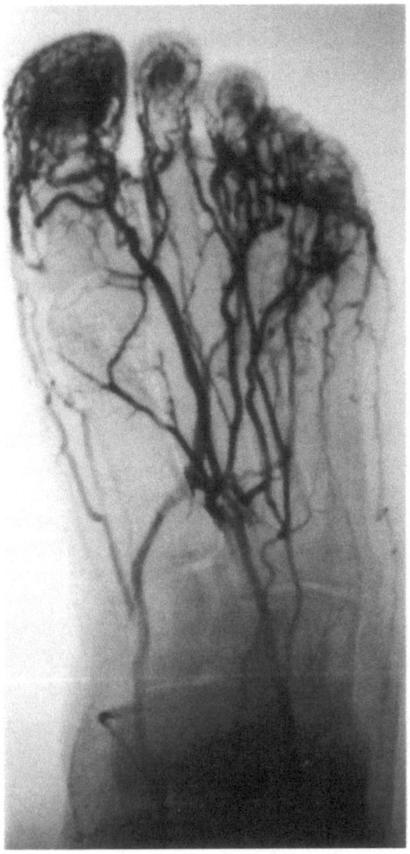

aii

ii. In another patient, a large and superficial dorsal first metatarsal artery is seen. This artery courses some distance lateral to the first metatarsal and arises from the dorsalis pedis artery.

b. *The plantar skin flaps are outlined.*

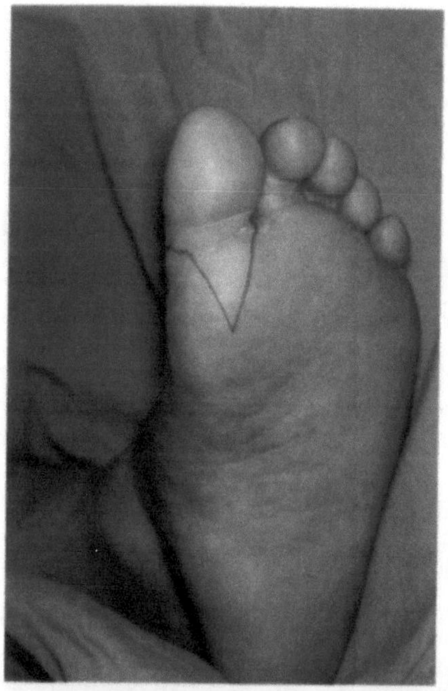

b

c. *The dorsal flap is planned* so that it is long enough to cover the vascular pedicle after the toe is transplanted. The dorsal and plantar flaps should allow primary closure of the foot wound without tension. Skin grafts and tension should be avoided in the foot because these will prolong healing time. A skin graft on the hand to cover areas of the transplant will heal well and cause little difficulty; this is particularly true on the radial side, where contracture is not a problem, but it is less desirable on the ulnar side. *A clay model*, which is very helpful in planning the flap (Figs. 4-8, 4-16, and 4-19), should include the flap of the first web space of the toe and mark the position of the vascular pedicle.

Prior to making the incision, the following should be clearly planned: (1) the site of osteotomy, (2) the site of the arterial pedicle, (3) the position of the superficial veins, and (4) the position and size of the skin flaps.

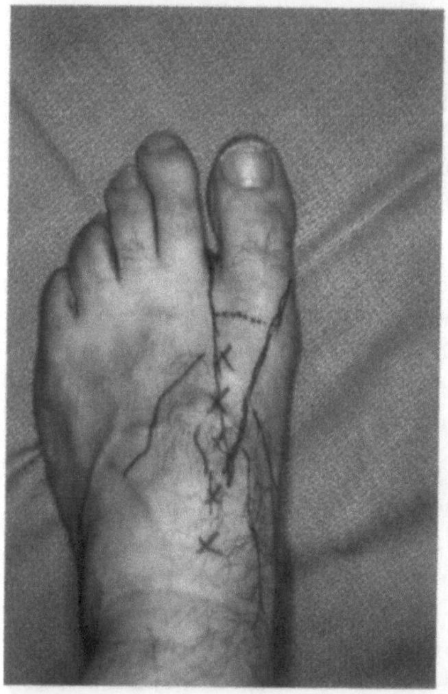

c

d. The dissection is performed under tourniquet control. The dorsal and plantar incision is made. An appropriate length of one of the large *subcutaneous veins* of the dorsal venous system draining into the saphenous system is dissected. Extra vein length is dissected to avoid any tension on the venous anastomosis, and extra vein should be taken if an interpositional vein graft is anticipated for the artery. The *extensor hallucis longus tendon* is dissected, depending on the length required in the hand, and the *extensor hallucis brevis* is shown approaching the long extensor. Beneath the extensor hallucis brevis is the neurovascular bundle, including the dorsalis pedis vessels and the deep peroneal nerve.

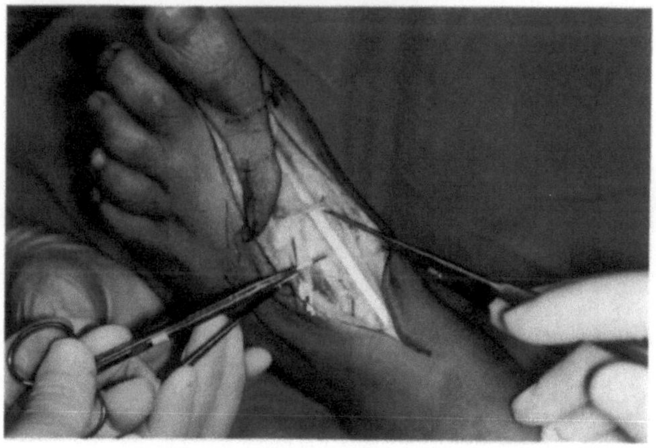

d

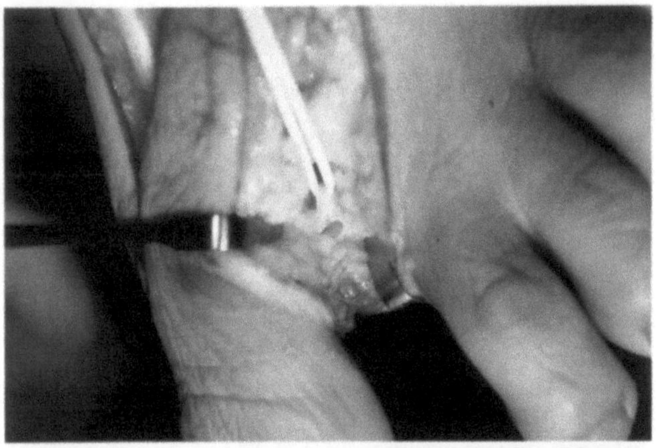

e

e. Next, the *first dorsal metatarsal artery* is dissected. Because the arteriogram demonstrated a plantar vessel, the artery is first dissected distally. The metatarsal artery has been tagged with a vessel loop just before it divides into branches that go to the great and second toes. The branch to the second toe is dissected and divided, and the branch to the great toe is retained. As the artery is dissected proximally, care is taken to dissect on the lateral aspect of this vessel to avoid injuring any branches from the artery to the toe or the dorsal skin flap. The artery may require dissection deep to the transverse metatarsal ligament, which is divided to complete the dissection (as in this patient). With a more dorsal vessel, dissection is dorsal to this ligament and can be carried back to the dorsalis pedis artery relatively easily. The plantar dissection is difficult, especially if the vessel curves under the metatarsal head. Often, an interpositional vein graft to the artery will be easier. (This option was chosen in this patient.)

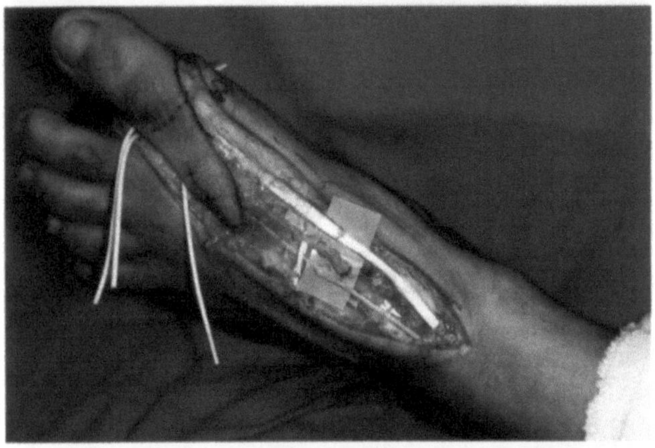

f

f. The venous tributary into the *saphenous venous system* is doubly ligated and divided. The *long extensor tendon* is also divided, and the deep peroneal nerve is dissected. **Prior to dividing any structures, the team dissecting the hand records the length of each structure required for the transplant.**

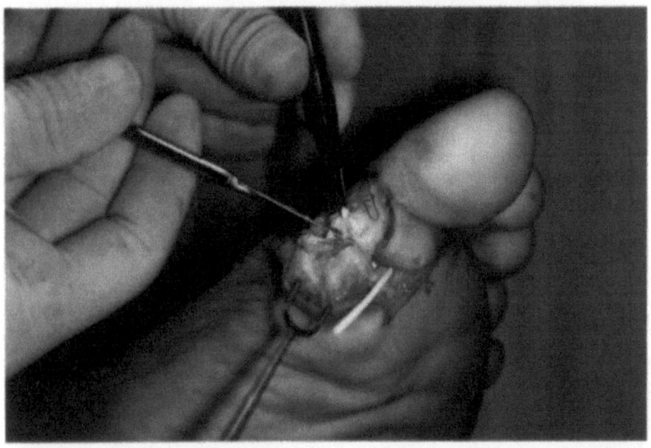

g

g. The plantar flap is elevated. The *medial digital nerve* is tagged with 6-0 silk suture and divided at a point determined by the length of nerve needed in the hand. The capsule of the metatarsophalangeal joint is now incised.

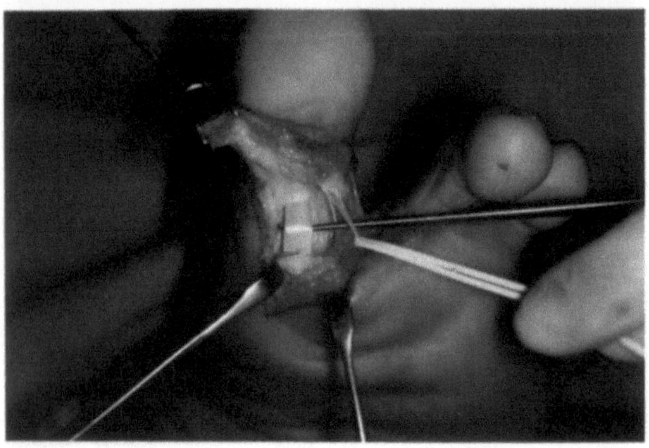

h

h. The *lateral nerve* is dissected proximally to the common digital nerve. If greater length is needed, this common digital nerve can be split, retaining the fascicles to the second toe. A long nerve for repair is thereby obtained while maintaining the nerve supply to the second toe. The *flexor tendon* is dissected. A more proximal plantar incision may be required to obtain a long flexor tendon. Often, approaching this tendon through an incision on the medial aspect of the foot is helpful. Dividing the tendon at the ankle is usually not successful in providing a longer tendon because of communications between the flexor tendons.

i. Once the capsule of the metatarsophalangeal joint is divided, the joint can be dislocated and the toe is then ready for the final stages of dissection. Seen from the dorsal aspect, the joint has been dislocated and all of the structures except the neurovascular pedicle have been divided.

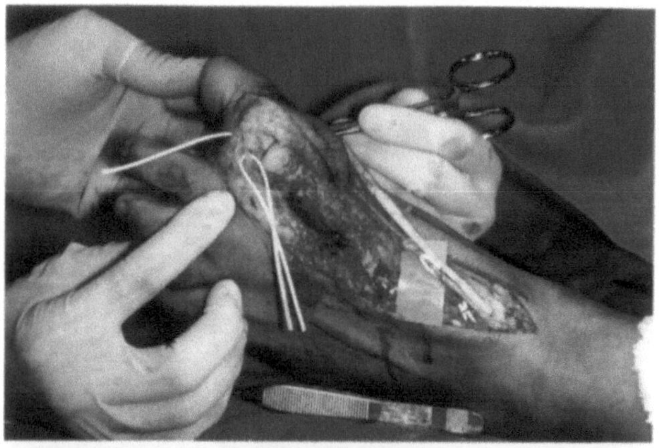

i

j. The plantar metatarsal artery is shown. This vessel is dissected proximally for several centimeters. All branches must be meticulously tied, using 6-0 silk for the larger branches and 9-0 nylon for any tiny ones. This measure helps to prevent later spasm of the vessels.

Before removing the toe, the leg tourniquet is released. This release ends the period of ischemia, giving the toe "a drink." Also, because only the vessels remain attached, the blood supply to the transplant is confirmed. It frequently takes as long as 15 to 30 minutes before the toe turns pink, generally because of spasm. Patient hydration and blood pressure must be good, and warm irrigation is used. A topical vasodilating agent such as bupivacaine hydrochloride (0.25%) is placed on the vessels. Under the microscope, the vessels are dissected and all tiny arterial branches are ligated.

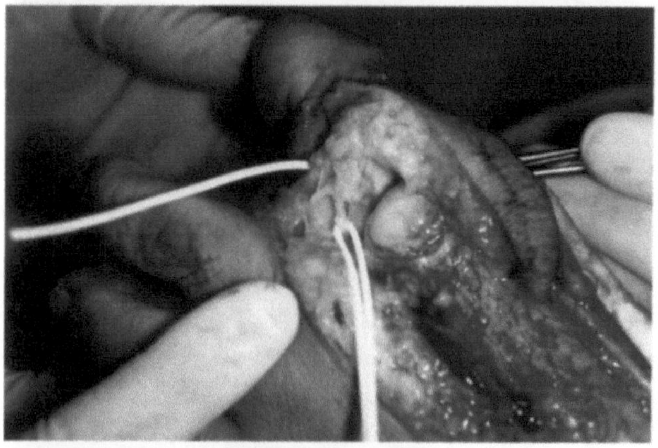

j

k. The toe is seen after removal. The artery (*on the blue background material*) is short and a reversed vein graft is anastomosed to the artery on a back table prior to placement on the thumb.

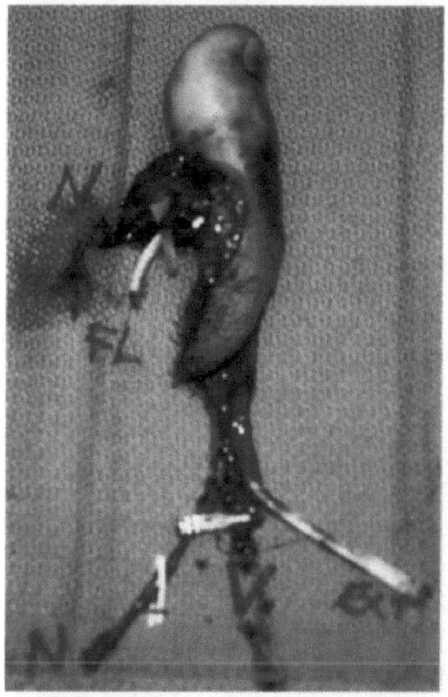

k

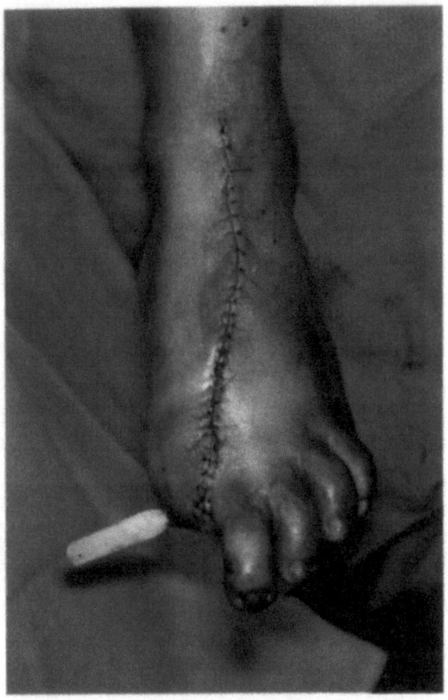

1

l. **Foot closure**. After the toe is removed, the position of the sesamoid bones is maintained and the dorsal aspect of the distal metatarsal is pared down if prominent; this sometimes facilitates closure and decreases tension on the medial skin flap. The ligament between the first and second metatarsals must be reconstructed using a strong, nonabsorbable suture. A suture around the first and second metatarsals may also be used to bring these two bones closer, and occasionally a Kirschner wire is temporarily inserted between the two metatarsals at an oblique angle to maintain their position. The foot is immediately elevated. The Penrose drain is removed after 24 hours.

Before receiving the toe, the following must be prepared in the *hand*: (1) the bone end to undergo osteosynthesis – methods of bone fixation include cross Kirschner wires, intraosseous wiring, or fashioning a bone peg from the thumb metacarpal to fit into the proximal phalanx of the toe (Sec. 4.4); (2) the flexor and extensor tendons – these should be repaired using a weave stitch, if possible, to provide the strongest tenorrhaphy; also, pulleys should be maintained if possible; (3) digital nerves; (4) arteries and veins; and (5) any contracture must be released and other reconstruction completed.

4.6.2 Toe Wrap-Around Procedure

(Morrison et al. 1980) (Fig. 4-21; see also Fig. 4-6)

The "wrap-around flap" consists of the soft tissue of the great toe as well as the toe nail. Bone support is provided by a bone graft from the iliac crest, although some surgeons include the distal phalanx of the great toe, which decreases the problem of iliac crest bone graft resorption. If this toe bone is used, then at least part of the toe must be removed. Reconstruction following the wrap-around technique produces a thumb that resembles its contralateral counterpart except that it only moves at the carpometacarpal joint. The whole great toe transplant is broader, but it restores good movement at the metacarpophalangeal and interphalangeal joints.

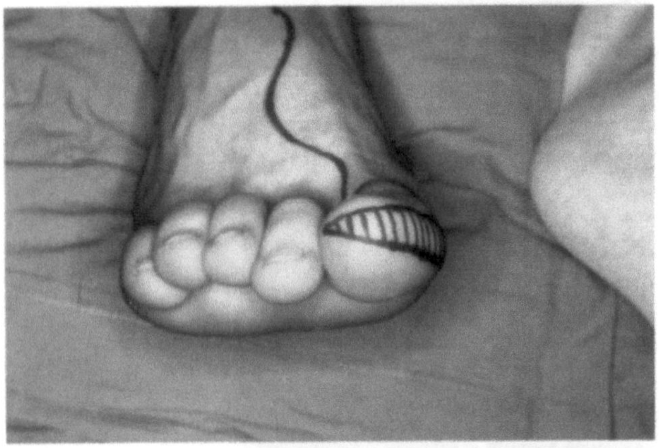

a

a. The flap is outlined on the great toe. The circumference of the opposite thumb is measured and the same measurement is made on the lateral aspect of the great toe. Because the great toe is about 20% larger than the thumb, a bridge of skin (*shaded area*) will remain on the medial aspect of the toe. If the toe nail is too broad, the incision should pass through the medial portion of the nail so that only the lateral two thirds of the toe nail is transplanted. The medial eponychium of the great toe is preserved to cover the area exposed by medial nail matrix and bed excision. (Courtesy of Hill Hastings II, MD.)

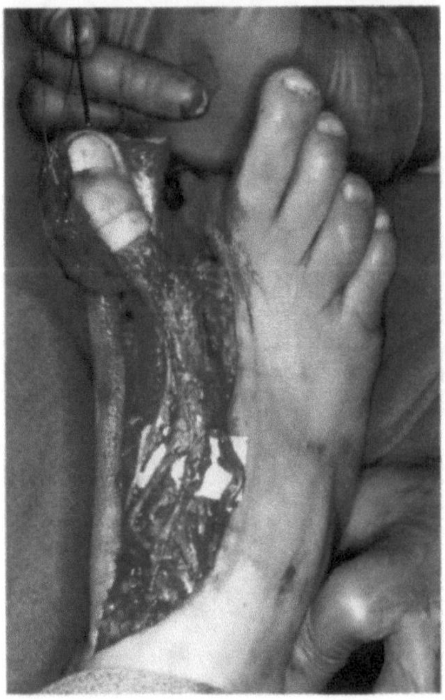

b

b. The vessels and nerves are dissected in a manner identical to that for standard great-toe transplantation; the dorsalis pedis artery, superficial vein, and deep peroneal nerve can be seen. The flap is then elevated over the dorsum of the toe, leaving paratenon intact. A portion of the distal phalanx may be taken with the transplant. Dissection under the nail must be deep enough to avoid damaging the germinal matrix.

c. A strip of skin remains with the toe. The defect is closed in the transplant, producing a thumb that has dimensions similar to its contralateral counterpart. The nail can be narrowed and the bone trimmed to the appropriate size. An iliac crest corticocancellous bone graft of appropriate length and width is wired onto the injured thumb metacarpal. The transplant is now wrapped around this bone. The distal phalanx of the toe is wired to the iliac crest graft. Each structure is repaired as in standard great-toe transplantation.

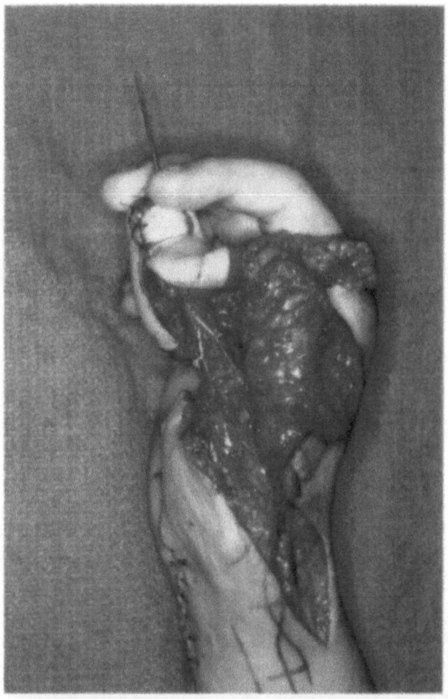

c

d. A diagram of the flap procedure on the left foot.
i. The incision is outlined.

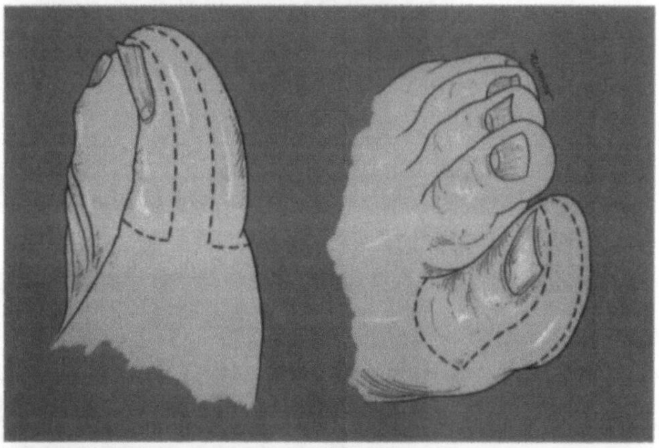

di

ii. If the nail is too broad, only a part of the nail is included.

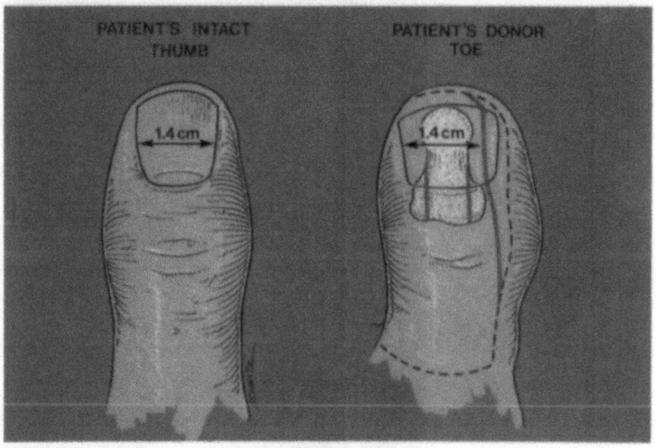

dii

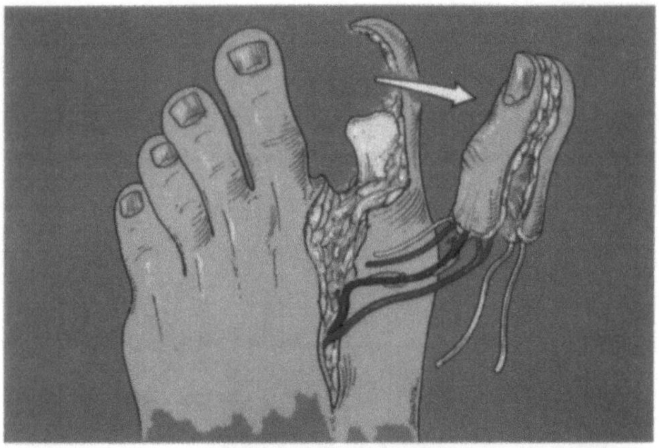

d iii

iii. The transplant includes the distal phalanx of the toe, the digital nerves, and the dorsal neurovascular bundle.

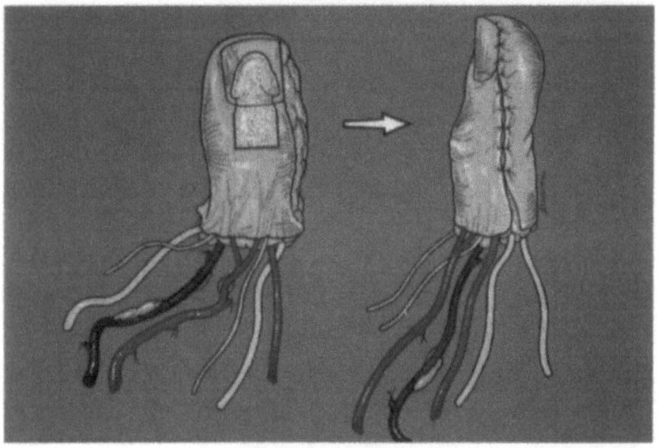

d iv

iv. The medial wound is closed, reconstructing a thumb that is slightly narrower than the great toe.

The **donor site** is treated by one of two techniques:

1. A cross-toe flap from the second toe is used to cover the dorsal aspect. Split-thickness skin graft covers the rest of the great toe and the plantar aspect of the second toe. The cross-toe flap is divided three weeks later. (The length of time in the hospital and morbidity in the foot are substantially greater with this technique.)
2. The proximal phalanx of the great toe is removed, allowing the remaining medial toe skin to cover most of the defect.

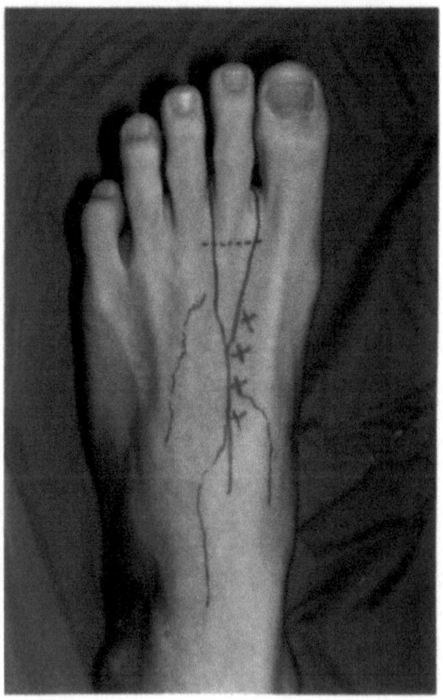

a

4.6.3 Second-Toe Transplantation

(Leung and Kok 1980, O'Brien et al. 1978, Wei 1983) (Fig. 4-22; see also Figs. 4-7 and 4-11)

a. The foot dissection must be carefully planned with regard to (1) right or left side, (2) size of the dorsal and plantar flaps, (3) vessels to be used, (4) site of osteotomy, and (5) method of osteosynthesis.

The *veins* are outlined. As with the great toe transplant, it is easiest to use the large subcutaneous dorsal venous arch which drains into the saphenous system. The *dorsal flap* should cover the entire vascular pedicle. The level of the second metatarsophalangeal joint is marked. A second-toe ray amputation with resection of the metatarsal near its base will provide the best functional and cosmetic result in the foot. One can therefore plan to remove skin back to this level for the cutaneous flap; this will be important once the toe has been transplanted and the pedicle needs to be covered. An arteriogram is used to assess the course of the *dorsalis pedis artery* and the *first dorsal metatarsal artery*. A Doppler study may also be helpful in demonstrating these vessels.

b. The *plantar flap* is planned in a similar way and should be of sufficient length to enable skin closure. The anticipated locations of the nerves are marked.

A clay model is very helpful in planning the skin incisions and marking out the site and position of the vascular pedicle. The model can also be brought up to the hand to assess length, rotation, and position of the transplant (Figs. 4-8, 4-16, and 4-19).

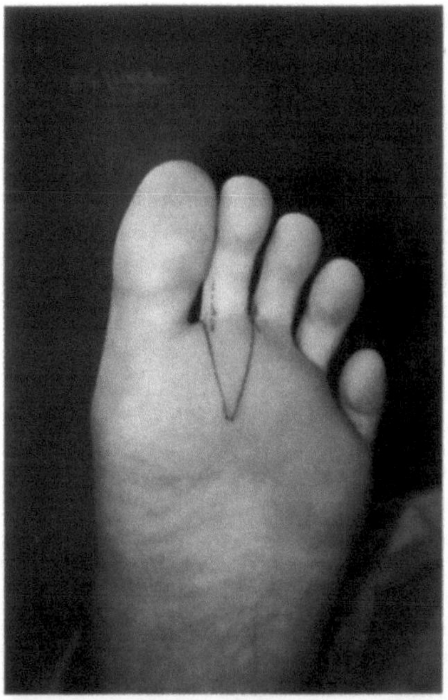

b

c. Under tourniquet control, the *venous system* is dissected, making sure to obtain an adequate length of one of the large veins that drain the toe and dorsal flap.

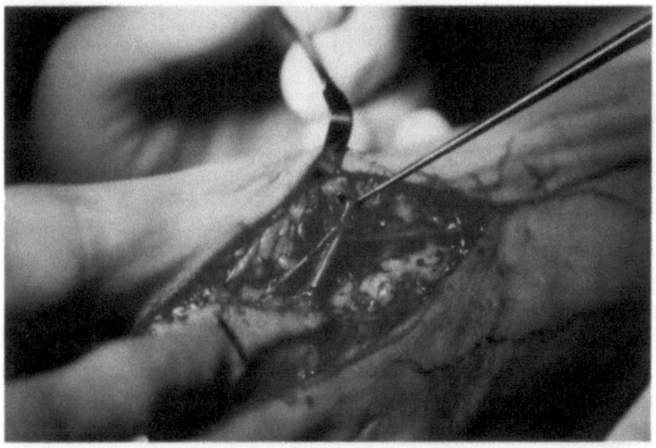

c

d. The *dorsalis pedis artery* is then dissected. The dissection is easy if a relatively large first dorsal metatarsal artery provides the primary arterial flow to the toe and is superficial. As this vessel approaches the web space, the branch to the great toe should be divided (*in the vessel loop*), leaving the circulation to the second toe intact. Sometimes, it is simpler to begin the dissection in the first web space distally, and then "connect" the proximal and distal dissections. When dissecting the *dorsal flap and dorsalis pedis artery* (*in the nerve hook*), care should be taken to extend the entire dissection deep to all the vessels, nerves, and extensor tendons, and not to separate the dorsal skin from any of its vascular connections. The *extensor tendon* is divided proximally, and if a dorsal nerve is available in the hand, the *deep peroneal nerve* traveling with the dorsalis pedis artery may be included in the transplant. It is extremely important during the dissection of the artery to ligate all branches of the vessel. If these branches are small, ligation should be done with 9-0 nylon. As stated before, this measure prevents spasm of the vessel later in the procedure.

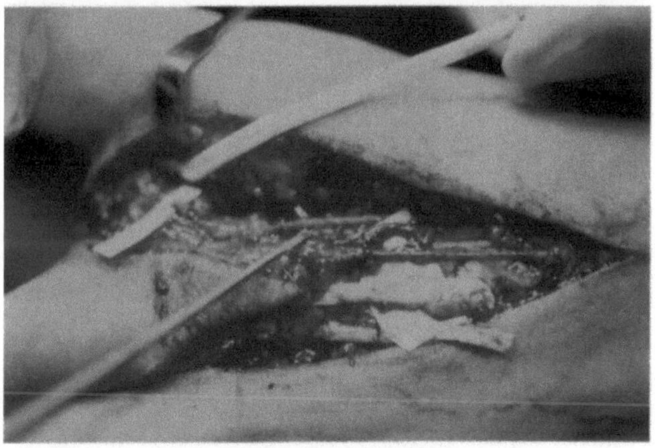

d

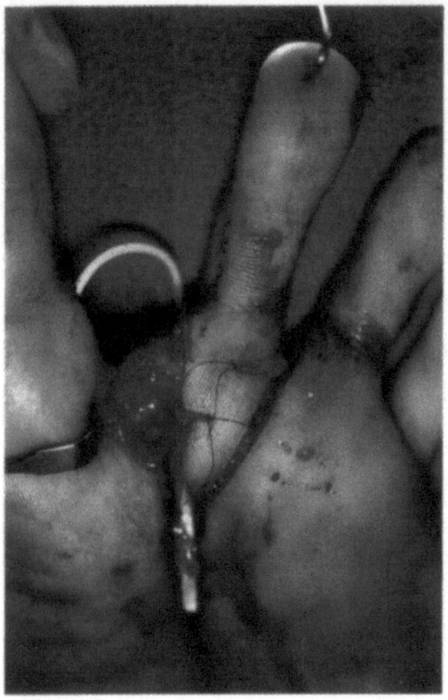

e

e. On the plantar surface, the *flexor tendon* is dissected and divided (Fig. 4-20 h). The *digital nerves* are dissected and tagged with 6-0 silk for later retrieval.

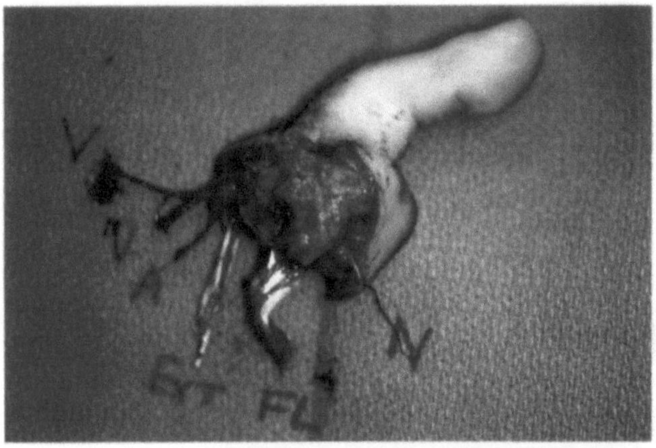

f

f. In this patient, the *toe* was removed and the capsule was divided at the metatarsophalangeal joint. The structures are shown.

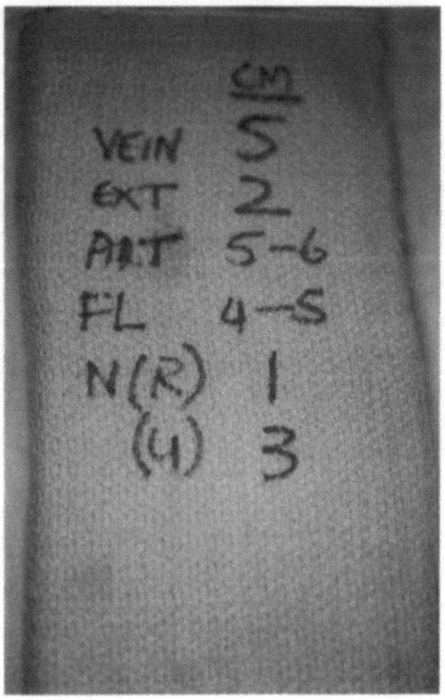

g

g. During the hand dissection, the required length of each structure should be recorded.

The toe is transferred to the *hand*. Various methods of osteosynthesis may be used (Sec. 4.4). With the distal interphalangeal joint in extension, a Kirschner wire is placed across the joint to avoid the problem of excessive flexion of the second-toe transplant. This wire is removed 2–3 weeks later. Tendon repairs are performed using a Pulvertaft weave stitch. This tenorrhaphy is strong enough to allow early range of motion. If possible, any pulleys in the A1 or A2 region proximal to the transplant should be retained because they will optimize ultimate motion. The nerves are then repaired using 9-0 nylon suture without tension.

4.6.3.1 Foot Closure

After second-toe or second metatarsophalangeal joint transplantation, ray amputation of the second toe usually produces the best functional and cosmetic result. The second metatarsal is divided back at the base, and the first and third metatarsals are approximated. A strong repair of the intermetatarsal ligament between these metatarsals is done, ensuring proper position, spacing, and rotation. Temporary Kirschner wires may be helpful, and routine skin closure without tension completes the repair.

4.6.4 Partial Toe Transplantation

(Foucher et al. 1980) (Fig. 4-23)

While various parts of the great or second toe can be used to reconstruct fingers, the procedure must be tailored to the specific needs of the injured digit. The distal phalanx along with its soft tissues, or soft tissue alone can be carried on the vascular pedicle. Either surface, plantar or dorsal, can be transplanted separately. The lateral half of the great toe and medial half of the second toe can be used as neurovascular transplants to resurface the palm or digits. This transplant can include a skin flap from the dorsum of the foot, making it a Y-shaped flap.

The sensory potential of such a flap is similar to that of skin following digital nerve repair. One can expect a good functional result because untraumatized nerve is sutured without any tension (Lipton et al. 1987, Poppen et al. 1983). This method enables reconstruction of the distal palm and adjacent web spaces of the fingers, and parts of the pulp of the fingers or thumb can be resurfaced with sensate skin. The donor site can usually be closed primarily, and the defect on the foot is slight. While many applications of this method exist, the following case is presented as a simple example.

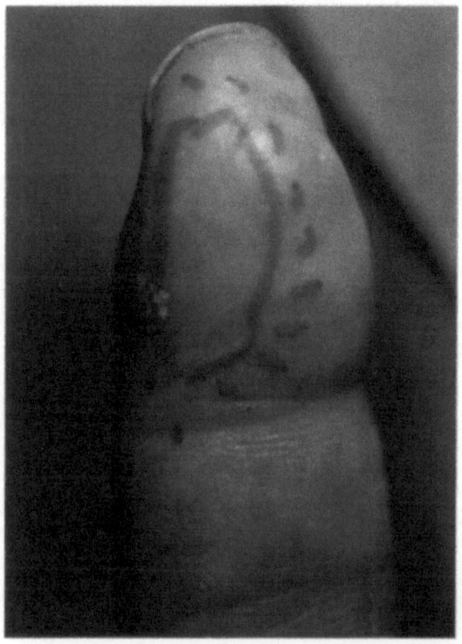

a

a. A 55-year-old man sustained a mangled laceration of the radial aspect of the distal phalanx of his index finger. An exquisitely tender neuroma resulted and a local flap failed to improve the condition. The neuroma was divided more proximally but the pain continued. He was referred to my care, unable to use the digit because of the severe pain. Although advised to undergo amputation, he strongly objected. Resurfacing of the sensitive distal pulp and nerve repair were planned as an alternative.

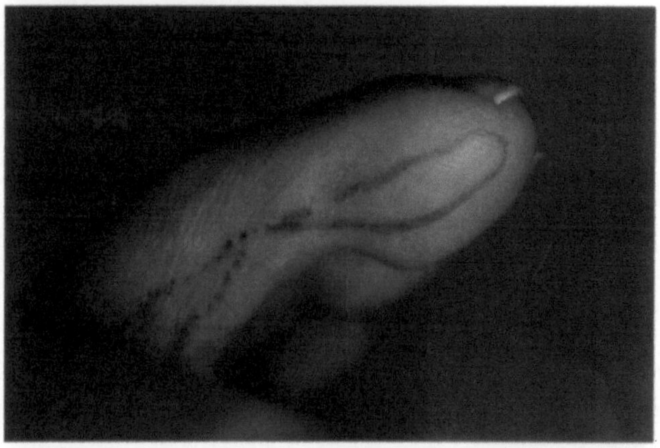

b

b. A neurovascular flap is outlined on the medial aspect of the second toe.

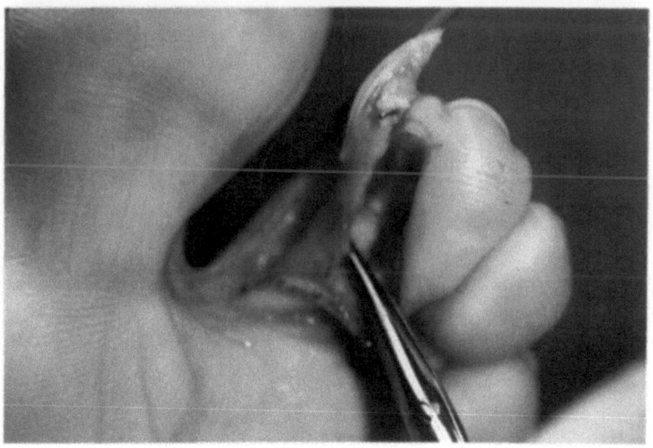

c

c. Under tourniquet control, the flap is elevated and the digital neurovascular bundle is dissected back to the base of the toe. This dissection includes a superficial vein.

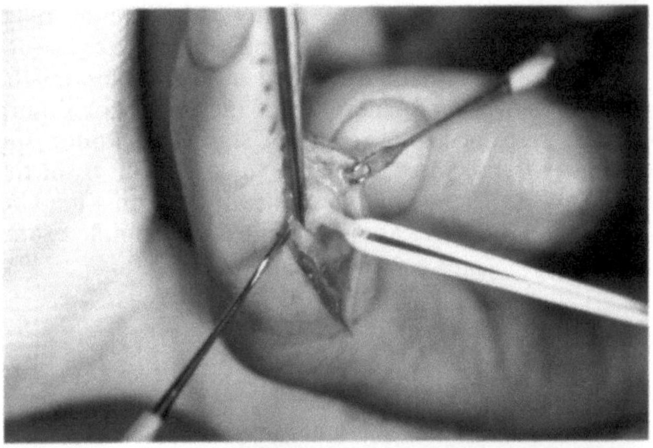
d

d. The neurovascular pedicle on the radial aspect of the index finger is dissected.

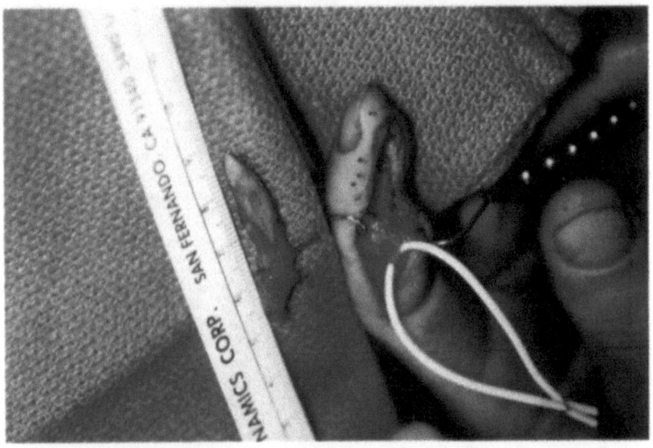

e

e. The transplant is taken from the toe after the pedicle has been carefully measured to make sure it is of adequate length.

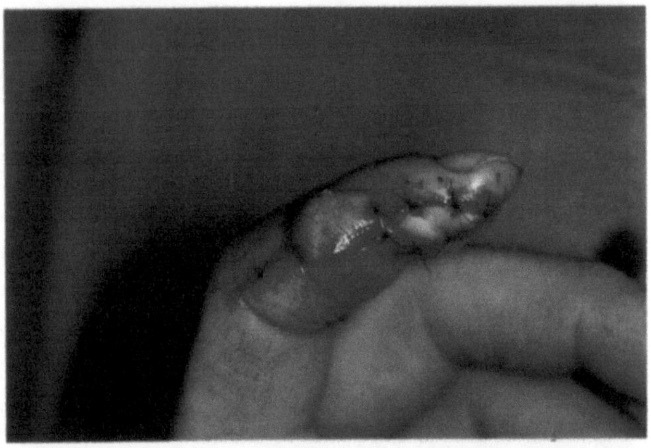
f

f. The transplant is sutured into place. Nerve and vascular repairs are performed proximally.

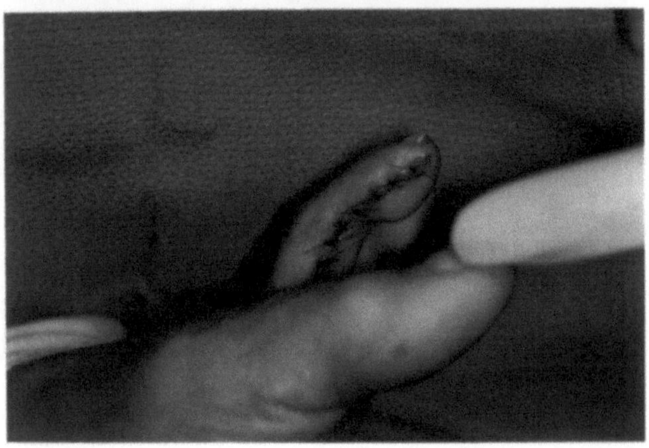
g

g. The toe defect is closed primarily. Total operating time: 3 hours.

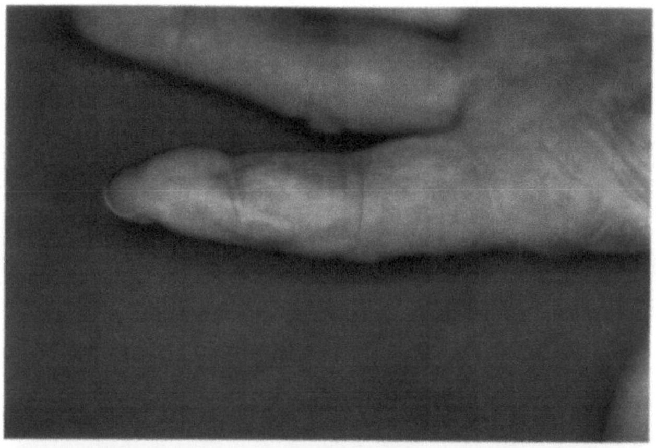
h

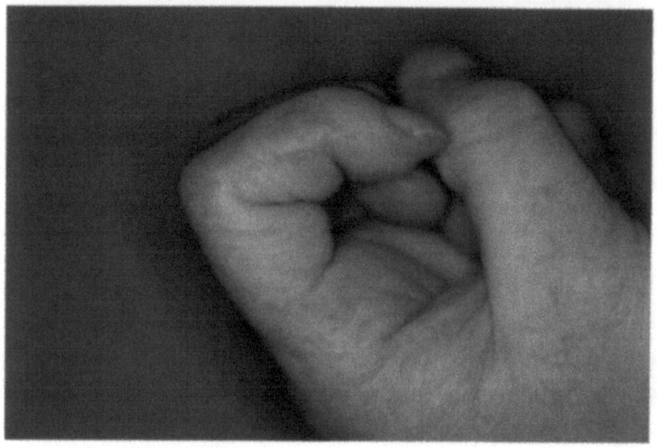
i

h and i. Good healing has been achieved with return of 5-mm two-point discrimination. The procedure enabled this patient to use his index finger.

4.6.5 Toe Joint Transplantation (Kuo et al. 1984, Mathes et al. 1980, O'Brien et al. 1978, Tsai et al. 1982)

4.6.5.1 Second Metatarsophalangeal Joint to the Metacarpophalangeal Joint of the Thumb
(Fig. 4-24; see also Fig. 4-19)

The metatarsophalangeal and proximal interphalangeal joints of the foot can be used to replace joints in the hand. Skin and/or tendon can be included for a composite transplant. Range of motion in these joints is generally no greater than 30–60°, making the procedure most useful in the thumb. Vascularized joint transplantation is indicated most clearly under the following circumstances: (1) for young patients in whom a silicone arthroplasty will not hold up to vigorous activities, and (2) for a joint that has been destroyed but where tendons remain intact. Continued growth is important in pediatric patients (Mathes et al. 1980, Tsai et al. 1982), who often achieve better range of motion than adults (Kuo et al. 1984, Mathes et al. 1980, O'Brien et al. 1978, Tsai et al. 1982).

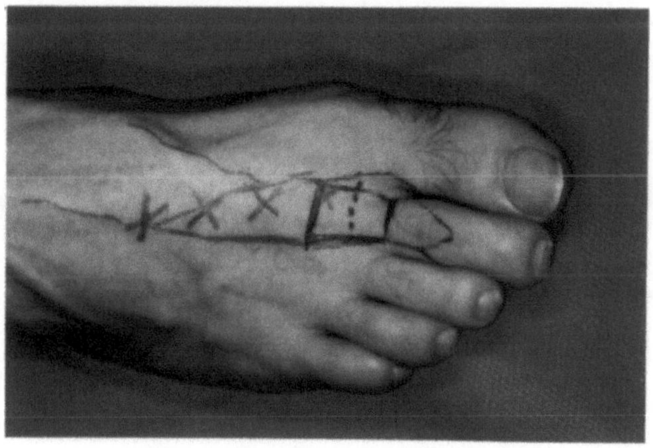
a

a. The *foot structures* to be transplanted must conform specifically to the requirements in the hand. Also, the *amount of bone* on either side of the joint is measured. Skin grafting should be avoided in the foot, so primary closure must be planned. The dorsalis pedis and first dorsal metatarsal vessels are palpated. An arteriogram and Doppler study are used to confirm the presence and position of the latter. The *dorsal veins* are outlined and the position of the metatarsophalangeal joint is marked.

The proximal interphalangeal joint of the toe has better flexion than does the metatarsophalangeal joint, but because a considerable amount of soft-tissue cover is needed in the web space and dorsum of the hand, the metatarsophalangeal joint was selected in this patient.

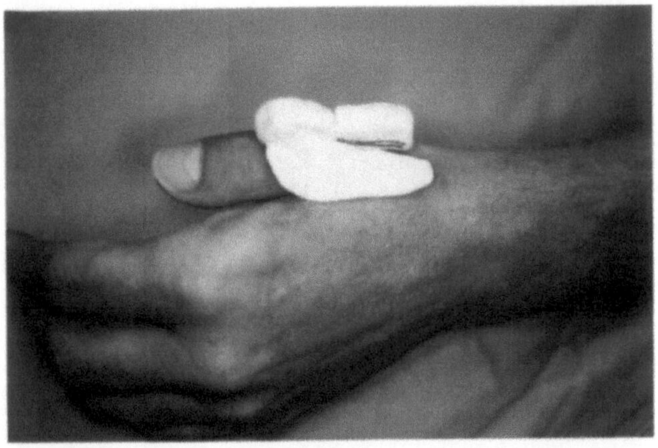

b

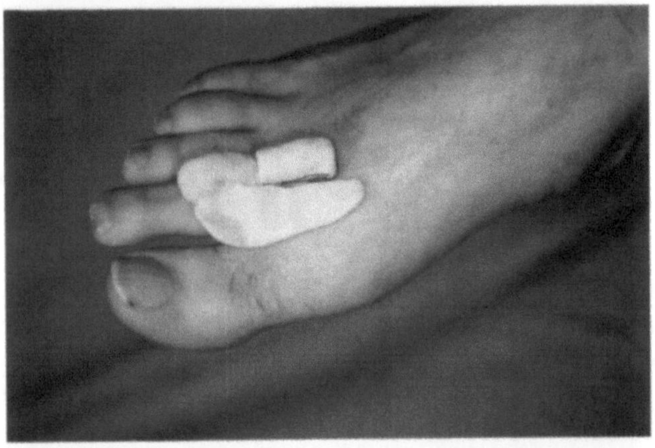

c

b and c. A clay model can be used to plan and measure the *skin flap* needed as well as the amount of bone and position of the vessels.

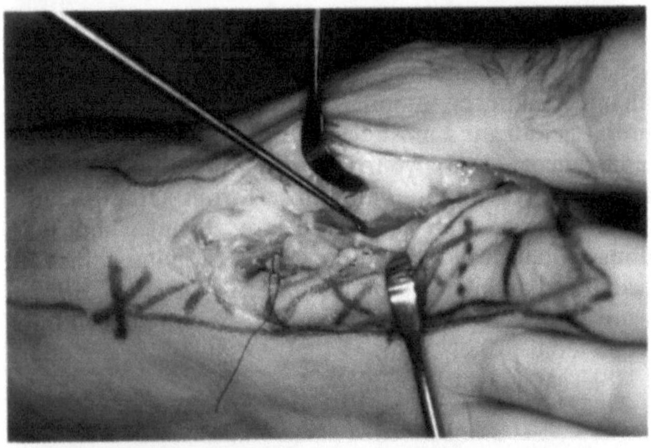

d

d. Under tourniquet control, a *dorsal vein* is dissected proximally; once the hand dissection is completed and the desired length of vein can be confirmed, it is divided. The *first dorsal metatarsal artery*, which emanates from the dorsalis pedis vessel, is identified (*in the nerve hook*) along with the deep peroneal nerve, just beneath the extensor hallucis brevis tendon. It is then dissected distally to the region just distal to the metatarsophalangeal joint. In this dissection, care is taken to dissect *only* on the medial side of the vessel so that any branches from the vessel to the soft-tissue flap, tendon, bone, or joint are retained. The vessel is then divided distally.

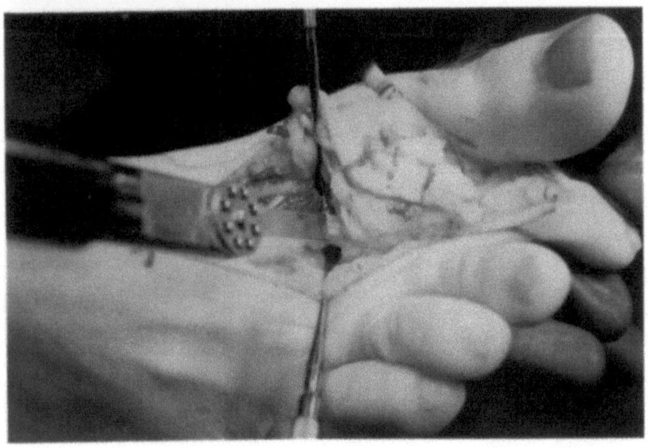

e

e. The *extensor tendon* is dissected proximal and distal to the skin flap and is included in the transplant. Dissection is then undertaken on the lateral aspect of the second metatarsal and metatarsophalangeal joint. Once the soft tissues have been dissected around the metatarsophalangeal joint, an oscillating saw is used to osteotomize the joint at the proximal and distal points that give the desired length. The vessels are divided and the joint is ready for transplantation (Fig. 4-19).

4.6.5.2 Toe Interphalangeal Joint Transplantation
(Wray et al. 1981) (Fig. 4-25)

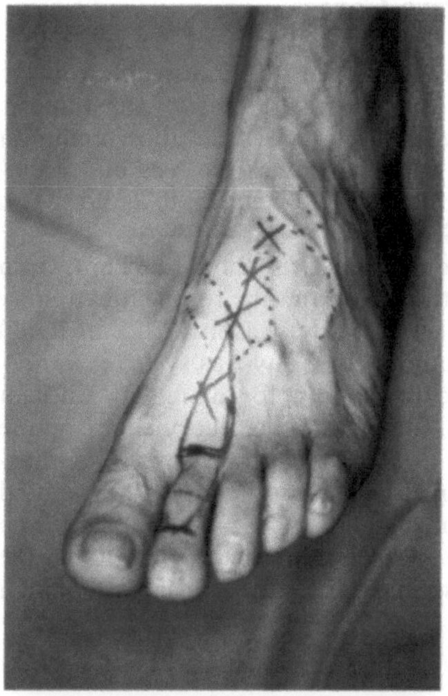

a

a. The dorsal skin island that will be required in the hand is outlined. The level at which osteotomy of the proximal and middle phalanges will be performed on either side of the proximal interphalangeal joint is estimated so that the transplant will fit the defect in the hand. The course of the dorsalis pedis and first dorsal metatarsal arteries is palpated and then confirmed by an arteriogram and Doppler study. The dorsal veins are outlined on the foot.

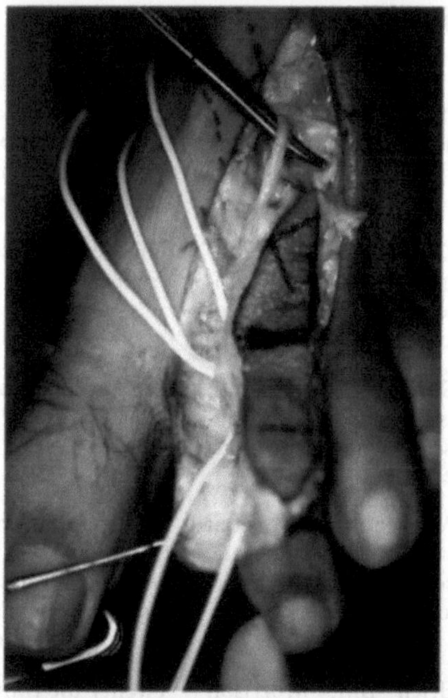

b

b. A large subcutaneous vein is dissected. The first dorsal metatarsal artery is dissected and is seen here being held up by the clamp. The branch of this artery to the great toe is divided. The first dorsal metatarsal artery must be dissected on its medial side to avoid injuring the vascular connections between it and the transplant.

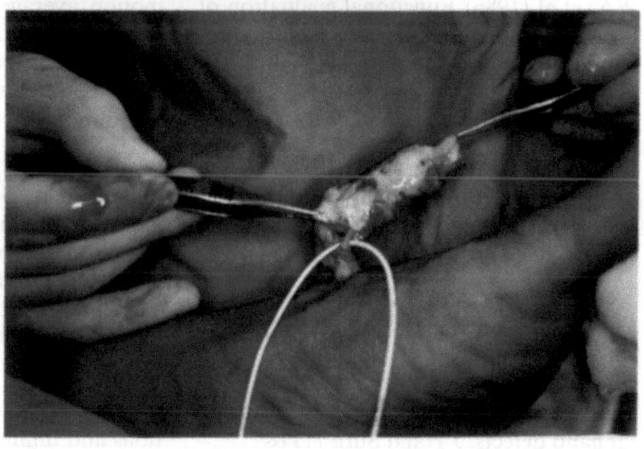

c

c. The osteotomy on either side of the interphalangeal joint is performed with an oscillating saw. The joint is ready for transplantation with only the vascular pedicle remaining intact. Good bleeding from both the skin margins and periosteum confirms good vascularity to the transplant.

4.7 Postoperative Care

The arteries and veins used in toe transplantation are generally large, so thrombosis at the site of anastomosis is unusual. *Spasm* in the artery is the most common vascular problem, which is why careful vascular monitoring is essential. Steps should be taken to avoid spasm if at all possible (Sec. 5.4.7).

The hospital room and patient should be kept warm at all times. Both the donor and the recipient extremity should remain well elevated. I use aspirin (325 mg daily) and dextran (30 cc/hour for 5 days) as systemic *anticoagulants*, and reserve heparin for extremely difficult vascular problems. Either a dermal fluorimeter or pulse oxymeter is used to *monitor vascularity* in the transplant. (The same methods and criteria should be used following toe transplantation as after replantation [Chapter 8].) The dermal fluorimeter quantitates the amount of fluorescein entering the transplant, while a pulse oxymeter gives continuous information and is entirely noninvasive.

The most important factor in postoperative care is quick and aggressive action should vascular problems arise. If corrective surgery is undertaken within the first several hours after arterial or venous thrombosis, the transplant can usually be salvaged. After approximately 7 days, gentle range of motion is initiated, beginning first with tenodesis exercises involving the more proximal joints, and later progressing to active motion at about 3 weeks. Postoperative therapy should be tailored to the individual; it should depend on the patient's need for motion and the type of tendon repair performed.

The *donor foot* is kept constantly elevated for a period of 2 weeks. Partial weight bearing is begun 4 weeks postoperatively, and, depending on the amount of swelling, an elastic bandage should be used for the first 6 to 8 weeks, especially when the foot is dependent.

4.8 Selected Bibliography

Cobbett JR (1969) Free digital transfer. Report of a case of transfer of a great toe to replace an amputated thumb. J Bone Joint Surg 51B:677

Great toe transplantation is described for the first time. One of the problems encountered years ago, i.e., vessel spasm, is still being experienced today. The nerves were not repaired primarily. It has subsequently become evident that the best ultimate results can be achieved if all structures are repaired at the initial operative procedure, obviating the need for subsequent reconstruction.

Doi K, Kuwata N, Kawai S (1985) Reconstruction of the thumb with a free wrap-around flap from the big toe and an iliac-bone graft. J Bone Joint Surg 67A:439

This report describes the procedure in ten patients. Results and complications are included.

Egloff DV (1984) Surgery of the Hand. Free Tissue Transfers by Nerve and Vascular Microanastomoses. Geneva, Editions Médecine et Hygiene

The vascular anatomy of the first web space is discussed.

Foucher G, Merle M, Maneaud M, et al (1980) Microsurgical free partial toe transfer in hand reconstruction. A report of 12 cases. Plast Reconstr Surg 65:616

Transplantation of parts of the great or second toe, including the pulp, the first web skin, part of the distal phalanx, and the vascularized toe joint, is described. These structures or various combinations are used for a variety of digital problems. A discussion of 12 cases includes some operative description and follow-up information.

Frykman GK, O'Brien BM, Morrison WA, et al (1986) Functional evaluation of the hand and foot after one-stage toe-to-hand transfer. J Hand Surg 11:9

Twenty toe transfers were followed up an average of 4.5 years later. Total active motion averaged 48° after toe-to-thumb transfer, and 106° after toe-to-finger transplantation. In 65%, two-point discrimination was less than 15 mm. The transferred toes decreased in bulk an average of 10%. Although 50% of the patients were unable to wear thongs, all wore normal shoes and foot morbidity was minor.

Furnas DW, Achauer BM (1983) Microsurgical transfer of the great toe to the radius to provide prehension after partial avulsion of the hand. J Hand Surg 8:453

A patient with carpometacarpal amputations is described in whom placement of the great toe onto the radius provided functional pinch. Removal of the great toe proximal to the metatarsophalangeal joint, as was done in this case, has not been popular because of the fear of compromising push-off and causing problems with ambulation. No such problem was encountered in this patient. The clinical problem presented has no other ready solution, making this technique an important one for rare cases of this kind. Details of the operative procedure are given.

Gilbert A (1982) Toe transfers for congenital hand defects. J Hand Surg 7:118

A series of toe transplants for treating congenital adactyly is described. Indications and timing are considered.

Gordon L, Buncke HJ, Alpert BS, et al (1984) Great toe-to-thumb transfer. Indications and results in 41 cases. In Buncke HJ, Furnas DW (eds) Symposium on Clinical Frontiers in Reconstructive Microsurgery, Vol. 24. St. Louis, Mosby, pp 239-246

This article discusses the indications for transfer of the great toe, and compares other methods of thumb reconstruction. The operative technique is described in detail, as is the preoperative planning and postoperative care. Functional results in terms of sensation, pinch, and grip strength are analyzed in the follow-up of 21 patients.

Gordon L, Leitner DW, Buncke HJ, et al (1985) Hand reconstruction for multiple amputations by double microsurgical toe transplantation. J Hand Surg 10A:218

The details of both sequential and simultaneous double toe transplantation are presented along with an analysis of the two procedures. One toe from each foot was taken, with the great toe being used for the thumb, and the second toe used for digital reconstruction. Simultaneous transplantation requires a larger operating team, a longer operating time, and somewhat greater risk, but total rehabilitation time, time away from work, and cost are all substantially less than if the procedures are done sequentially.

Gordon L, Rosen J, Alpert BS, et al (1984) Free microvascular transfer of second toe ray and serratus anterior muscle for management of thumb loss at the carpometacarpal joint level. J Hand Surg 9A:642

This article describes an approach to the difficult reconstruction of the thumb that has been amputated at the carpometacarpal joint. The operative procedure for microvascular second-toe transplantation with the second metatarsal, followed by second-stage microneurovascular transplantation of serratus anterior muscle, is detailed. The specific indications for this procedure are described, and a comparison with other techniques is included. A case report with follow-up information on function, grip strength, pinch strength, and sensation is given.

Gu YD, Wu MM, Zheng YL, et al (1985) Vascular variations and their treatment in toe transplantation. J Reconstr Microsurg 1:228

The vascular variations found in 160 patients who underwent toe transplantation are analyzed in detail, and treatments are suggested. When the first dorsal metatarsal artery is absent or has an inadequate diameter for second-toe transplantation, use of the plantar metatarsal artery or the second dorsal metatarsal artery is proposed. Venous variations are also discussed.

Kuo ET, Ji ZL, Zhao YC, et al (1984) Reconstruction of metacarpophalangeal joint by free vascularized autogenous metatarsophalangeal joint transplant. J Reconstr Microsurg 1:1

Six cases of metatarsophalangeal joint transplantation are described. The anatomy and vascular supply to the metatarsophalangeal joint are detailed. In the cases involving the metacarpophalangeal joint of the thumb, good results were achieved, but joint motion in the other fingers was approximately 30°. Motion was 90° in one case – an excellent result which I have not yet been able to duplicate in any patient.

Leung PC, Kok LC (1980) Transplantation of the second toe to the hand. A preliminary report of sixteen cases. J Bone Joint Surg 62A:990

Second-toe transplantation to replace either an amputated thumb (nine cases) or a finger (seven cases) is described. Details of the surgical technique are presented and anomalies of the first metatarsal space vascularity are mentioned.

Leung PC, Wong WL (1983) The vessels of the first metatarsal web space. An operative and radiographic study. J Bone Joint Surg 65:235

The anatomy of the first web space, with emphasis on the variability of the first dorsal metatarsal artery, is described in cadaver dissections. An understanding of this anatomy is essential for the surgeon embarking on a toe transplantation procedure.

Lipton HA, May JW Jr, Simon SR (1987) Preoperative and postoperative gait analyses of patients undergoing great toe-to-thumb transfer. J Hand Surg 12A:66

Gait was studied prospectively in 12 patients who underwent microvascular great toe transplantation. Only one patient had a change in motion with reduction in ankle plantarflexion on push-off. Velocity, cadence, step length, and step width did not change significantly. Only two patients had symptoms, which were mild.

Lister GD, Kalisman M, Tsai TM (1983) Reconstruction of the hand with free microneurovascular toe-to-hand transfer. Experience with 54 toe transfers. Plast Reconstr Surg 71:372

The method of preparation, surgical technique, and postoperative management in 24 cases of thumb reconstruction are described (the great toe was used in 13 cases, and the second toe was used in 11 cases). In 13 cases of transmetatarsal amputation, reconstruction was accomplished by combined second- and third-toe transplantation. Other treatment options are evaluated.

Mathes SJ, Buchanan R, Weeks PM (1980) Microvascular joint transplantation with epiphyseal growth. J Hand Surg 5:586

The continued growth of epiphyses is essential for successful toe and joint transplantation in pediatric patients. In this case report describing the transplantation of the second metatarsophalangeal joint to the metacarpophalangeal joint of the long finger, a 2.5-year follow-up evaluation confirmed growth of the revascularized epiphyses.

May JW, Daniel RK (1978) Great toe to hand free tissue transfer. Clin Orthop 133:140

The technique of great-toe transplantation is clearly described. The anatomy of the vasculature in the first metatarsal space suggests a higher incidence of superficial first dorsal metatarsal artery (78%) than has subsequently been found by others (Leung and Wong 1983, Wu et al. 1980).

May JW, Smith RJ, Peimer CA (1981) Toe-to-hand free tissue transfer for thumb construction with multiple digit aplasia. Plast Reconstr Surg 67:205

The indications for using the great toe to construct an opposable thumb in multiple digital aplasia is described. This article covers preoperative planning and surgical technique.

Meals RA, Lesavoy MA (1983) Hallux to thumb transplant during ankle disarticulation for multiple limb anomalies. JAMA 249:72

This is a case report of a 10-year-old boy with four anomalous limbs who had his left great toe transplanted to the left hand for use as a thumb. Simultaneously, he underwent an ankle disarticulation to improve his lower extremity function. While no active motion was achieved in the thumb, three-point grasp of light-weight objects was possible after surgery.

Michon J, Merle M, Bouchon Y, et al (1984) Functional comparison between pollicization and toe-to-hand transfer for thumb reconstruction. J Reconstr Microsurg 1:103

This retrospective study comparing pollicization with great- or second-toe transplantation for various hand defects has important practical implications. For patients who were missing the thumb but had four normal fingers, pollicization provided the best sensibility and mobility. Power was better after great-toe transplantation than after pollicization or second-toe transplantation. Pollicization in cases of relatively greater loss depended on the mobility of the proximal interphalangeal joint, the sensibility of the transferred digit, and the quality of the nontransferred digits.

Morrison WA, O'Brien B McC, MacLeod AM (1980) Thumb reconstruction with a free neurovascular wrap-around flap from the big toe. J Hand Surg 5:575

The technique of placing an iliac crest bone graft to lengthen the amputated thumb and then covering this graft with a wrap-around flap of soft tissues from the great toe is presented along with five case summaries.

O'Brien BM, Gould JS, Morrison WA (1984) Free vascularized small joint transfer in the hand. J Hand Surg 9A:634

Seven patients, including four children, underwent vascularized joint transplantation. The metatarsophalangeal joint (four cases), proximal interphalangeal joint (two cases), and proximal interphalangeal joint of a useless finger (one case) were used to reconstruct proximal interphalangeal and metacarpophalangeal joints in the hand or thumb. Stability, absence of pain, and continued growth occurred in six of the seven patients. Range of motion ranged from 15–50°.

O'Brien B, MacLeod AM, Sykes PJ (1978) Microvascular second toe transfer for digital reconstruction. J Hand Surg 3:123

The technique of second-toe transplantation is described in two patients. In one patient who had sustained an amputation of all four fingers at the metacarpophalangeal joint level, the toe was placed in the index finger position. In the other patient, whose ring finger was reconstructed after it had been amputated at the proximal interphalangeal joint, the procedure must be considered to have been primarily cosmetic.

Poppen NK, Mann RA, O'Konski M, et al (1981) Amputation of the great toe. Foot Ankle 1:333

Gait is analyzed after removal of the great toe.

Poppen NK, Norris TR, Buncke HJ (1983) Evaluation of sensibility and function with microsurgical free tissue transfer of the great toe to the hand for thumb reconstruction. J Hand Surg 8:516

This article analyzes the results in a series of great toe transplantations. Subjective assessment by the patient, objective measurements of pinch and grip, and details of the patients' work histories are given.

Tsai TM, Jupiter JB, Kutz JE, et al (1982) Vascularized autogenous whole joint transfer in the hand. J Hand Surg 7:335

Reconstruction of the metacarpophalangeal and proximal interphalangeal joints of the finger and thumb is described in six patients who underwent proximal interphalangeal joint transplantation from the toes. Details of the anatomy, surgical technique, and results are presented.

Wei W (1983) Keys to successful second toe-to-hand transfer. A review of 30 cases. J Hand Surg 8:902

This article analyzes the technical factors involved in successful toe transplantation, and should be useful to those preparing for this procedure. Anatomic variations are emphasized. Wei found the dorsalis pedis to be absent in 4% of the patients, and to have an abnormal origin in 5%.

Wilson CS, Buncke HJ, Alpert BS, Gordon L (1984) Composite metacarpophalangeal joint reconstruction in great toe-to-hand free tissue transfers. J Hand Surg 9A:645

This article describes composite joint reconstruction in toe transplantation using the joint surfaces of the proximal phalanx of the toe and the metacarpal of the thumb.

Wray RC, Mathes SM, Young VL, et al (1981) Free vascularized whole joint transplants with ununited epiphyses. Plast Reconstr Surg 67:519

Foot-to-hand joint transplantation is described in two patients. In one, the metatarsophalangeal toe joint was used, and the proximal interphalangeal toe joint was used in the other patient. Nonvascularized joint transplantation, epiphyseal transplantation, and vascularized joint transplantation are discussed.

Wu JB, et al (1980) The distribution of arteries supplying the dorsum and planta of the foot. Acta Anat Sinica 11:13

Arterial anatomy and its variations in 100 cadaver feet are described in detail. The dorsalis pedis was absent in 4% of the feet; it originated from the fibular artery in 3%, and from the perforating branches of the tibial or fibular arteries in 2%. The first dorsal metatarsal artery arose dorsally in 51%, and from the plantar aspect in 49%. In most cases, the first dorsal metatarsal artery lay within the first interosseous muscle. It was subcutaneous in only 11%.

Zhong-Jig, Ho GH, Chen TCH (1984) Microsurgical reconstruction of the amputated hand. J Reconstr Microsurg 1:162

Sixteen cases of toe transplantation for hand reconstruction after uni- and bilateral amputation are described. One prerequisite of reconstruction was possession of a forearm at least two thirds of its original length. Artificial metacarpals were used in conjunction with the toe transplants.

5 Replantation

5.1 Indications

In the 1970s, when the possibilities for replantation were relatively unexplored, this procedure was thought to be appropriate only for clean-cut, "guillotine-type" amputations. Within 5–10 years, however, many adventurous attempts accomplished the salvage of avulsed or mangled parts. More cautious surgeons objected, citing poor ultimate function following such injuries. Uncertainty and controversy abounded, and the distinction between the kind of injuries that should be replanted and those that should be amputated was unclear. Eventually, many replantation centers generated reports of large series of patients, and these reports began to clarify the indications for replantation (Chow et al. 1979, May et al. 1982, O'Brien et al. 1974, Tamai 1982, Urbaniak et al. 1985, Weiland et al. 1977). While these indications continue to evolve and do depend partly on the experience, skill, and opinion of the surgeon, each injury can be analyzed with regard to some basic prognostic features.

One must individualize the decision of whether or not to replant a part in each case by considering **personal factors**.

Occupation and hobbies. The need for five-fingered activities such as using a keyboard or playing a musical instrument must be assessed. Some patients may require a strong tubular grasp. Also, the need to return to work as soon as possible may be a relative contraindication for replantation, which requires many months of therapy to achieve a satisfactory result.

Personal preferences. Cultural pressures may influence the priority of restoring an amputated part. Each individual views the loss of a body part differently. The longer hospital stays (7–10 days) and rehabilitation period (2–6 months) are the reasons that some patients prefer amputation closure. It should be remembered that amputation closure does not necessarily solve or end the patient's problem. Neuroma formation, skin adherence or sensitivity, poor sensation, lack of dexterity, or poor pinch and grasp can all complicate single- or multiple-digit amputations.

The **patient's general condition**, both physical and mental, must be considered. When *other major injuries* contraindicate the replantation of digits, the latter assumes secondary importance. *Mental status* is always a difficult factor to assess in the emergency situation, as patients who are unstable or depressed may respond to psychiatric treatment and return to a productive life. For this reason, psychiatric factors alone should very seldom contraindicate replantation. I would proceed with replantation under most circumstances, except where chronic or permanent psychiatric illness makes cooperation with the rehabilitation program impossible. It is important to discuss these factors with the patient's mental health care professional.

The following approach to the indications for replantation relates **site and type of injury** to the likely functional outcome.

5.1.1 Single-Finger Amputations (Phelps et al. 1978, Urbaniak et al. 1985)

Single-finger replantation should be performed for the occasional patient who has strong cosmetic, psychologic, or cultural reasons for wanting the procedure done. Certain functional considerations may be important, such as if the patient is a performing musician or uses a keyboard as part of his or her occupational duties. Single-digit replantation should only be attempted with the following considerations kept in mind regarding level of injury.

5.1.1.1 Distal Phalanx

The *digital artery* trifurcates between the distal interphalangeal joint and the base of the nail. In general, arterial anastomoses are possible proximal to this trifurcation, but replantation of an amputated fingertip is difficult if it is to be performed distal to a point 2–3 mm proximal to the base of the nail. In distal am-

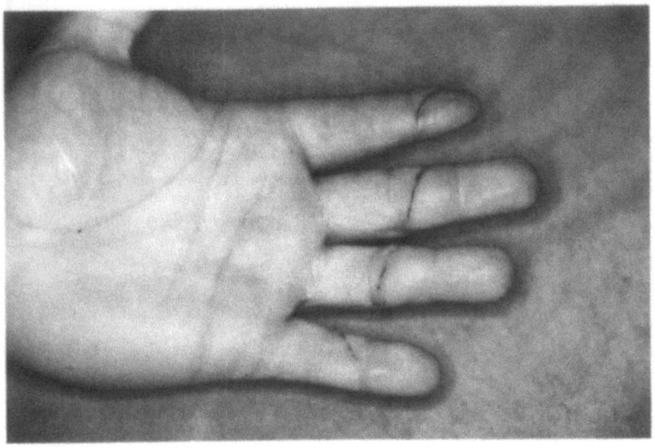

a

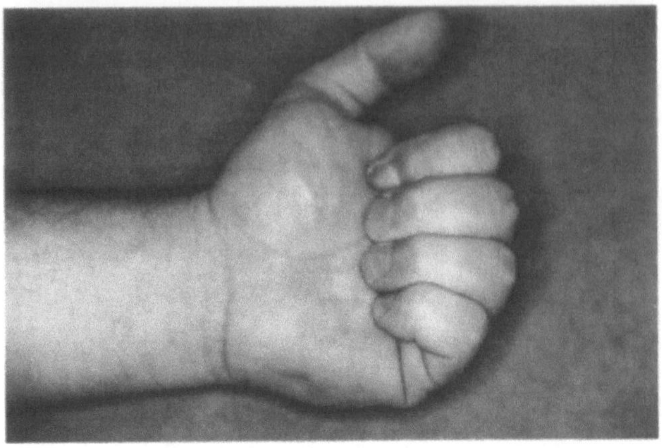

b

Fig. 5-1. a. In a single-finger injury, an amputated distal phalanx should be replanted only if the patient has a specific cosmetic or functional need to engage in five-fingered activities, such as playing a musical instrument or using a keyboard. More commonly, replantation of the distal part of a finger is indicated when it is part of an injury involving multiple fingers. This patient had devascularizing injuries of all four fingers. Survival of any of them was uncertain. **b.** The functional result is good. The patient uses the index finger for pinch against the thumb and for grip. He has some hypersensitivity in his finger, which is not unusual for parts replanted at this level.

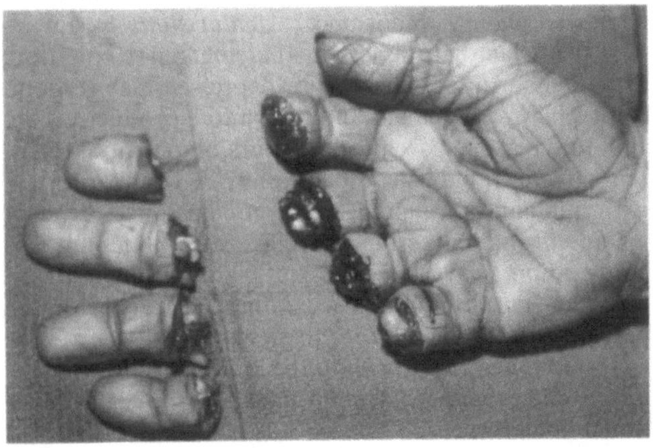

a

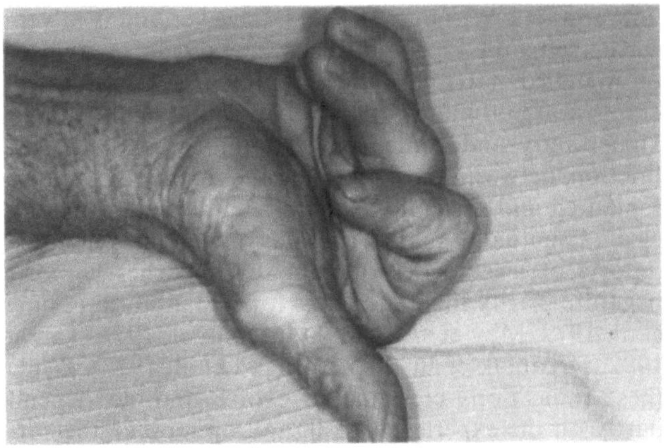

b

Fig. 5.2. a. This patient amputated all four fingers. Only the amputation of the index finger was distal to the proximal interphalangeal joint. **b.** The index finger flexes well at the proximal interphalangeal joint compared with the long, ring, and small fingers, which were amputated proximal to the flexor digitorum superficialis insertion. (All fingers in a *multiple finger amputation* should be replanted, but *single-finger amputations* should only be considered for replantation if they are distal to the flexor digitorum superficialis insertion.)

putations it may be difficult to find an adequate vein in the amputated part, and several techniques may be used to provide *venous drainage* (Sec. 5.4.9).

If adequate vessels and nerves can be found, replantation of a distal phalanx may restore good finger function. The *extensor tendon* is difficult to repair at this level and the flexor is far stronger – a situation that results in a mallet deformity of the distal phalanx. For this reason, if a good extensor tendon is not present, the flexor digitorum profundus should not be repaired; instead, the distal interphalangeal joint should be pinned in extension so that the joint will become fairly stiff.

Even though pinning of the fracture and joint and repair of the digital artery and nerves can be accomplished in well under 2 hours, such distal replantation is only indicated in patients who have a specific functional or cosmetic need for five fingers. More frequently, replantation at this level is indicated after multiple digit amputations (Fig. 5-1).

5.1.1.2 Between the Proximal and Distal Interphalangeal Joints (May et al. 1982)

Digits that are replanted distal to the flexor digitorum superficialis tendon insertion will develop good function because the proximal interphalangeal joint is intact. If this joint moves normally, the only loss of motion is at the distal interphalangeal joint (Fig. 5-2). Also, if the nerves are not severely damaged, good sensation can be expected following revascularization and

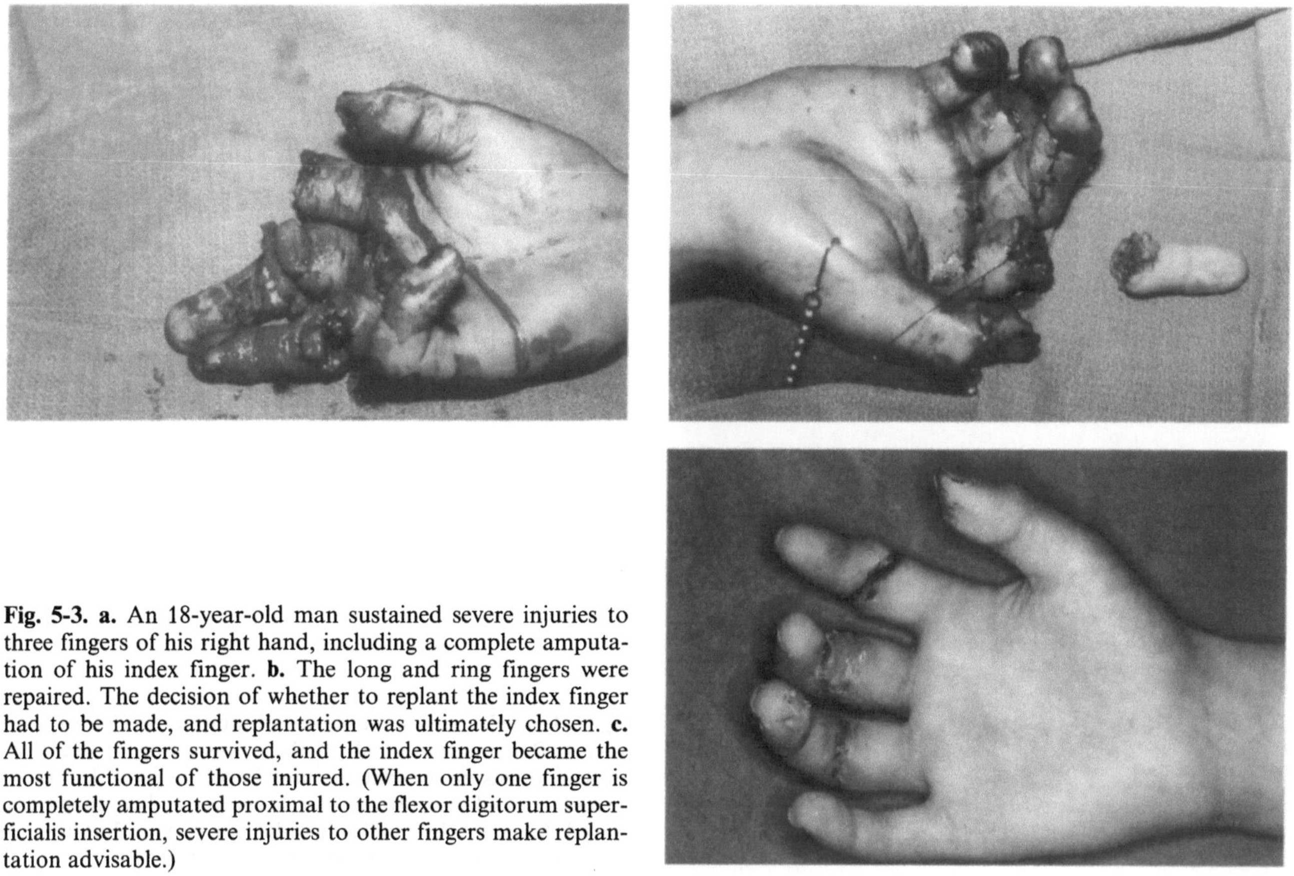

a b c

Fig. 5-3. a. An 18-year-old man sustained severe injuries to three fingers of his right hand, including a complete amputation of his index finger. **b.** The long and ring fingers were repaired. The decision of whether to replant the index finger had to be made, and replantation was ultimately chosen. **c.** All of the fingers survived, and the index finger became the most functional of those injured. (When only one finger is completely amputated proximal to the flexor digitorum superficialis insertion, severe injuries to other fingers make replantation advisable.)

nerve repair. The degree of sensation should approximate that after simple nerve repair in this region.

5.1.1.3 Proximal to the Proximal Interphalangeal Joints (injury to the flexor digitorum superficialis, or disruption of the proximal interphalangeal joint) (Fig. 5-17b).

Replanting a digit in which both the flexor digitorum superficialis and profundus have been divided or the proximal interphalangeal joint itself has been disrupted will seldom result in good active motion at the proximal interphalangeal joint. Tendon adherence in the pulley region between the distal palmar crease and the proximal interphalangeal joint is well known to those who treat tendon lacerations, and it is an even greater problem following replantation. Poor motion at the proximal and distal interphalangeal joints severely compromises finger function. Especially if the other fingers move normally, the replanted finger will be conspicuous and cumbersome, so single-digit replantation proximal to the proximal interphalangeal joint is almost always contraindicated.

If one finger is amputated and an adjacent finger has a tendon or nerve injury, the amputated digit is no longer classified as a "single-finger amputation." A finger with tendon and nerve injury may become stiff, and the replanted digit may indeed be more useful than the one with the somewhat less apparent injury. In this situation, therefore, the amputated digit should be replanted and the injuries to the adjacent finger repaired (Fig. 5-3).

5.1.2 Multiple-Finger Amputations

Considerable disability results from the loss of more than one finger, so when multiple fingers are amputated or injured, they should be replanted. In general, as many fingers as are amputated should be replanted, even if they are proximal to the proximal interphalangeal joint, because one can never be certain of the survival of any replanted part (Fig. 5-4). The digits should be replanted even if they are severely crushed or avulsed and considerable shortening is required. The results of replantation, even if it means having stiff fingers, are usually better than the results of any other, later reconstructive option.

If only one or two fingers are replantable, I tend to place these toward the ulnar side of the hand. If they are placed in the index and long finger positions, large object grasp may be compromised if they become stiff. I prefer to place them in the ring and long finger positions to restore both large and small object grasp.

5.1.3 Thumb Amputations (Chow et al. 1979, Komatsu and Tamai 1968, Vlaston and Earle 1986)

Of all replantation efforts, the best functional results are achieved in the thumb. Thumb loss can represent

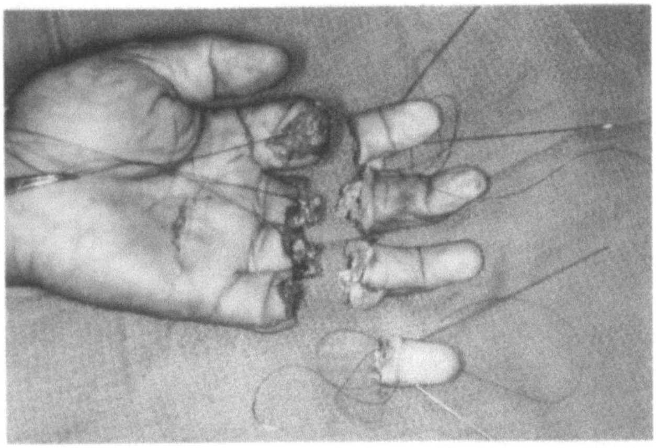
a

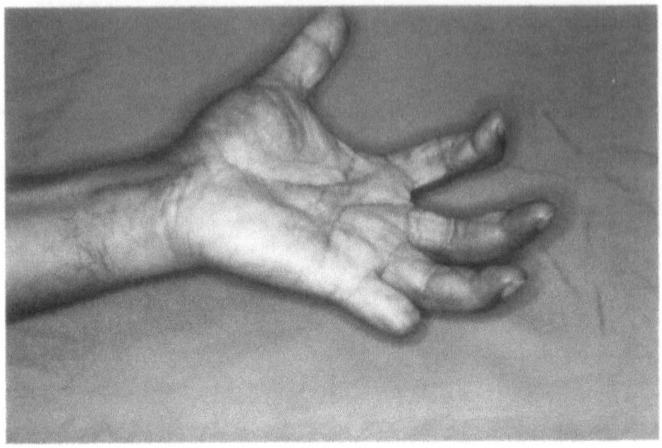
b

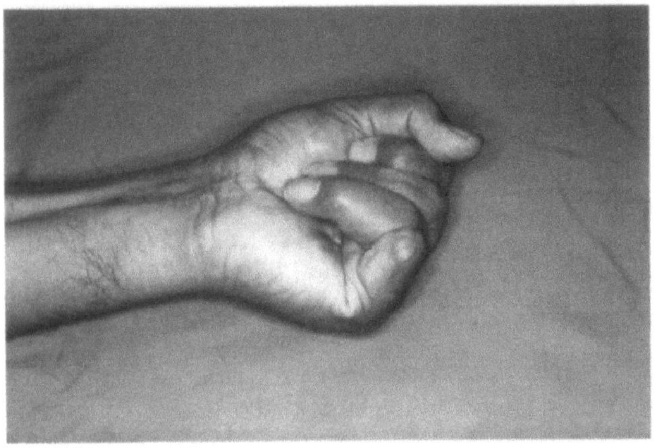
c

Fig. 5-4. a. This patient sustained an amputation of all four fingers. Replantation of all of them was planned. (Because one cannot ensure survival, as many fingers as possible should be replanted.) The neurovascular structures and tendons were tagged. **b** and **c.** The small finger did not survive, but a good functional result was achieved in the other three.

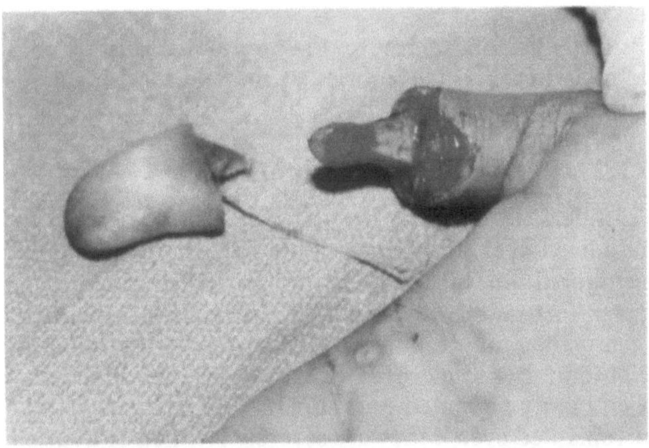
a

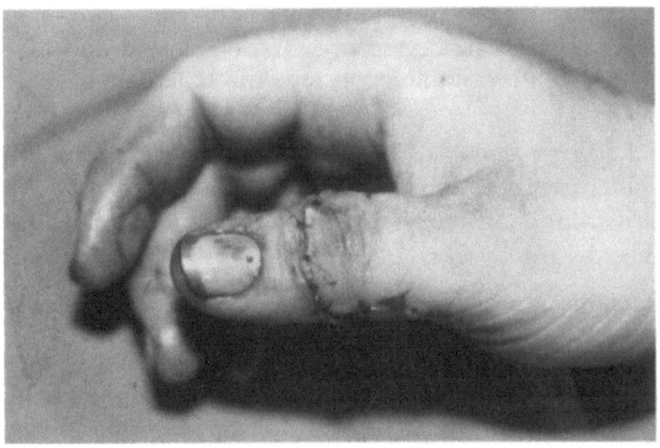
b

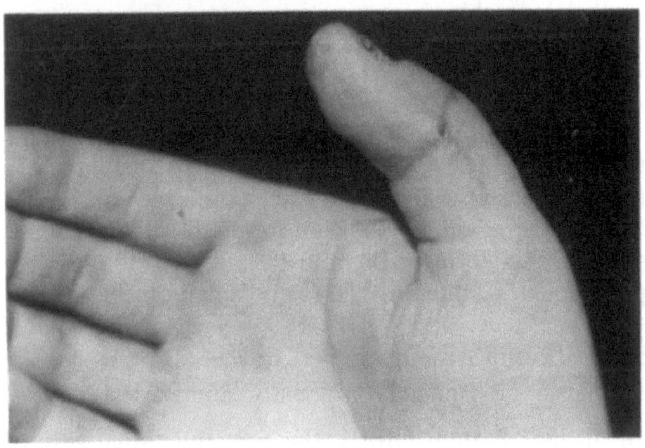
c

Fig. 5-5. a. This avulsive injury of the soft tissues of the distal phalanx of the thumb left the entire skeleton, including that of the distal phalanx, intact. **b.** Using vein grafts for arterial and venous repair, the thumb was replanted. **c.** A good functional and cosmetic result was achieved. The patient required subsequent nerve grafting 5 months after the replantation to restore functional sensation.

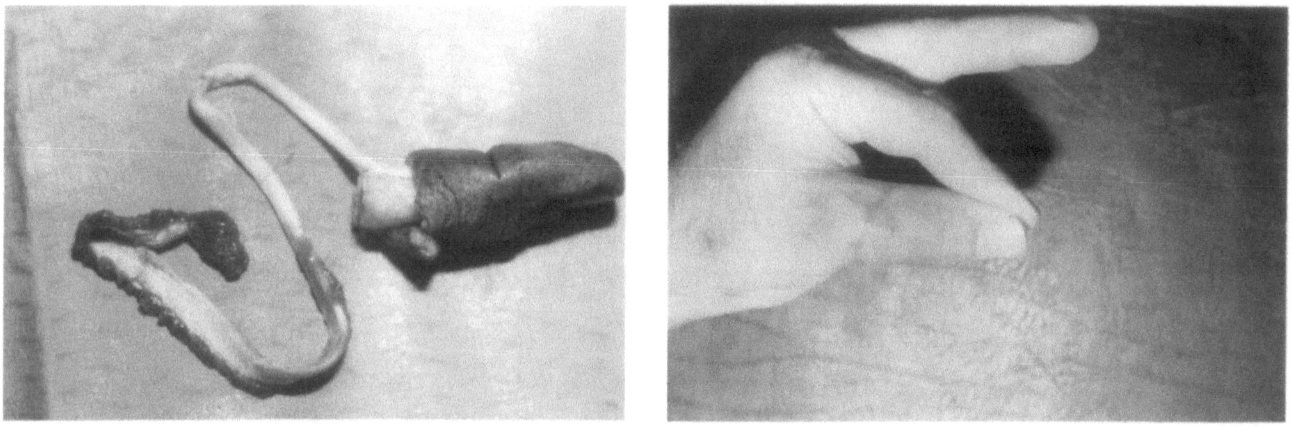

a b

Fig. 5-6. a. This avulsive amputation of the thumb involved the flexor pollicis longus at the musculotendinous junction. The thumb was replanted, using vein grafts for both arterial and venous repair. **b.** The replantation was performed without flexor or extensor tendon repair. The interphalangeal joint was pinned and subsequently became stiff. The patient has excellent function in his thumb and no further reconstruction was required. (If the extensor tendon cannot be repaired in a thumb or finger replant at the distal joint, the long flexor should not be repaired because a mallet deformity will result. Loss of motion at the metacarpophalangeal or interphalangeal joint is not as important in the thumb as it is in the fingers.)

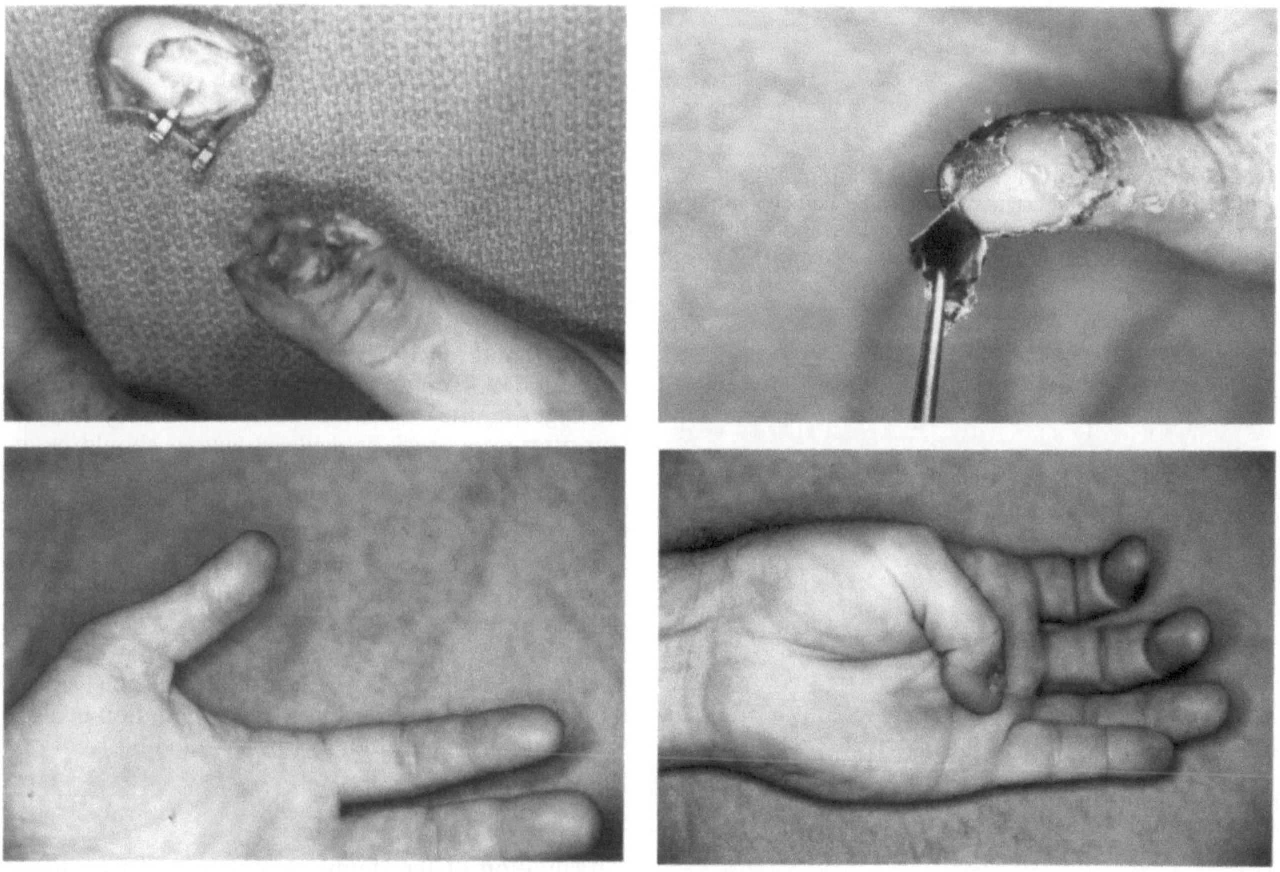

a b c d

Fig. 5-7. a. The distal half of the distal phalanx of this thumb was amputated in a saw accident. A small digital artery was dissected at the level of the digital artery trifurcation, and replantation was performed by anastomosing this small artery. Venous drainage was achieved through partial nail plate removal (Sec. 5.4.9). **b.** Five weeks later, the superficial skin was removed, revealing a viable, pink thumb. **c** and **d.** The functional result is good, the thumb having protective sensation but no hypersensitivity.

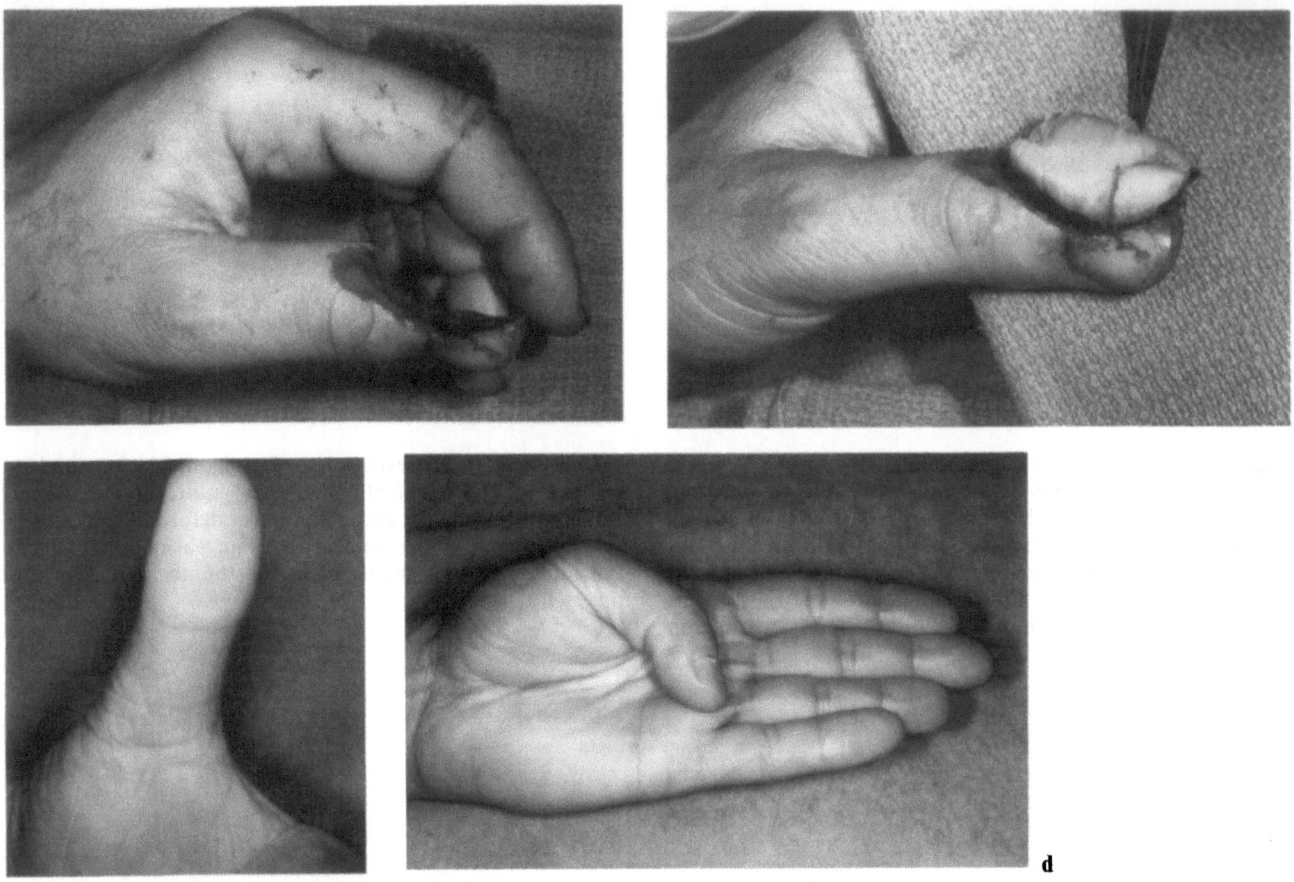

a b c d

Fig. 5-8. a. This sharp, longitudinal amputation of the thumb would have required substantial shortening had replantation not been possible. **b.** The ulnar digital artery and nerve were repaired. (This artery is almost always substantially larger than the radial digital artery of the thumb.) Part of the nail plate was removed for venous drainage (Sec. 5.4.9). **c** and **d.** The result is excellent.

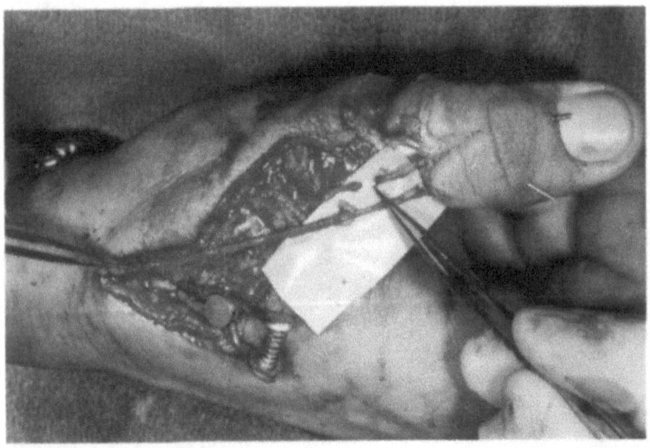

Fig. 5-9. Following an avulsive injury of this thumb, vein grafts were used for both arterial and venous repair. The distal anastomoses were performed on a separate table prior to replanting the thumb. The artery was sutured end-to-side to the radial artery (*seen in the clamp*) on the dorsal aspect of the first web space.

a loss in hand function of up to 40%, so the indications for thumb replantation are as strong as those for multiple-finger injuries. As with multiple-finger injuries, repair after even *crush* or *avulsion injuries* should be attempted because such efforts will often result in salvage (Fig. 5-5); this is particularly true because the demands for motion at the interphalangeal joint of the thumb are less than those at the proximal interphalangeal joints of the fingers, so even a stiff or shorter thumb is likely to function adequately (Fig. 5-6). The presence of a nail and pulp in the thumb is important and enhances function considerably. Replantation should therefore be attempted even if the amputation is distal to the interphalangeal joint (Figs. 5-7 and 5-8).

5.1.4 Avulsive Digital Injuries

Replantation of the thumb or multiple fingers should be performed, even if the injury was avulsive. Following such injuries, *vein grafts* should be used routinely to bypass the length of vessel damaged by the stretching injury (Vlaston and Earle 1986) (Fig. 5-9).

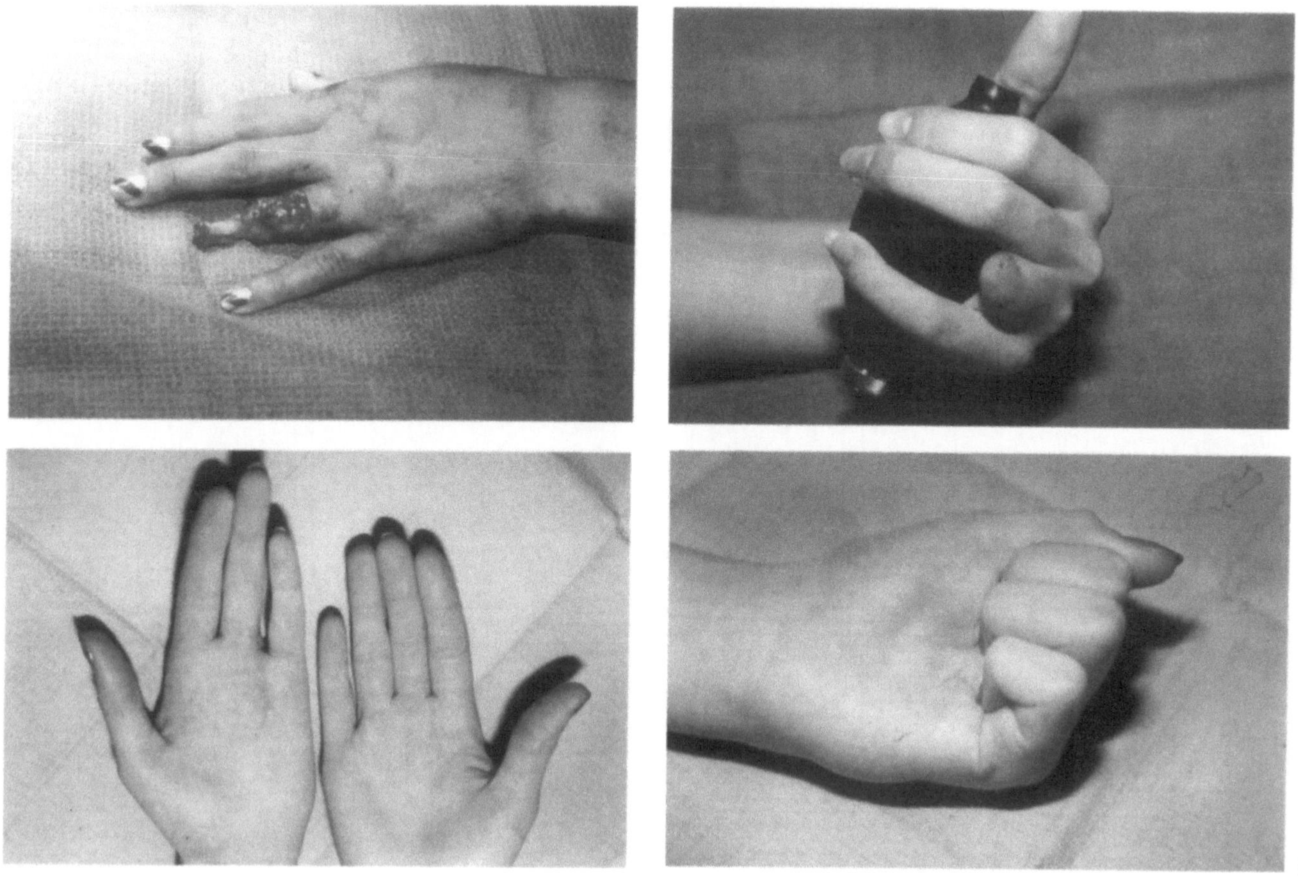

Fig. 5-10. a. After a ring avulsion injury, the digit in this 12-year-old girl was not replanted. **b.** Substantial cosmetic and functional deficit resulted. **c** and **d.** The hand has good function and appearance. (Ray transfer of the small finger to the ring finger position is a useful alternative in many such cases.)

Single-finger avulsive injuries such as *ring avulsions* present a problem with regard to indications (Urbaniak et al. 1981). Devascularizing injuries with partial degloving can usually be salvaged with good function and appearance. When the finger has been completely amputated and the amputated part includes the distal phalanx along with the skin of the entire finger, a good result is less likely. Many such injuries are amenable to later ray amputation and transfer, with good cosmetic and functional results (Fig. 5-10). This option may be preferable to replantation. It should always be understood that replantation in this situation is difficult and may involve extensive rehabilitation and several operations. Nevertheless, a good functional outcome can sometimes be achieved (Figs. 5-11, 5-12, and 5-31). Mature judgment is required in deciding whether to replant single-digit avulsive amputations.

5.1.5 Transmetacarpal, Wrist, and Forearm Amputations (Chow and Bilos 1979)

The disability after the loss of a hand is obvious. If at all possible, hand and forearm amputations should be replanted. When the amputation is proximal to the midpalmar crease, there are no pulleys at the site of tenorrhaphy, and the resultant range of motion is usually good (Fig. 5-13); when the amputation is more proximal in the forearm, the considerable muscle damage that has been sustained results in poorer finger motion (Fig. 5-14).

The more proximal the amputation, the more aware one must be of the *ischemia time*. When there is a substantial amount of muscle in the amputated part and it remains ischemic for more than 4–6 hours, muscle necrosis may present such life-threatening problems as myoglobinuria, acute tubular necrosis of the kidney, and clostridial and other infections. A replantation attempt is therefore contraindicated when the duration of warm ischemia is more than 3–4 hours. If the amputated part has been kept cold for a part of this time, however, the limit of tolerable ischemia may have been extended to 5–6 hours.

Placement of Scribner shunts can be performed as soon as the patient arrives at the replantation center; this ends the period of ischemia and allows replantation to proceed safely (Fig. 5-15a).

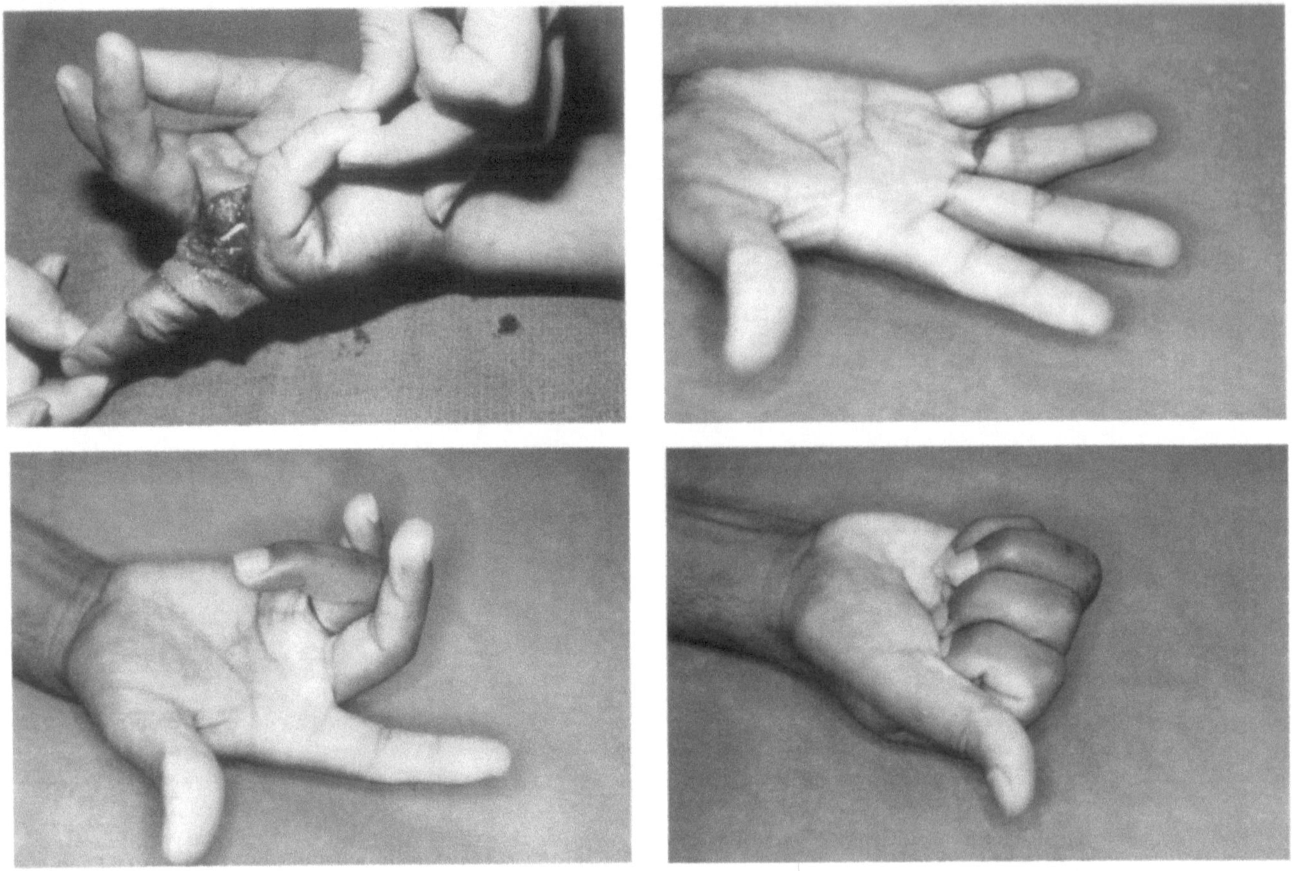

a b c d

Fig. 5-11. a. This ring avulsion injury degloved the soft tissues to the level of the distal phalanx and devascularized the digit. Revascularization was performed with the use of vein grafts. **b–d.** Good extension and independent flexion of the finger was achieved, but, although sensation was adequate for function, the patient continued to have discomfort in the digit 2 years after replantation. He nevertheless was able to perform heavy work.

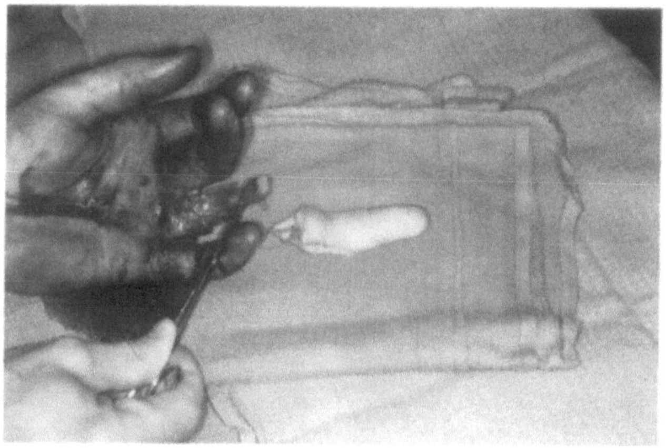
a

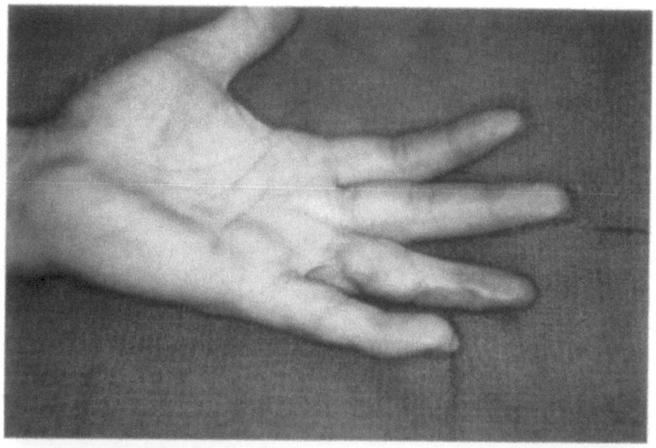
b

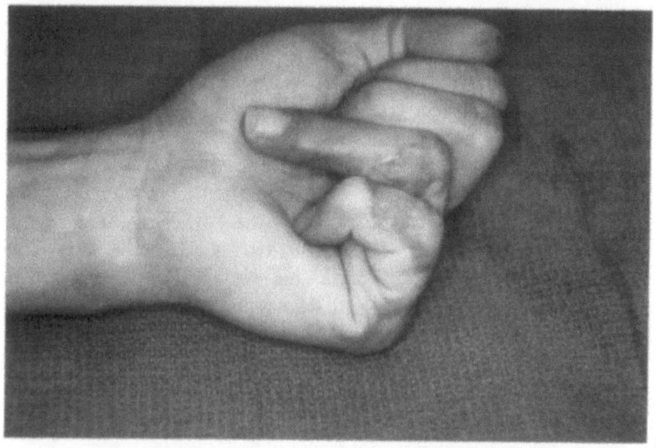
c

Fig. 5-12. a. This guitarist sustained a ring avulsion injury. After considering all of the treatment options, he wanted the finger to be replanted. Vein grafts were used. **b.** Adequate vascularity and sensation were restored. **c.** The patient has good motion at the proximal interphalangeal joint, but a mallet deformity developed distally. This prevented his playing the guitar until a fusion of the joint in a more extended position was done.

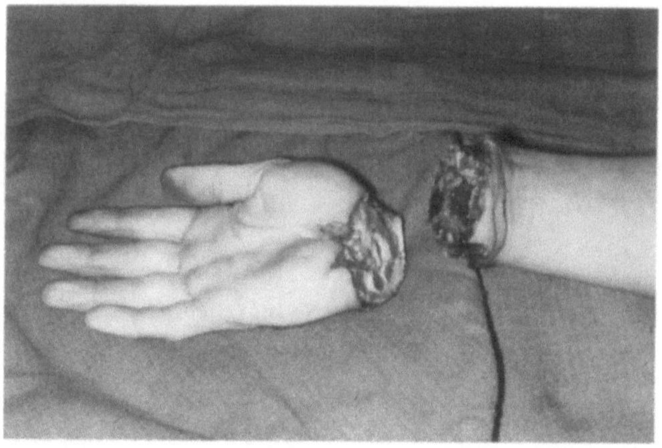
a

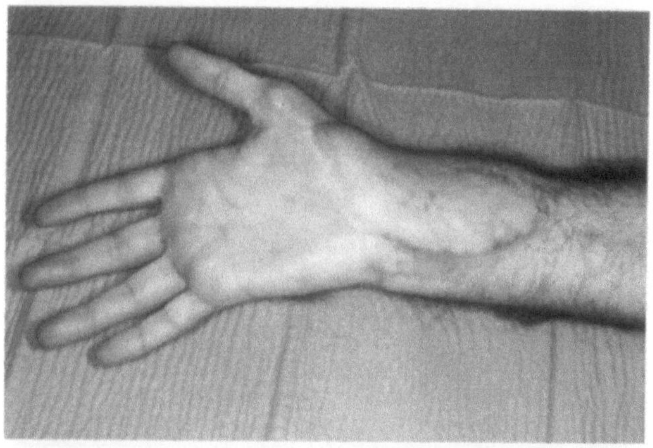
b

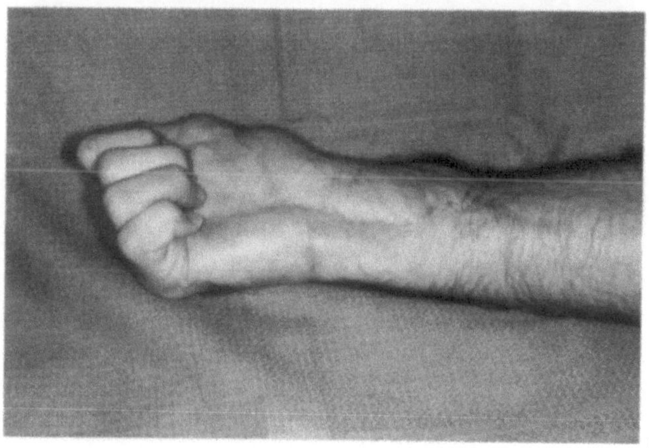
c

Fig. 5-13. a. A hand that was sharply amputated at the wrist was replanted. **b** and **c.** Good tendon gliding can be achieved following replantation at this level, and this patient regained excellent flexion and extension; nerve function in this hand was a greater problem, however. Because return of thenar innervation was absent, a subsequent opposition transfer was needed. Sensation with 15-mm two-point discrimination was restored in some fingers. (Sensation in this situation is generally poorer than it would be following digital replantation.)

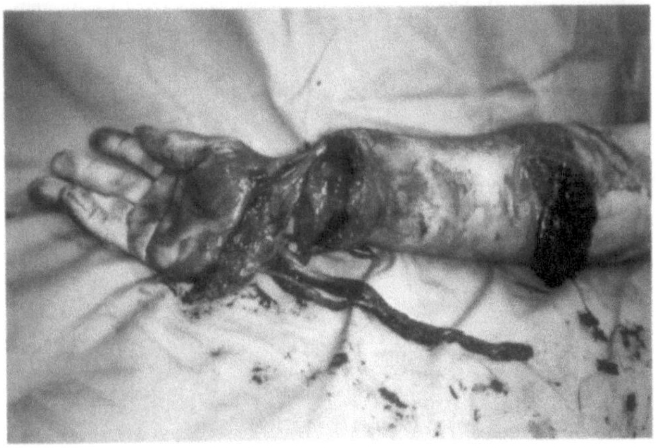
a

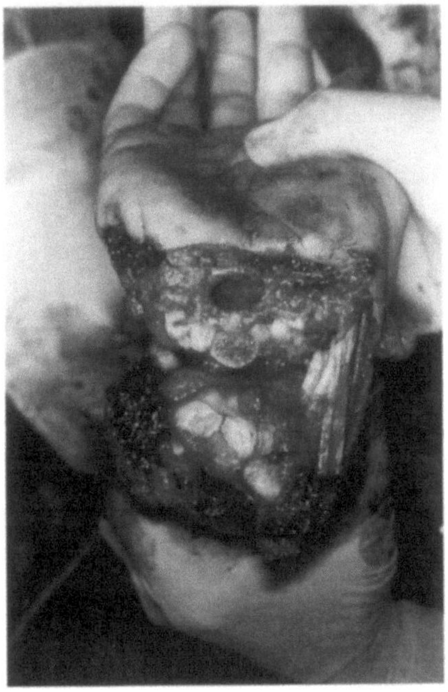
b

Fig. 5-14. a. This patient suffered an avulsive partial amputation at wrist level when he caught his hand in an industrial ice-crushing machine. Despite the avulsive nature of the injury, revascularization was successful. (Most amputations at this level should be replanted because of the marked disability that results from amputation of an entire hand. Also, fasciotomy of all forearm and hand compartments is essential when a crush injury is followed by ischemia.) **b.** The amputation cut through the carpus. The empty carpal tunnel is seen. Initially, the carpus was pinned; this was followed 6 months later with wrist fusion. **c** and **d.** An adequate result was achieved, with functional sensation and grasp (Fig. 2-2).

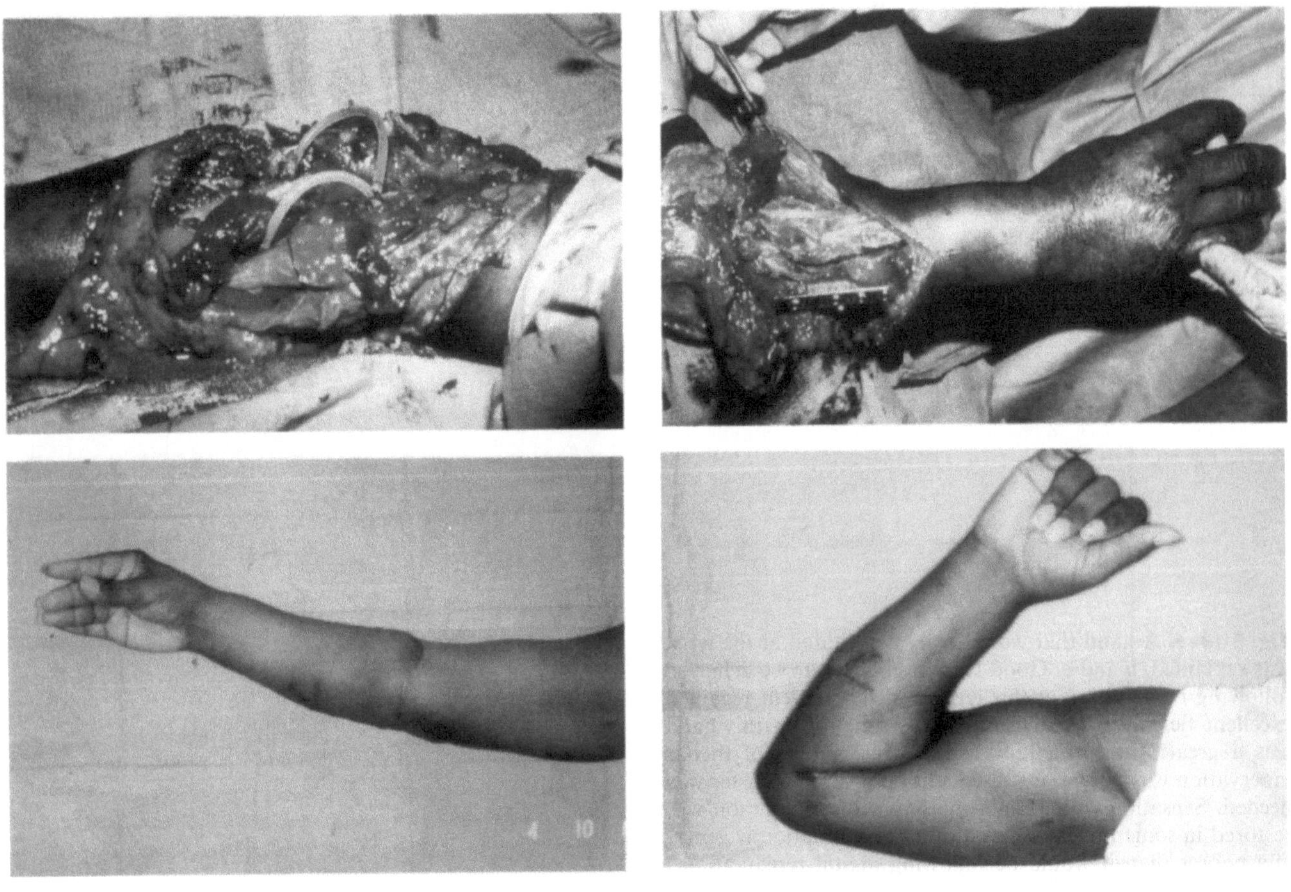
a b c d

a 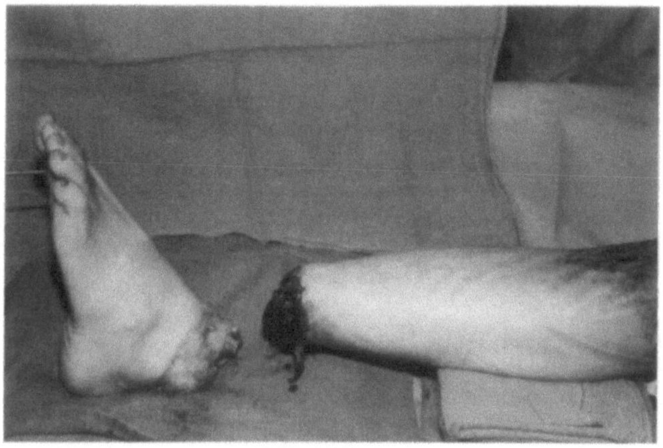 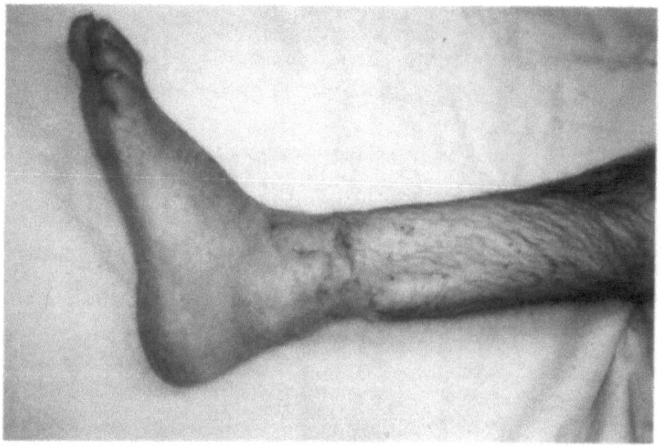 b

Fig. 5-16. a. This sharp amputation just proximal to the ankle required only 2 cm of shortening, and the posterior tibial nerve was in good condition on both sides of the amputation. Under these circumstances, replantation of a lower extremity is reasonable. **b.** An adequate functional result was achieved with protective sensation on the sole of the foot and a stable ankle. The patient walks with an imperceptible limp, and he has mild pain.

5.1.6 Above-Elbow Amputations (Malt and McKhan 1978, O'Brien et al. 1974)

Children fare better than adults following replantation at any level. Their regenerative potential is well known to hand surgeons, and justifies a limb salvage attempt that may not be appropriate in an older individual. Above-elbow amputations fall into this category. In adults, replantation above the elbow may be considered if there is a reasonable possibility of salvage and later function of the elbow. An attempt at salvage is justified when one considers the functional difference between an above-elbow and a below-elbow prosthesis.

In many situations, replantation above the elbow is doomed to a poor functional outcome, with the patient undergoing multiple procedures over a period of several years. Faced with that option, the patient would be far better served by closure of the amputation stump. Replantation is contraindicated in the presence of crushed or injured muscle, extensive nerve damage, or concomitant brachial plexus injury or avulsion (Fig. 5-17a).

◁

Fig. 5-15. a. This patient suffered an amputation at the proximal forearm level in a car accident. Because the patient arrived 4 hours after the injury, vascular shunts (Sec. 5.4.1) were used to connect the proximal with the distal vessels and end the period of ischemia in the amputated part. **b.** The shunts were retained while irrigation, debridement, bone fixation, and tendon repair were done. Thereafter, vein grafts were used to repair the radial and ulnar arteries. **c** and **d.** A good functional result with good extension and flexion of the elbow and good flexion of all but the small finger was achieved. The patient desired no further reconstruction. Sensation in the fingers was protective.

5.1.7 Multiple-Level Amputations (Fig. 5-17e)

Successful replantation is improbable if longitudinal structures have been injured at multiple levels. Although vascular repair can technically salvage an extremity damaged in this way, nerve and tendon function is unlikely to be satisfactory.

5.1.8 Lower-Extremity Amputations

Because lower-extremity prostheses function excellently, the indications for replantation are far narrower than those for amputated upper extremities. Replantation of the lower extremity should only be attempted under the following circumstances: (1) in cases of clean-cut amputation, (2) where less than 3–4 cm of shortening is required, (3) in the distal third of the leg or around the ankle, and (4) if there is good-quality nerve tissue for repair (Figs. 5-16 and 5-17c and d).

5.2 Contraindications (Fig. 5-17)

1. *Severity of damage.* Replantation is not feasible after multiple-level injuries, in cases of severe upper-arm injury that involves the brachial plexus or has other serious nerve damage, or where there has been severe vessel damage (Fig. 5-17).
2. *Ischemia time.* Even though there have been anecdotal reports of digital replantation after ischemia times of 24 hours or longer, the duration of ischemia should be kept as short as possible. With amputations proximal to the ankle or wrist, 6 hours of ischemia is the upper limit for safe replantation because muscle tissue is present in the amputated part (Sec. 5.1.5).
3. *Single-digit amputations.* Replantation of digits

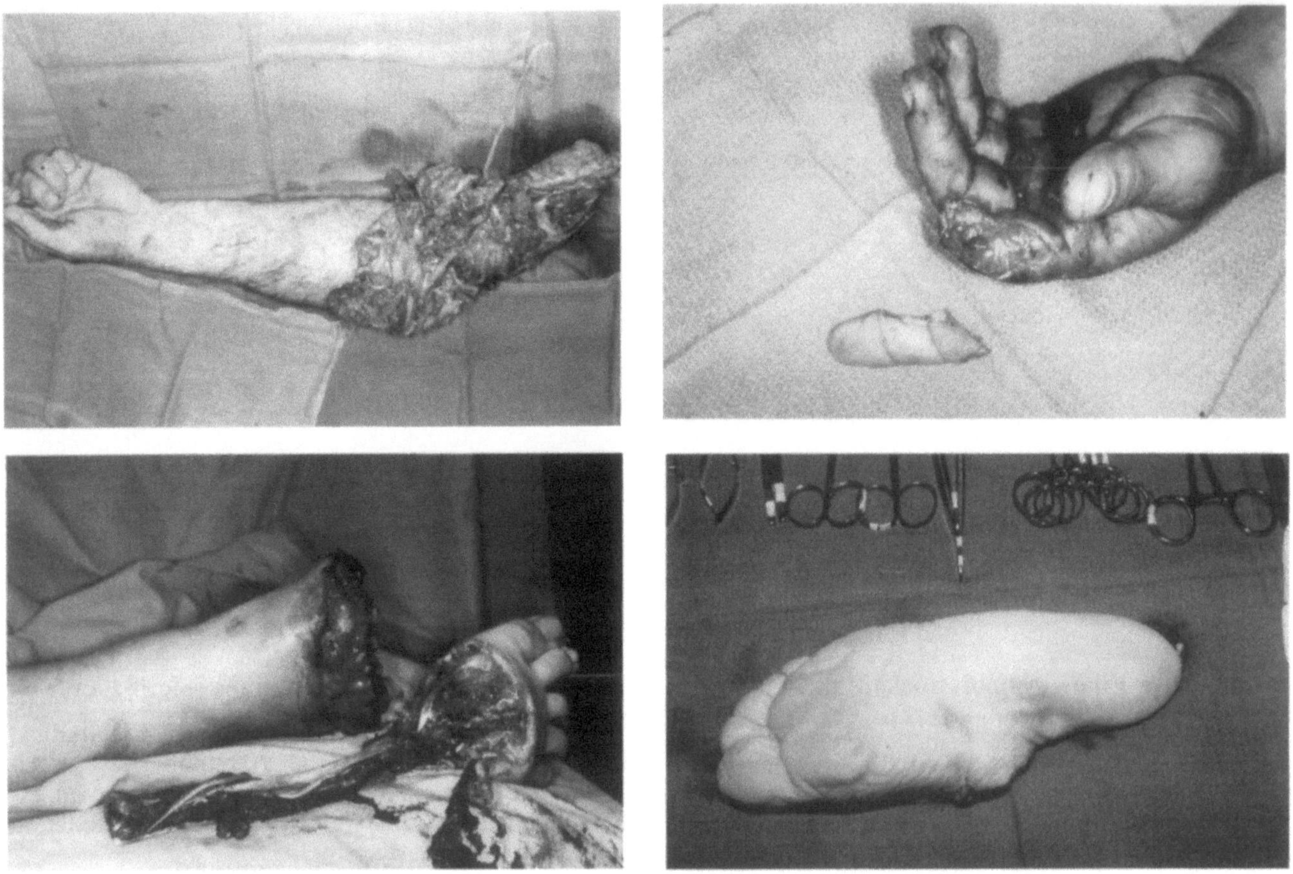

a b c d

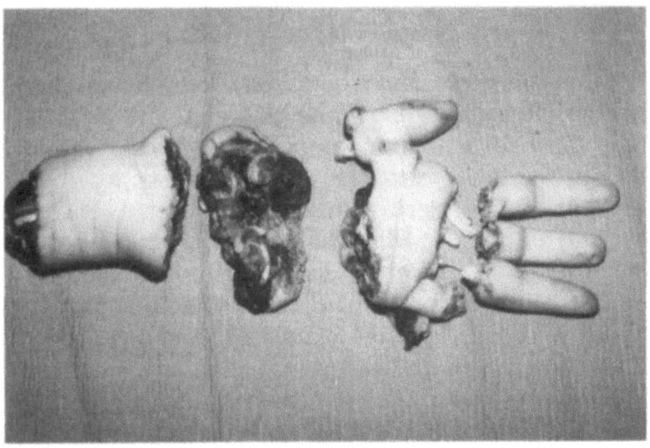

e

Fig. 5-17 a–e. The following injuries should not be replanted: **a.** Injuries that involve avulsion of major nerves of an extremity, such as the brachial plexus. **b.** Amputations of a single finger proximal to the flexor digitorum superficialis tendon insertion, or where the proximal interphalangeal joint has been severely damaged – with poor motion at the proximal interphalangeal joint, the finger is likely to be an obstacle to good hand function (Fig. 5-2). **c.** Crush or avulsion injuries of the lower extremity – if replanted, these parts will function poorly. **d.** Injuries in which the vessels have been avulsed. The "ribbon sign" results from hemorrhage along the course of a vessel and reflects avulsive damage to it. This sign is a predictor of failure of vascular repair, and can be seen in this foot. It will also be apparent following similar injuries in fingers. **e.** Multiple-level injuries – because these require multiple arterial, nerve, and tendon repairs, the ultimate function will not be adequate.

should not be performed when the amputation is proximal to the flexor digitorum superficialis insertion, or when there is severe injury to the proximal interphalangeal joint.

In my experience, *age* has not been a contraindication to replantation (Sekiguchi and Ohmori 1979). Some motivated senior citizens have done excellently in using their replanted parts, so motivation is more important than age. Unfortunately, this factor is difficult to assess in the emergency situation.

5.3 Emergency Department Care

The UCSF Hand and Microsurgery Service suggests the following protocol for the emergency department management of patients with amputated and/or devascularized parts.

1. **Stabilize the patient**. Start a large-bore intravenous line and administer a cephalosporin intravenously. Give tetanus prophylaxis as needed. Do not give the patient anything by mouth.

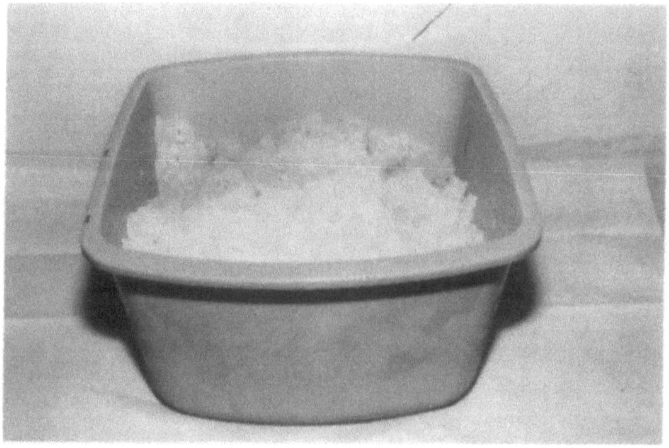

Fig. 5-18. Amputated fingers should be placed in a slightly moist sponge which is then placed in a dry, clean container. This container, in turn, is placed in a larger one containing ice. The amputated parts are not placed in direct contact with the ice, and dry ice is never used. In partial amputations, a plastic bag containing crushed ice is placed around the devascularized part. Crushed ice will conform to the contour of the amputated part better than ice cubes.

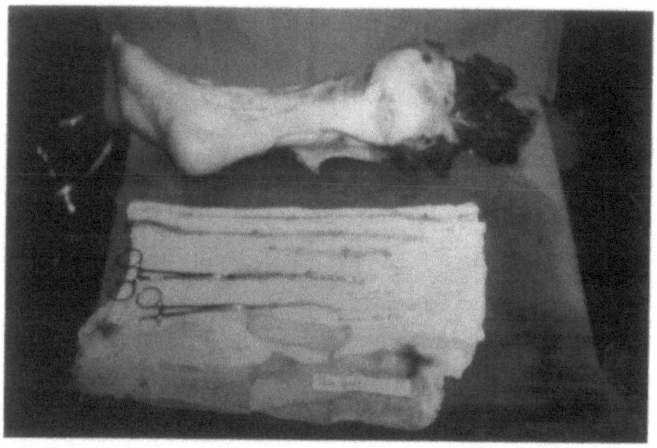

Fig. 5-19. Any amputated part that is not replantable should be used for "spare parts." This leg was not replantable, but nerve, vessel, and skin grafts were harvested to repair other injuries. Tissue transplants can also be harvested, often from donor sites that are not normally available; for example, when a foot cannot be replanted, the sole can be used as a free tissue transfer, or multiple toes can be combined with skin flaps.

2. **Prepare the amputated or devascularized part.** Cool the amputated part with regular ice as follows: If *completely amputated*, place the part in a dry container, and put this container in a larger one filled with ice (do not use dry ice) (Fig. 5-18). If *incompletely amputated*, dress the injured extremity, apply a splint, and surround it with a plastic bag containing crushed ice.
3. **Care of the injured extremity.** Wrap the wound in a bulky, soft dressing that has been soaked with an antibacterial preparation, and apply a splint.

5.4 Surgical Technique – General Considerations

5.4.1 Initial Preparation

As the patient and operating room are being prepared for surgery, additional surgeons should begin *preparing the amputated parts*. The amputated part is thoroughly irrigated and debrided, and each structure is tagged. Indeed, if multiple digits have been amputated, each one can be prepared by a different surgeon before the patient even arrives at the operating suite. Also, vein, nerve, or skin grafts can be harvested from nonreplantable parts (Fig. 5-19). In the operating room, the microscope is tested and adjusted, an appropriate mattress (e.g., an eggshell or other design appropriate for long operations) is positioned, and the room is warmed.

An axillary block *anesthetic* may be adequate for short procedures but is often inadequate for operations lasting longer than 4–6 hours. Although it has the benefit of sympathetic blockade, many patients become restless or anxious and begin to move, whereupon a general anesthetic becomes necessary. For this reason, if an operation lasting many hours is anticipated, a general anesthetic is given initially.

The patient is given intravenous *antibiotics* (a *cephalosporin*) at 6-hour intervals throughout the procedure. For extremely contaminated wounds or those involving a considerable amount of ischemic muscle tissue, *tobramycin* is added to combat any gram-negative organisms. Other antibiotics may be necessary, depending on the circumstances of the injury. Following muscle ischemia and revascularization, it is important to maintain good renal flow and urine alkalinization. Intravenous *sodium bicarbonate* is administered for this purpose. In these situations, the patient's blood potassium, electrolytes, pH, and P_{CO_2} are carefully monitored. Also, urine is tested for myoglobinuria, and a urinary catheter must be placed.

As was mentioned, the *duration of ischemia* is of critical importance when muscle tissue is involved. This crucial period can be ended by using a *Scribner shunt* to restore blood flow to the amputated or devascularized part (Figs. 5-15 and 5-20). If the duration of ischemia has been very long, the shunt can be placed when the patient reaches the emergency department, but it is more safely done immediately after the patient arrives in the operating room. The smallest size Scribner shunt adapter is sutured into the proximal and distal arteries, and the communicating tubing is connected. The adapters and tubing are tied securely into place in the vessel. Once the shunt has been placed, the surgeon must remain with the patient. Should the tubing disconnect, dangerous bleeding will result because the vessel will be unable to retract. The muscle is allowed to bleed

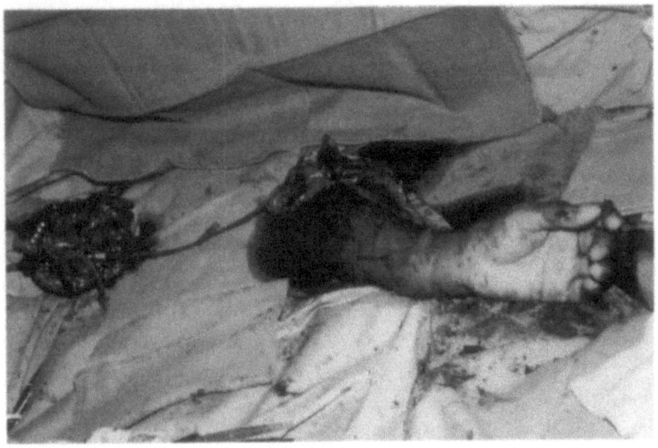

Fig. 5-20. This amputation above the elbow was temporarily revascularized with a shunt; this ended the period of ischemia and allowed bone fixation, debridement, and tendon and nerve repair to be done prior to the vascular anastomoses.

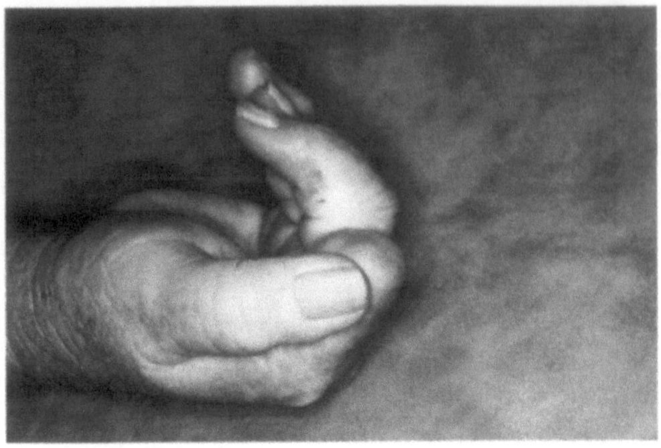

Fig. 5-21. Digital transposition provided fingers with intact proximal interphalangeal joints and some motion 6 weeks after injury (see also Fig. 5-32).

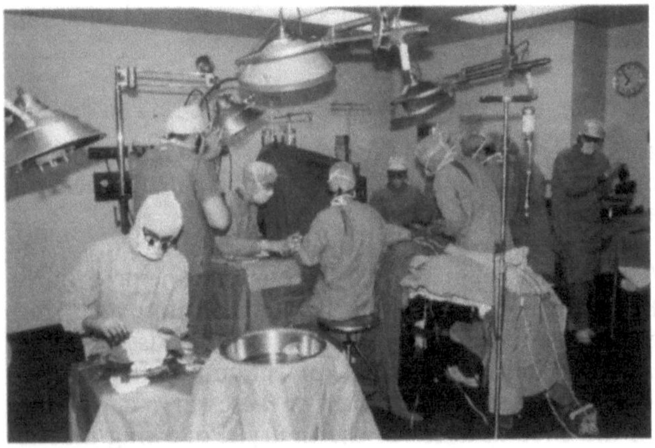

Fig. 5-22. Following amputation of both hands at the wrist level, replantation in this patient required four operating teams. While two surgeons prepared the amputated parts, two other teams prepared the amputation stumps. (Most replantation cases can be performed by a single surgeon and an assistant with equipment that is standard for most operating rooms. Some injuries, however, require the presence of expert surgeons over a course of many hours, and this can only be accomplished through a carefully coordinated effort. This photograph was taken during my fellowship at Massachusetts General Hospital [Courtesy of Richard J. Smith, MD†].)

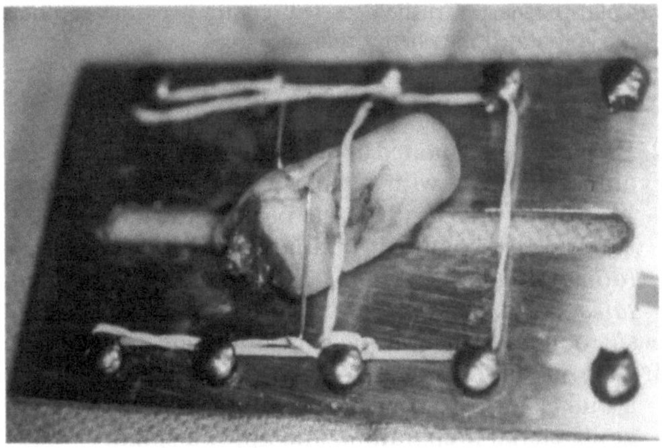

Fig. 5-23. This "digit board" holds an amputated finger in place so that a single surgeon can dissect and tag its structures (courtesy of Elaine Chiu). An incision is made just dorsal to the neurovascular bundle. Grayson's ligaments are incised, and both *digital nerves and arteries* are dissected and tagged with 6-0 silk suture. The *flexor and extensor tendons* are located and tagged with 3-0 or 4-0 nylon, and the *phalanges* are prepared for replantation. This preparation may require either wiring the loose pieces or shortening.

from the venous side for 15–20 minutes, and blood administration is usually required during this period. Venous egress releases many of the metabolites present in the muscle and ends the period of ischemia while the vessels are further dissected, debridement is completed, and bone fixation is accomplished.

Shortly after the operation begins, the regimen of *anticoagulation* is decided upon (Sec. 5.5.2). I use heparin only for severe crush or avulsion injuries. More routinely, low-molecular-weight dextran is given (a bolus of 50 cc is followed by administration at a rate of 30 cc/hour). Excessive bleeding can result from dextran, and is directly related to dosage. For children, I prefer heparin over dextran because the effect of the dose can be more accurately monitored.

5.4.2 Procedure Planning

The surgeon should carefully examine the injury and the amputated parts, and devise a general operative

† Deceased.

plan. First, the decision of whether to replant the amputated part must be made, and then the position the part should occupy must be considered. Transposition of digits is often beneficial (Figs. 5-21 and 5-32). If the thumb is too badly damaged for replantation, priority should be given to placing a digit in the thumb position. Salvage of a finger with an intact proximal interphalangeal joint is also a priority, and may be an indication for digit transposition. Replantation should start with the ulnar digits, and if only one or two digits are to be replanted, they should be in the long or ring finger position. This arrangement enables both large and small object grasp, which may not be possible if the digit is placed in the index finger position and later becomes stiff.

5.4.3 Debridement and Tagging

Two surgical teams can work simultaneously – one to prepare the injured extremity, and the other to prepare the amputated parts (Fig. 5-22).

The *wounds* are thoroughly debrided of necrotic and potentially infected tissue, and irrigated until clean. If the amputation is through the distal part of the forearm and divides the muscles in their distal third, it is likely that the distal segment of muscle will be devascularized. Despite revascularization of the amputated part, circulation to the distal part of each muscle is frequently intramuscular and not segmental, so the distal muscle remains devascularized. The distal muscle stumps should therefore be debrided.

The *injured extremity* is similarly prepared, and nerves, vessels, and tendons are tagged (Fig. 5-4). The fractured bone is prepared for fixation. Transposition of vessels from one finger to another is often a useful technique, depending on the pattern of the injury. Transposition of nerves is also sometimes helpful but is less desirable because cortical reorientation in older individuals will usually be incomplete.

Structures in the *amputated part* are tagged. It is sometimes difficult to position the finger, especially when no assistant is available for that purpose, so we have fabricated a small "finger holder" (Fig. 5-23). Exposure is accomplished through a longitudinal incision just posterior to the midaxial line (Nissenbaum 1980). This incision exposes the neurovascular bundles and allows elevation of a palmar and dorsal flap. The dorsal flap is elevated off the extensor apparatus, exposing the deep surface of the subcutaneous tissue of the dorsal skin. The veins of the finger can be identified on the deep surface of this dorsal flap and tagged with 6-0 nylon suture. The palmar flap is elevated. Grayson's ligament is divided, thereby exposing the digital arteries and nerves. Several veins are tagged with 6-0 silk suture, and the divided ends of the tendons are tagged with 4-0 nylon (Fig. 5-4). The bone is prepared for osteosynthesis by removing any devascularized fragments. Occasionally, bone shortening is necessary if the bone is severely comminuted or to allow nerve repair. If vessels have been damaged, vein grafts are used to compensate for any deficiency. After they are tagged, the digits are put back on ice.

5.4.4 Vein Grafts (Biemer 1981, Cooney 1978, Jupiter 1986) (Figs. 5-9, 5-31, and 5-33)

After a crush or avulsion injury, vein grafts should be planned. The best grafts for this purpose are taken from the dorsum of the foot, where veins of various sizes are generally present. To help mark out the course of available veins, the thigh tourniquet is raised to a pressure between systolic and diastolic, thereby making the available veins stand out. Veins in the distal part of the dorsum of the foot are usually of an appropriate size for use in replacing digital vessels, while veins at the ankle or proximal foot are best for forearm arteries and veins. One end of the harvested vein should be marked so that the vein can be appropriately reversed for arterial repair. One of the most common technical errors made by the inexperienced replant surgeon is the failure to liberally use vein grafts in replacing damaged arteries and veins.

5.4.5 Osteosynthesis (Gordon and Monsanto 1987, Ikuta 1978, Nunley et al. 1987, Tupper 1978, Urbaniak et al. 1978)

It is becoming increasingly evident that early postoperative range-of-motion exercises are important if good mobility is to be restored following replantation. I begin the patient on range-of-motion exercises as soon as swelling and healing permit. This point is usually reached within the first week after surgery. The exercises must begin well before osseous healing has occurred, which places several demands on bone fixation techniques.

Stable fixation is essential for stability in the angular and rotatory planes. The fixation techniques used **must not involve the proximal or distal joints** because these must be allowed mobility. Any technique used must lend itself to **fairly rapid execution** in order to minimize the period of warm ischemia. There is often poor vascularity in the region of the amputation, so bone healing is often slow; this is particularly true if vein grafts have been used to bridge segments of damaged vessels because the small branches to the tissues that normally would have supplied the area of the fracture have been lost. When this circumstance is encountered, a method must be chosen in which **the hardware can be retained** for several months while rehabilitation proceeds.

As the bones are prepared or the intraosseous wires are placed, it is helpful to place the bone ends through a piece of glove rubber or elastic bandage to protect the soft tissues (Jupiter 1986).

The following osteosynthesis techniques are the most commonly used in replantation (Fig. 5-24).

1. *Cross Kirschner wiring.* In this technique, crossed

Kirschner wires are driven retrograde into the amputated part. The fracture is reduced and the Kirschner wires are then driven proximally. This technique is quite simple and quick. Fixation is only fair. The disadvantage is unavoidable involvement of the surrounding soft tissues, which makes early mobilization difficult. In addition, it is difficult to avoid immobilizing adjacent joints, especially if they are near the amputation site.

2. *Intraosseous wiring* (Gordon and Monsanto 1987). This technique has many advantages: the adjacent joints are left mobile, even if the amputation is close to the joint; good fixation is achieved in all planes; and the wires need not be removed, thereby providing long-term fixation.

   A 24- or 26-gauge wire is passed through drill holes made proximal and distal to the fracture. The fracture is reduced and the wires are twisted tight. Several patterns of application can be used, depending on the soft-tissue exposure and lines of force in the particular bone. Care must be taken to provide fixation in all three planes, i.e., sagittal, coronal, and rotatory. The most frequently used patterns of application are coronal and sagittal wiring. Several other patterns are shown in Fig. 5-24.

   Intraosseous wiring can be combined with a variety of other techniques. For example, a single or cross Kirschner wire configuration can be combined with coronal or sagittal intraosseous wiring. For comminuted bones, circumferential wiring is sometimes useful as an initial step, followed by any of the various techniques described.

3. *Tension-band wiring* (Khuri 1986). This technique provides good fixation and resists angulation into flexion at the fracture site. As stress into flexion is applied at the fracture, the dorsal wire tightens and resists this force. The disadvantage is that the Kirschner wires often have to pass through the dorsal extensor apparatus, and when these wires are removed, the optimal fixation provided by the technique is lost.

   Two parallel and longitudinally oriented Kirschner wires are passed across the fracture site on the dorsal aspect of the phalanx, the metacarpal, or the wrist. Depending on the site, a 20- to 26-gauge wire is passed across the bone distally and brought in figure-of-eight fashion around the Kirschner wires as they exit the bone (Fig. 5-24e). This technique may be used successfully for fixation at the wrist level (Fig. 5-22) or for smaller bones in the hand. It is particularly useful for the fusion of small joints in the hand.

4. *Plating* (Nunley et al. 1987). The use of small plates is effective in stabilizing transverse fractures of the metacarpals and proximal phalanges. I also use plates in the forearm and humerus. Plates provide solid fixation, even for slow-healing fractures, and simplify dressing changes and postoperative therapy. With appropriate debridement and irrigation, the infection rate following plating is extremely low.

5. *External fixation*. This technique is reserved for situations where extensive bone loss requires later bone grafting.

Primary silicone arthroplasty can replace a joint that is completely destroyed if the wound is relatively clean. However, stiffness results from periarticular swelling and fibrosis, and seldom from incongruity of the joint surfaces. Primary silicone arthroplasties have therefore not been effective in providing good mobility.

5.4.6 Tendon Repairs

Flexor tenorrhaphy is performed with 3-0 or 4-0 nylon suture. Any of the standard tendon suturing techniques (e.g., the modified Kessler, the Kleinert, or the Bunnel stitch) can be used. If tendons are being transferred or if there is enough tendon length, a weave stitch should be used because it provides the strongest repair.

In my experience with late tendon reconstruction, I have often found the flexor digitorum superficialis and flexor digitorum profundus to be markedly adherent following replantation in "zone 2", making tenolysis difficult. In *zone 2*, therefore, I repair the flexor digitorum profundus alone. In *regions without pulleys*, such as the metacarpal region or the wrist, I repair both tendons. Occasionally, transfer of the flexor digitorum superficialis tendon proximally to the flexor digitorum profundus tendon distally may be useful.

Tendons that have been *avulsed* from their musculotendinous junctions do poorly because of edema and fibrosis. Following this kind of tendon avulsion, bleeding into the forearm can occur, and monitoring for compartment syndrome is important, especially if the patient is receiving anticoagulants. If the *flexor pollicis longus* has been avulsed, a tendon transfer may restore flexion at the interphalangeal joint of the thumb. The brachioradialis tendon is most frequently used for this purpose. More commonly, a fusion of the interphalangeal joint of the thumb is preferable. Initially, pinning of the interphalangeal joint suffices, and, if necessary, a formal fusion procedure can be done at a later date. *Silicone tendon rods* for later tendon grafting are not useful in the acute replant situation because infection, exposed wounds, and poor passive range of motion of the joints limit the benefits of the technique.

5.4.7 Arterial Repair

It is important to anastomose a *normal vessel* proximally to a normal vessel distally. Careful scrutiny of the intima under high-power magnification is essential. Some surgeons place great emphasis on a strong "*spurt" of blood* from the proximal artery. While this strong spurt is reassuring, spasm of a quality vessel can limit the force of this blood spurt from the proximal vessel. Yet, if uncertainty persists, it is always best to resect a greater amount of vessel and replace the injured vessel with a reversed vein graft. In general, the distal artery will be of adequate quality just distal to the *first*

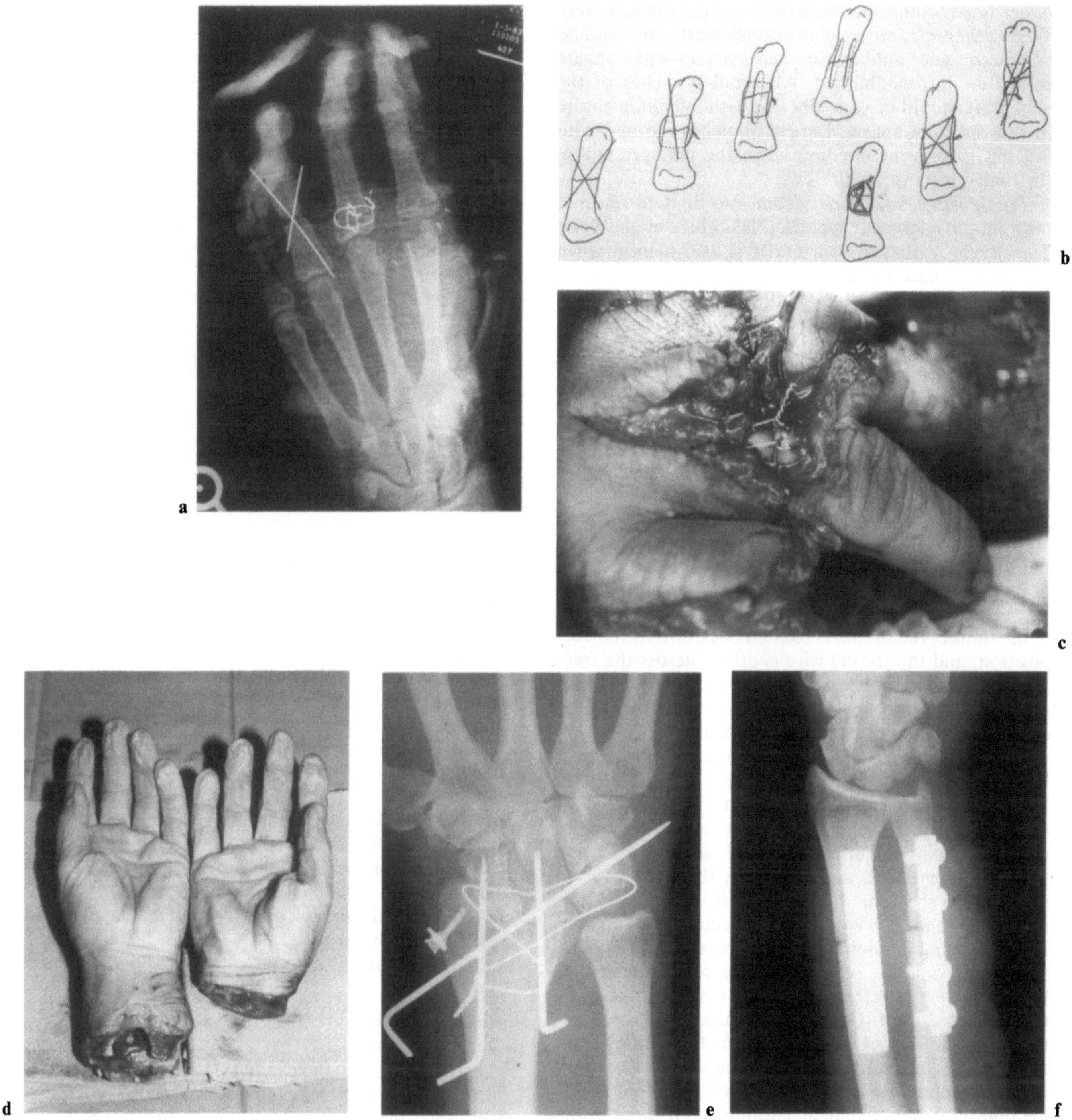

a b c d e f

Fig. 5-24. a. Three fingers had been amputated in this patient. The ring finger was amputated at the *midportion of the proximal phalanx*, and cross Kirschner wires were used for fixation. The long finger was amputated *very close to the metacarpophalangeal joint*. In order that this joint be left free after fixation, sagittal and coronal intraosseous wiring was used to provide stabilization. The index finger was amputated *through the metacarpophalangeal joint*. A primary silicone prosthesis was placed in an attempt to retain function in this joint. (In my experience, such prostheses have not been successful in retaining good joint mobility. It is not the joint surfaces that limit motion following replantation, but *capsular and periarticular fibrosis* and *tendon adherence*, and these are not affected by silicone arthroplasty.) **b.** Any of several patterns of intraosseous wiring combined with Kirschner wiring can be used. **c.** The fractures in this amputation just distal to the metacarpophalangeal joint were fixed with two intraosseous wires which provided both angular and rotatory fixation (Fig. 5-22). **d.** This patient sustained amputations of both hands. **e.** In the amputation that occurred through the wrist, AO figure-of-eight tension band wiring was used in combination with cross Kirschner wires. **f.** In more proximal amputations, plating is the best method of fixation. Plates provide stability and do not impede mobility, rehabilitation, or dressing changes. Except for the most contaminated wounds, the infection rate following plating appears to be no greater than that occurring with other fixation techniques. Meticulous debridement and irrigation are always essential, however.

intact branch (and vice versa for the proximal vessel). When *vein grafts* are used as arterial grafts, they should be placed under mild tension because they will elongate once flow is reestablished. All small branches of the vein graft should be carefully tied with 9-0 nylon suture to prevent later spasm. Larger branches are tied with 6-0 silk to prevent bleeding when the pressure within the lumen increases with flow.

Transposition of arteries from one digit to another may simplify vascular repairs (Nakamura et al. 1980). The use of Y-shaped vein grafts is also helpful when one is fortunate enough to find such a graft at the donor site (Jones and Jupiter 1985, Pho et al. 1979).

Positioning an amputated thumb for the arterial repair is particularly difficult. The ulnar digital artery of the thumb is considerably larger than the radial, but it cannot be easily exposed from either the palmar or the dorsal surface. This problem is greatly simplified by using one of several positioning techniques. A single longitudinal Kirschner wire is placed across the interphalangeal joint and fracture, and a second oblique wire is positioned at the fracture site, ready to be passed across it. The thumb is placed in a supine position if the ulnar artery is approached from the palmar side, or pronated if this artery is approached from the dorsal side. The vein graft is anastomosed to the ulnar artery in the thumb, the thumb is rotated back into the correct position, and the second wire is driven across the fracture. Alternatively, one can suture a vein graft to this ulnar digital artery prior to replacing the thumb (Pho et al. 1979, Shafiroff and Palmer 1981).

Once resection back to the normal artery or vein has been accomplished and the vessel is irrigated with heparin (100 units/cc) prior to the anastomosis, the vessel ends are dilated gently and the repair is done. I generally repair the artery first, followed by the nerve that accompanies it, and then turn the hand over to anastomose the vein. If possible, all repairs are done under *tourniquet control*. This approach has two virtues. First, bleeding is minimal and the repairs can be done simply and quickly. Second, the hyperemic phase after the tourniquet is released may improve circulation to the replanted digit. Once the tourniquet has been released, it should not be reinflated in the face of fresh anastomoses, as stagnant blood at the site of these anastomoses can initiate thrombosis. Therefore, with multiple-digit amputations, all anastomoses but those in the initial digit are generally performed with the tourniquet deflated.

Following vascular repair, the restoration of distal circulation may be slow. The rate at which circulation is restored may depend on the duration of ischemia. Failure to restore flow in the face of patent anastomoses may result from distal capillary and cellular damage that was probably caused by prolonged ischemia. Other causes of slow return of circulation must be considered, the most common being vessel spasm.

I take the following steps when spasm is thought to be responsible for inadequate distal flow:

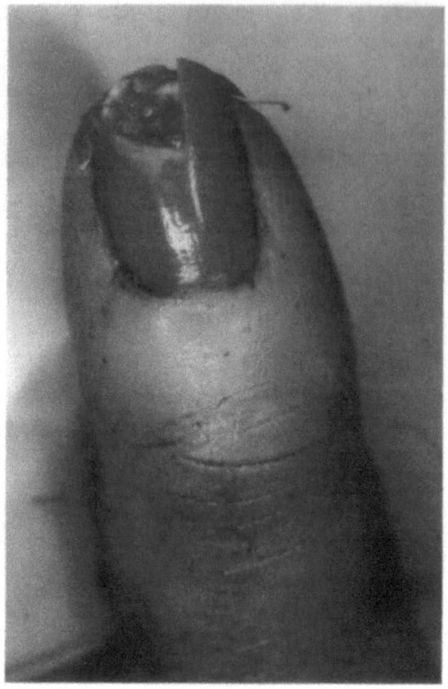

Fig. 5-25. Removal of a small part of the nail allows bleeding from the nail bed. If this area dries out, more nail can be removed.

Local Measures

1. A patency test is performed to ensure that the anastomosis is open.
2. Using a 25-gauge needle, topical bupivacaine HCl is delivered under mild pressure along the course of the vessel into the adventitia.
3. Under high-power magnification, the adventitia of the vessel is dissected and removed, and any untied small branches are ligated (even the tiniest of these can produce spasm).
4. Topical papaverine HCl is administered.
5. If available, the vessel on the opposite side of the digit is anastomosed.
6. Finally, a longer vein graft is used and the repair is redone.

Systemic Measures

1. One must make sure that a vasodilating anesthetic is being used, and one can also consider using chlorpromazine (an α-blocker) or isoxsuprene (a β-stimulant) (Sec 5.5.2). These latter two agents are more often used postoperatively.
2. Other systemic measures such as maintaining warm ambient temperature, irrigating with warm saline, and maintaining adequate blood pressure may also improve peripheral circulation and diminish vessel spasm.

5.4.8 Nerve Repairs

The nerve repair will largely dictate the functional outcome of the procedure. Nerve repairs should be done as carefully as vascular repairs, using 9-0 or 10-0 nylon suture. If mild tension is present, 8-0 suture can be

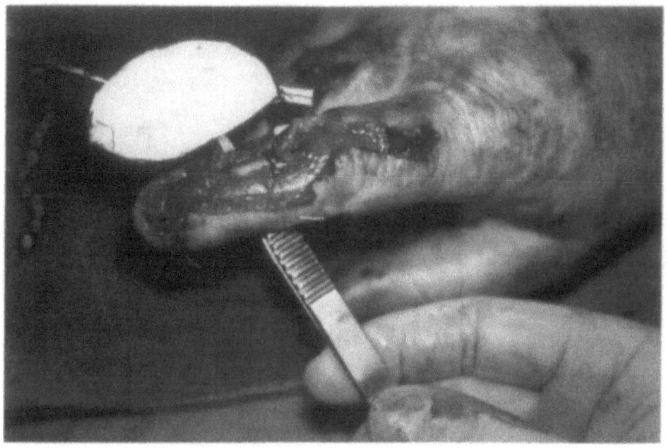

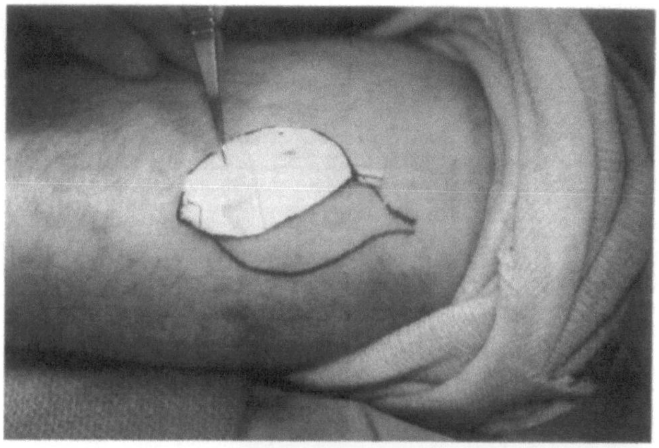

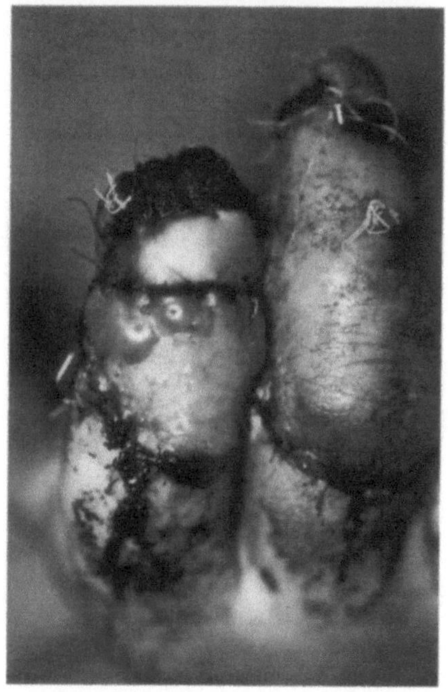

Fig. 5-26. a. This saw injury denuded the soft tissues on the dorsum of the finger. All of the fingers were badly damaged, so salvage of as much length of this index finger as possible was desirable. A vein was dissected proximally and distally, and the size of the planned flap was measured. **b.** The flap was centered over a vein in the proximal forearm. **c.** The flap is seen just proximal to a full-thickness skin graft. Despite initial congestion, the flap survived while the skin graft was lost. Enough length of the digit was salvaged for good pinch.

placed in the epineurium to hold the nerve together while 9-0 or 10-0 is used for subsequent stitches. I do not use primary nerve grafts because survival of the replant cannot be ensured. If the nerve is too badly damaged for repair, delayed nerve grafting 3–4 months after the replantation should be planned.

5.4.9 Venous Repairs

The dictum often quoted describes the use of two veins for each artery that has been anastomosed. If a good venous repair is accomplished with normal-looking vessels, a single vein will suffice. Indeed, it may be preferable to have a single well-repaired vein with a high rate of flow rather than multiple veins with relatively lower rates of flow. Vein grafts should be used as liberally to replace damaged segments of vein as they are to replace damaged arteries.

When performing very distal digital replantation, a vein may not be found in the amputated part, and yet venous egress must be accomplished. Several techniques can be used for this (Sec. 5.5.2).

5.4.10 Soft-Tissue Cover

Skin closure must be loose and involve as few stitches as possible. *Split-thickness skin grafts* are helpful and should be used liberally. They can successfully cover most soft tissues, including vascular grafts and anastomoses. An attempt should be made to cover tendons and fractures with full-thickness skin.

A flap containing a vein can be used to cover *dorsal or palmar finger wounds* (Yoshimura et al. 1987). Such a flap is particularly useful when a vein graft will be needed anyway. The vein graft is harvested from the proximal forearm with overlying skin, and grafted into the vein(s) of the finger (Fig. 5-26). On the *palmar surface*, skin defects can be covered with a similar flap, reversed, and anastomosed at the proximal and distal ends to a digital artery, or proximally to a digital artery and distally to a vein (Fig. 5-27). Of these combinations, the flap connected to a vein proximally and distally is the one least likely to fully survive, but it is useful if the underlying injuries preclude the use of a vein graft covered with a split-thickness skin graft.

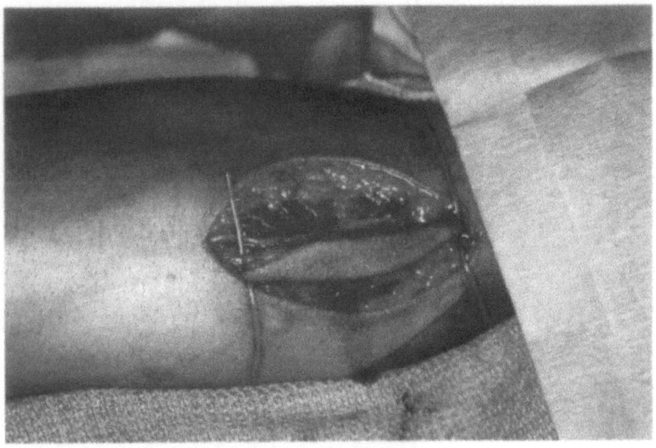

a

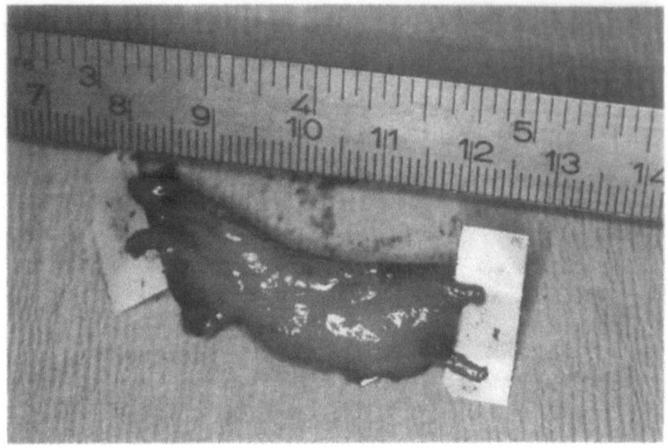

b

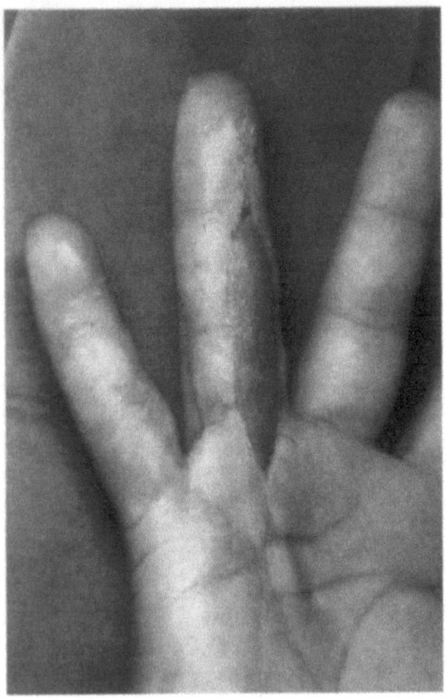

c

Fig. 5-27. a. This flap was centered over a forearm vein. The connections between the vein and overlying skin were carefully preserved. **b.** The deep surface of the flap is shown. **c.** The flap was reversed and interposed into the proximal and distal digital artery. The flap provided good cover over the extensive palmar digital wound.

In amputations proximal to the wrist where there has been some muscle ischemia, routine *fasciotomy* should be performed in the forearm, including both the volar and dorsal compartments (Fig. 5-28). These fasciotomy wounds should be left open and treated with skin grafting 3-4 days later or when the swelling has subsided.

5.5 Postoperative Care

Postoperatively, the patient should be in a heated room with the replanted part positioned well above the heart.

5.5.1 Dressings

Dressings should be applied extremely loosely. I use the following regimen: (1) Initially, antibiotic ointment is placed on the wounds to prevent adherence of the dressings. (2) Petrolatum gauze is then applied. Because such gauze can become caked with blood and cause constriction, it should be placed longitudinally and not circumferentially. (3) A bulky, soft dressing is then placed on both the palmar and dorsal surface, followed by a dorsal positioning splint. In the recovery room, dressings are often split down to the skin to prevent any possibility of constriction, and then loosely taped. It is important that the dressing provide warmth and allow access to the fingertips, which require monitoring.

The first dressing change can produce anxiety in the patient, which, in turn, can cause vascular spasm. If possible, the first dressing should be left in place for 4 to 5 days and then changed under adequate analgesia and sedation; this is done as a precautionary measure to avoid spasm, especially in children. A custom-made, low-temperature thermoplastic splint is then fabricated so that range-of-motion exercises can be initiated.

a 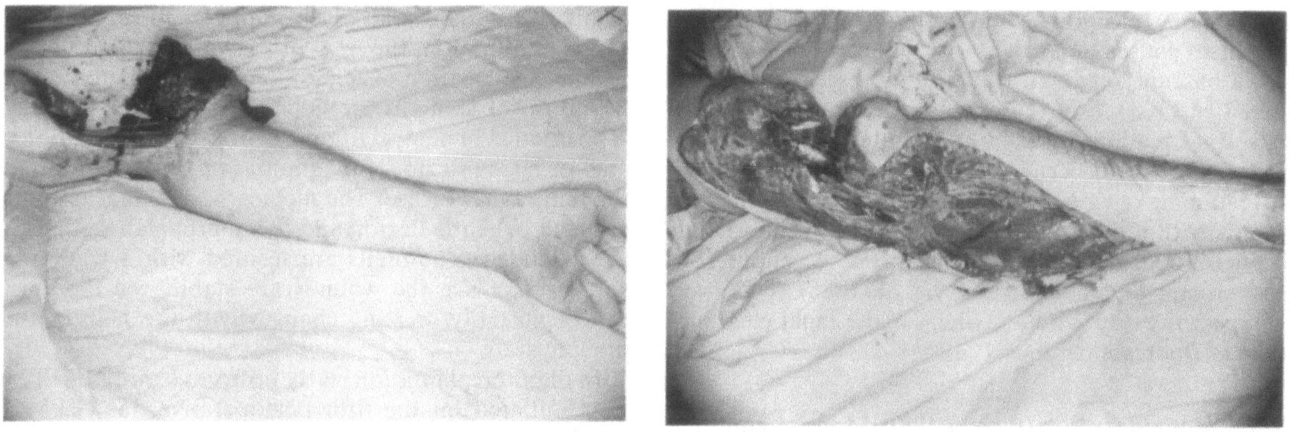 b

Fig. 5-28. a. This partial amputation of the upper arm was the result of a motorcycle accident. The forearm was ischemic for 4 hours afterward. **b.** The vessels were exposed and the muscle bulged as the fascia was incised. (It is extremely important to perform a fasciotomy of all compartments in all cases where the forearm muscles have been ischemic for more than 1 hour.)

5.5.2 Postoperative Medications

Each replantation center has its own protocol regarding anticoagulants and other medications. My protocol consists of the following:

1. *Aspirin*, 325 mg daily.
2. *Dextran*. A loading dose of 50 cc intravenously is used at the beginning of the procedure. Thereafter, 30 cc/hour is given for 5–7 days.
3. *Heparin* is used in crush or avulsion injuries. After administering a loading dose of 5000 units intravenously, 1000 units/hour is given. The dose thereafter depends on the partial thromboplastin time, which is maintained at 1.5-2 times the normal value. (Heparin is never used for microvascular free tissue transplants because the large surface area of the donor site has a great potential for hematoma formation.)
4. *Chlorpromazine HCl* (5–10 mg orally every 8 hours) is used as a peripheral vasodilator only if spasm is troublesome.

In amputations at the middle or distal phalangeal level where a usable vein cannot be found, venous drainage is effected by partial nail plate removal and bleeding from the nail bed (Fig. 5-25) (Gordon et al. 1985). In this technique, a wedge of nail is removed, intravenous heparin is administered, and a heparin pledget is applied to keep the nail bed moist. This pledget is changed every 20–30 minutes. Continuous, slow bleeding from the nail bed occurs for 3–4 days. After this period, venous channels form between the replanted part and the rest of the finger, and bleeding from the nail bed diminishes. If the digit becomes congested again, more nail plate is removed. The chance of such congestion is the reason only part of the nail is removed initially.

Other techniques to accomplish venous egress, such as leeches or bleeding from the suture lines, are used by some surgeons after replantation at this level. Leeches have the disadvantage of being socially objectionable, and there are difficulties with locating a reliable source of supply. Because they come in contact with the patient's blood, questions of parasite, bacteria, or virus transmission must be raised. Nevertheless, they are a useful option if venous congestion cannot be treated by other methods.

5.5.3 Monitoring

There are many methods of confirming circulation to the fingertips. Indeed, an experienced observer is probably as good as any monitor, using the signs of capillary return, turgor, color, and temperature. The dusky, swollen appearance of a congested digit, or the empty, wrinkled pallor of arterial compromise can usually provide an accurate clinical assessment. Frequently, however, the signs are less dramatic, especially early in the sequence of vascular problems. Also, it is often difficult to have an experienced observer available on a 24-hour basis.

The *ideal monitor* should be noninvasive, continuous, quantitative, reliable, sensitive, and specific. The *pulse oxymeter* (Fig. 8-2a), which meets all of these requirements, operates by measuring the level of saturated hemoglobin. A drop in pressure below 90 mm Hg indicates arterial occlusion. With venous occlusion, a further drop will occur approximately 1 hour after the problem arises. This apparatus is available in most anesthesia and cardiac care departments.

If a pulse oxymeter is unavailable, the *dermal quantitative fluorimeter* can substitute, but it has two disadvantages. First, the reading is taken every 2 hours and is therefore not continuous. Second, it requires a 1-cc intravenous injection of fluorescein, which occasionally produces nausea or an allergic reaction. With this method, a baseline reading is taken. Fluorescein is then injected intravenously (1 cc for an average-size adult). A second reading is taken 10 minutes later. A rise of at least 30% will occur if arterial circulation is intact. A reading taken 1 hour after injection will show a slow runoff with a decrease in the fluorescein value. If this decrease does not occur, the diagnosis of venous congestion can be made (Graham et al. 1985). This cycle is repeated every 2 hours, which is the renal clearance time of fluorescein.

5.5.4 Reexploration (Biemer 1981, Moneim and Chacon 1985)

When there is evidence of arterial or venous thrombosis, the part should be reexplored immediately. Patients are given nothing by mouth for 24 hours after surgery because of the possibility that reexploration may be necessary. If arterial or venous thrombosis is diagnosed early enough (within 1–2 hours), the other vessel (artery or vein) may still have flow. Heparin is useful in preventing thrombosis in these vessels. While many medications such as heparin and streptokinase have been advocated for the treatment of thrombosis, they are rarely indicated or effective when used alone. Reexploration is the only method that will provide reliable salvage. A salvage rate of 60–70% can usually be achieved with the use of vein grafts if the vascular problem is detected early enough.

5.5.5 Hand Therapy and Rehabilitation Program – by Pam Silverman, O.T.R.

The hand therapist becomes involved in the rehabilitation program within the second or third day after surgery. The therapist and surgeon review the structures that have been repaired, the level of the fractures, the nature of the injury, and then discuss any precautions that must be observed in the initial management. The first dressing is generally changed about 4–5 days after surgery. This dressing change should be done sooner if there has been excessive bleeding or if there is any question that the dressing is constrictive. In cases where the amputation was proximal to the wrist and there is a large amount of muscle tissue in the replanted part, dressings should be changed daily because swelling and muscle necrosis predispose the patient to infection and subsequent vascular problems. Regular dressing changes allow an early diagnosis of such problems.

0 to 10 Days (Acute Phase)

Once it is removed, the bulky, soft dressing is replaced and the therapist carefully designs and fabricates a static dorsal positioning splint. In the initial evaluation and treatment planning, the therapist must take into account the stability and level of the fracture, the level of the amputation, the level of the vascular and neural repairs, the location of tendon repair, and the type and condition of skin closure and any grafting. The wrist is positioned in neutral for more proximal amputations, and in slight flexion for amputations at or distal to the midpalmar crease. The metacarpophalangeal joints are held in gentle flexion and the interphalangeal joints are extended. The digits are secured with a wide and soft strap. Once the wounds are stable, the therapist can begin daily dressing changes with the help of the nursing staff.

In digital replantation, early protective motion (EPM I) is initiated on the fifth postoperative day. EPM I consists of simple tenodesis exercises, with gentle wrist flexion. This position allows the metacarpophalangeal joints and interphalangeal joints to gently extend. The wrist is then brought to a neutral position with simultaneous flexion at the metacarpophalangeal and interphalangeal joints.

10 Days to 3 Weeks

At this point, the next stage of early protective motion (EPM II) is begun. EPM II involves the following: (1) The wrist is positioned in *neutral* and the fingers are brought into an *intrinsic-plus* position, with the metacarpophalangeal joints flexed and the interphalangeal joints extended. The patient is asked to *hold* this position. (2) From the above *intrinsic-plus* position, the digits are carefully placed in a *claw* or *intrinsic-minus* position, with the metacarpophalangeal joints in extension and the proximal interphalangeal and distal interphalangeal joints gently flexed. The patient again holds this position. Edema and pin placement may initially limit these positions.

Certain precautions must be taken:

1. Proximal interphalangeal joint flexion should be limited to 60° if there is a zone 2 extensor tendon repair. The extensor tendons generally function poorly following replantation in this region, and there is often an excessive pull of the flexor tendons, causing a late flexion contracture of both the proximal interphalangeal and distal interphalangeal joints. Tenolysis of the extensor tendons is difficult and often unrewarding. For this reason, the extensor tendons should be favored and flexion of the fingers limited.
2. If there is a nerve or vascular repair at the proximal interphalangeal joint level, motion should be limited to approximately 30° of extension until about 3 weeks, at which time it is safe to proceed without risk of damage.
3. The claw position is begun as a passive exercise. It progresses to an active exercise at approximately 10–14 days.
4. If the level of tendon repair is distal to the proximal interphalangeal joint and the flexor tendon has been repaired, the dorsal blocking splint should be com-

bined with a palmar platform splint; this discourages development of a mallet finger, and flexion/extension should be limited to approximately 10° at the distal interphalangeal joint. In zone 2 injuries, more distal interphalangeal joint motion is permissible, but only if the finger is maintained in extension between hand therapy sessions.

3 to 8 Weeks

The range-of-motion exercises are continued, with passive and active composite motion permitted at approximately 4 weeks. In addition, dynamic splinting with rubber bands is also instituted at about 4 weeks, with alternating composite extension and flexion. These splints are frequently needed following digital replantation to increase composite passive motion. Muscle reeducation, activities that promote dexterity, and progressive resistive exercises are begun at about 8 weeks.

Other aspects of hand function receive attention, depending on the particular needs of the patient. *Edema control* with retrograde massage, compressive wrapping, and contrast baths are begun at approximately 3 to 4 weeks. Vascular supply and pain must be monitored. The edema control techniques may also decrease pain. If *desensitization* is necessary, vibration techniques and dowels are useful. Compression gloves can be prescribed after 8 weeks.

As wound care, motion, and attention to hand function continue, many other facets of the patient's rehabilitation program must be considered. The patient's reaction to injury and motivation are perhaps the most important factors in the rehabilitation process. *Psychologic supportive* measures are extremely important. Early reintegration of the individual back into the workplace is particularly helpful in this regard, especially if the employer can provide a light-duty position. Anything that brings the patient closer to functioning as he or she did prior to the injury is beneficial. Work hardening programs, job retraining, and dominance change must all be considered at the appropriate time.

Any *reconstructive surgery* is generally undertaken once hand swelling and inflammation have resolved. This resolution generally takes about 6 months. Finally, the "team approach" in handling these complex injuries can markedly improve the result. It is therefore important to include family and other support systems as well as insurance companies, rehabilitation nurses, and vocational counselors in the rehabilitation program.

5.5.6 Late Reconstruction (Figs. 5-29 and 5-30)

To restore the best possible function, later reconstruction is often necessary. It is important to wait for all inflammation and swelling to subside before proceeding; this usually takes about 6 months, but it may be longer if foreign material is present, if there has been infection, or in cases of crush injury. The most common reconstructive procedures are tenolysis, tendon reconstruction, and nerve grafting (Fig. 5-29). If tenolysis is not possible and tendon grafting is necessary, two-stage reconstruction is almost always needed because of the magnitude of these injuries and their propensity for scarring (Fig. 5-30).

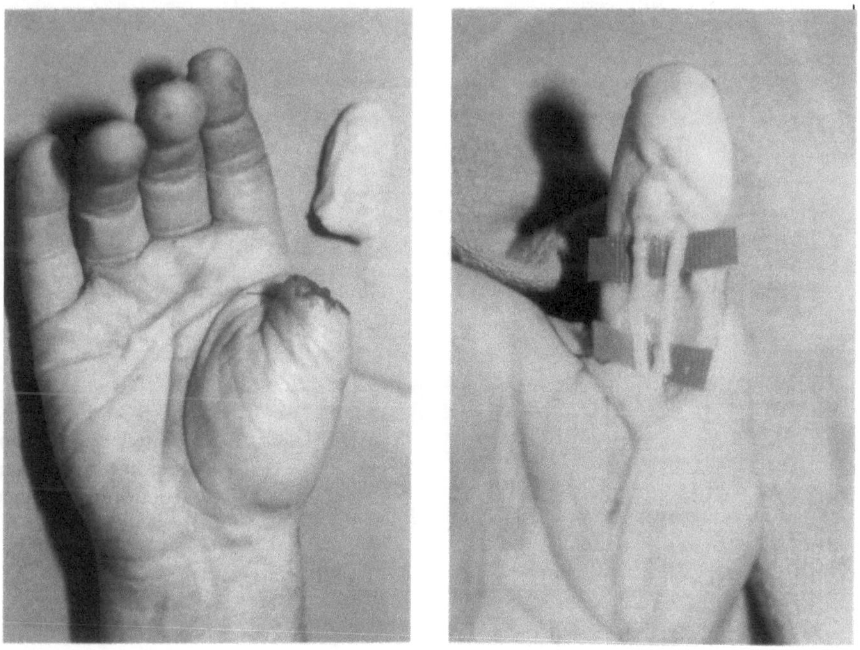

Fig. 5-29. a. This sharply amputated thumb was replanted. **b.** Two nerve grafts were performed to improve sensation. **c** and **d.** Good mobility and 8-mm two-point discrimination were achieved (see next page).

a b

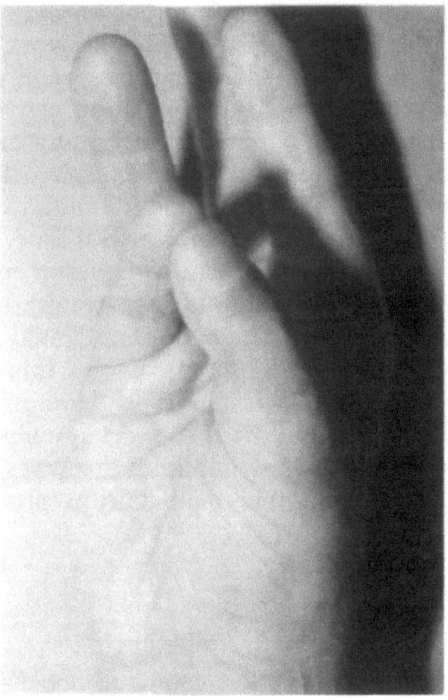

c

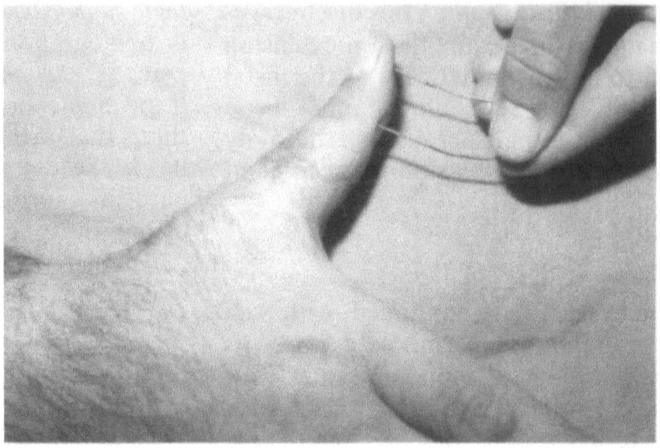

d

Fig. 5-29c, d

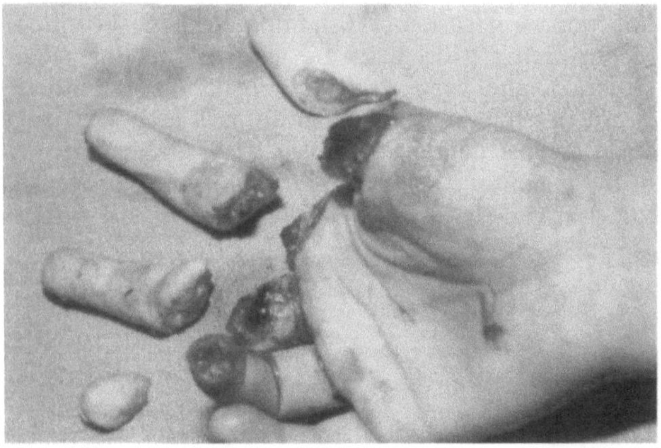

a

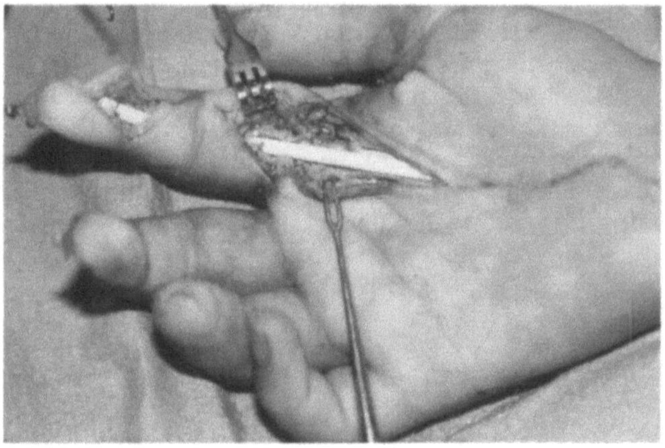

b

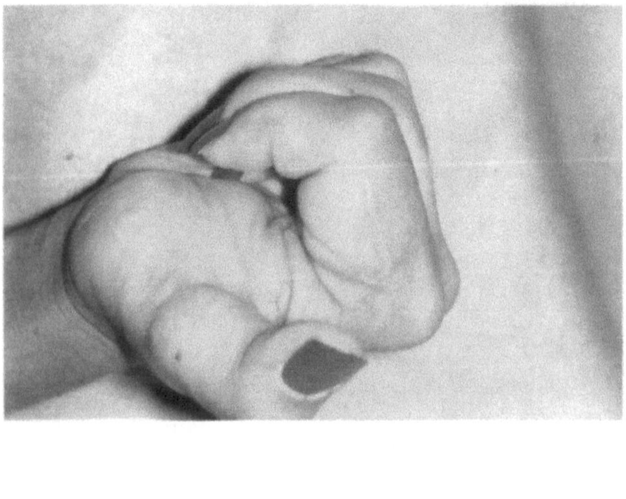

c

Fig. 5-30. a. This patient's thumb and three fingers were amputated by a tile-making machine. **b.** Poor flexor tendon excursion required tendon reconstruction. (A two-staged reconstruction using silicone rods is almost always needed following these injuries.) **c.** A good functional result was achieved.

5.6 Surgical Technique

5.6.1 Thumb Replantation (Fig. 5-31)

a. This 35-year-old patient was involved in a roping accident and sustained an amputation of the thumb at the interphalangeal joint level. Because this was an avulsive injury, vein grafts were planned.

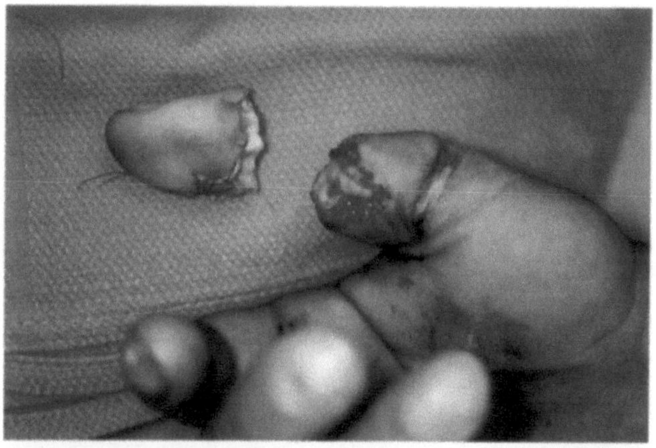

a

b. The radial artery is palpated and marked on the dorsal aspect of the hand between the first and second metacarpals. The veins are outlined; these are planned as the recipient vessels.

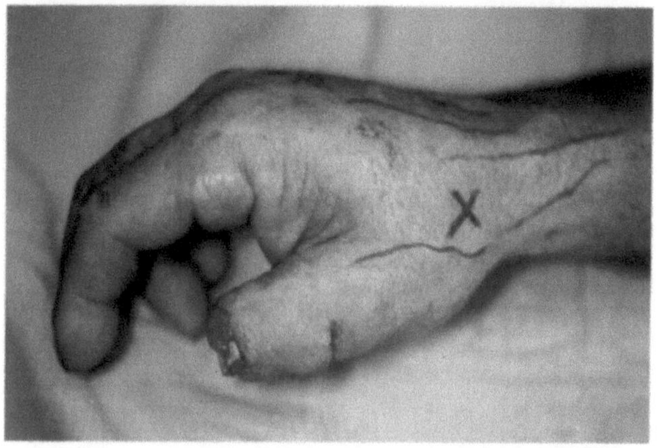

b

c. The amputated part is prepared by tagging the *digital artery and nerve* on both sides and dissecting a dorsal vein.

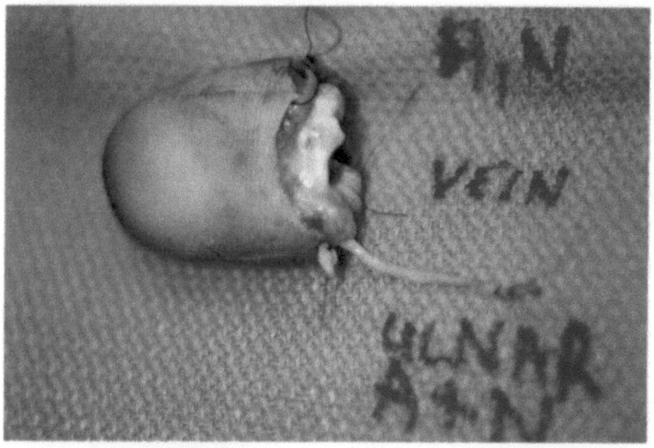

c

d. A vein graft is harvested from the foot and taken to another table where it is sutured to the *ulnar digital artery* and a dorsal vein. In the thumb, the ulnar digital artery is always much larger than the radial artery.

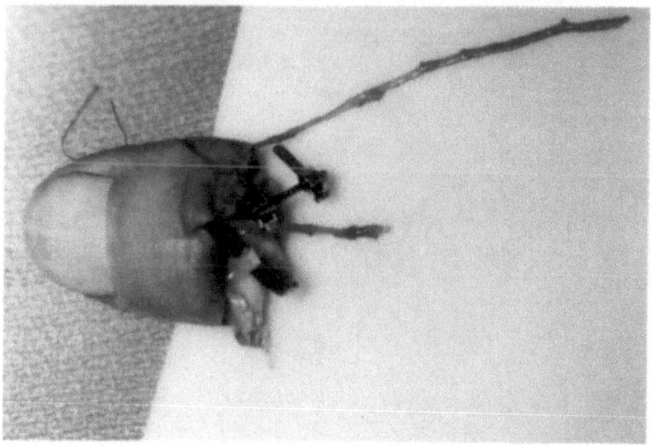

d

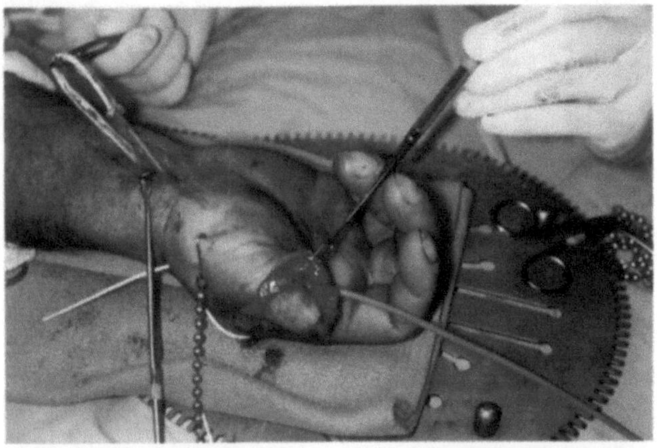

e

e. The *extensor pollicis longus* and *flexor pollicis longus* are identified. The flexor pollicis longus is sutured to a catheter and delivered into the distal wound. The digital nerves are also dissected and tagged on the palmar surface.

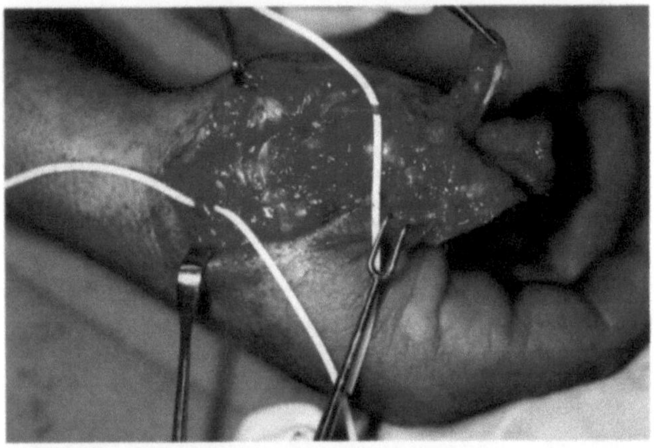

f

f. Three structures are dissected and tagged on the dorsal surface: (1) the radial artery, (2) a dorsal vein, and (3) the extensor tendon.

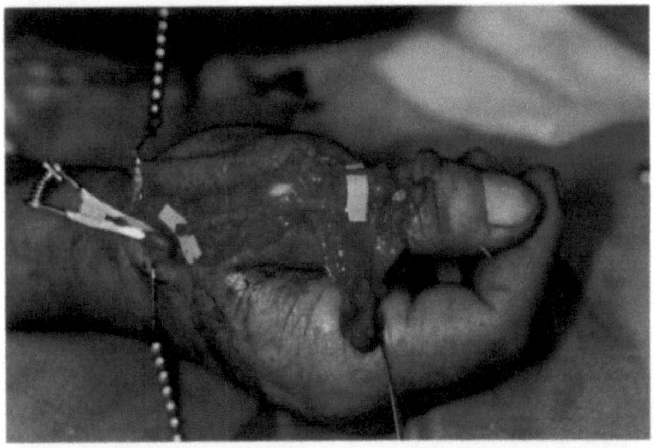

g

g. Thumb fixation is performed with cross Kirschner wires passed retrograde into the amputated part, which is then positioned on the amputation stump. The Kirschner wires are then passed proximally into the proximal phalanx. Next, the dorsal vein is repaired. The vein graft connecting the ulnar digital artery to the radial artery is then anastomosed end-to-side to the radial artery. The skin is closed loosely.

5.6.2 Digital Replantation

(Fig. 5-32; see also Fig. 5-21)

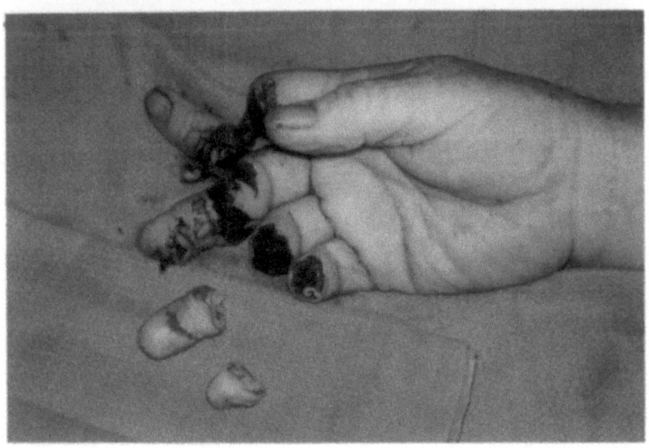

a

a. A 45-year-old man sustained a saw injury to all of the fingers of his right hand. After inspecting the amputated part, it is evident that the artery of the amputated small finger is injured too distally for replantation, but the proximal interphalangeal joint in this finger is intact on the hand. The index finger is too badly damaged to salvage. The overall situation makes digital transposition advisable in order to salvage as many fingers with intact proximal interphalangeal joints as possible.

b. The index finger is inspected and the distal part is found to have an adequate neurovascular bundle, but the damage proximally precludes its replantation.

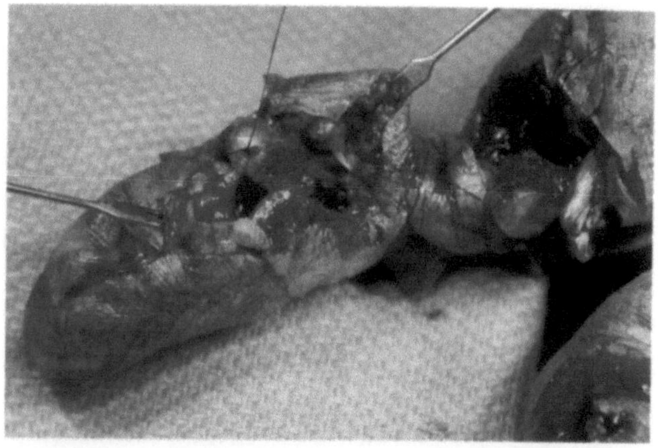
b

c. The amputated index finger is dissected through an incision just dorsal to the neurovascular bundle. The nerve can be seen with the artery just dorsal to it.

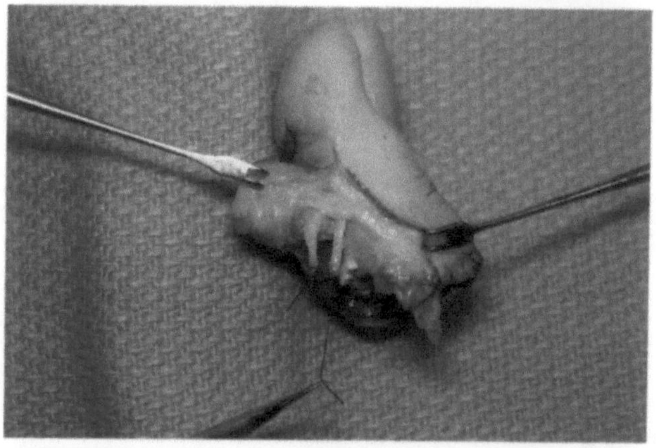
c

d. The dorsal skin flap is then raised off the extensor tendon, and, on inspection of the deep surface of this flap, veins can be identified. A vein has been dissected and tagged.

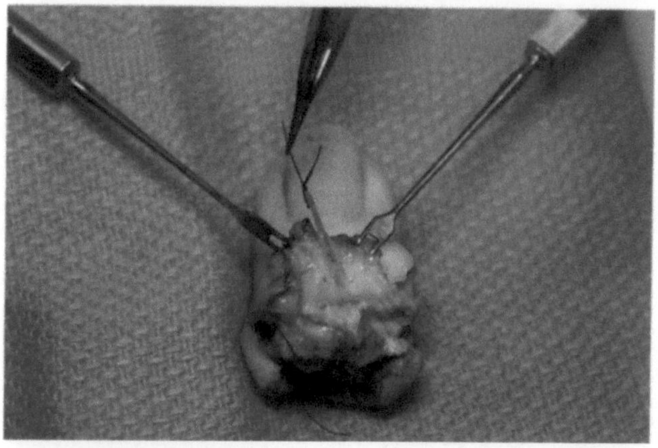
d

e. The neurovascular bundles are identified in the amputation stumps. The artery and nerve are dissected through incisions just posterior to the midaxial line. The arteries and nerves are tagged with 6-0 silk suture. The flexor and extensor tendons are also identified. An incision at the midpalmar crease may be necessary to identify the flexor tendon and deliver it into the distal wound. These tendons are then tagged with 3-0 nylon.

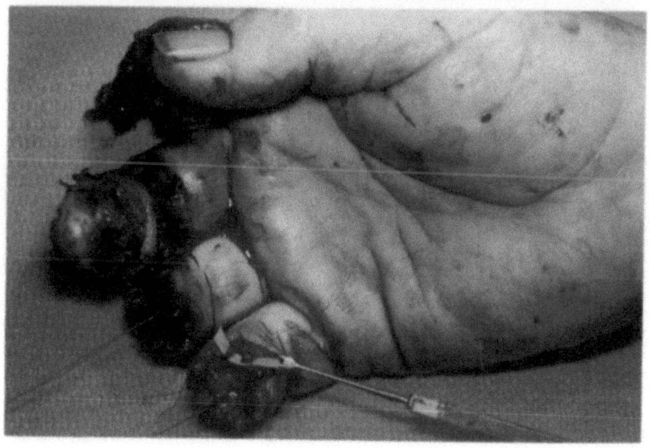
e

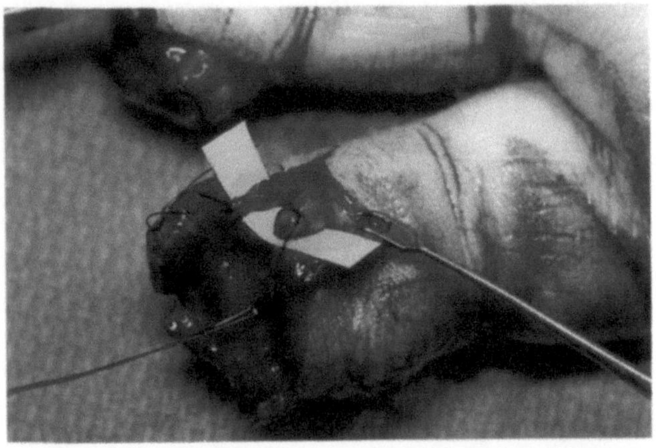
f

f. A close-up of these structures.

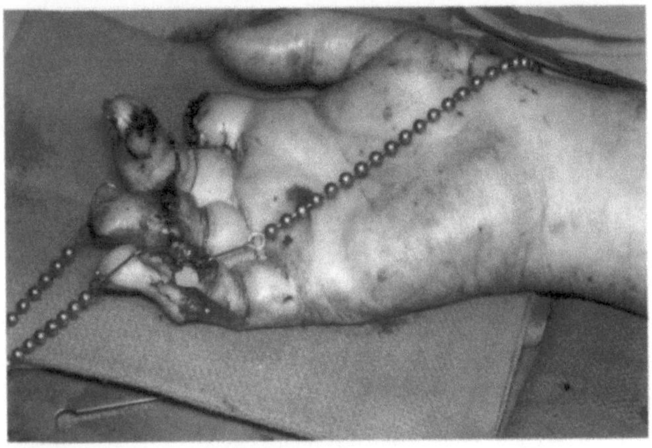
g

g. Appropriate retraction is important and the fingers are positioned so that exposure is not impeded.

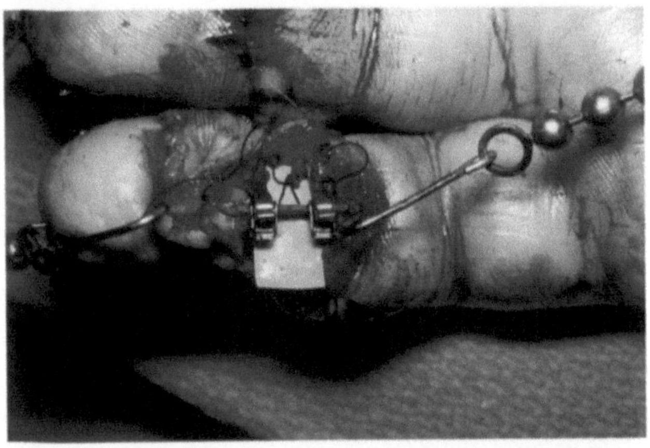
h

h. The bone fixation is accomplished (Sec. 5.4.5) (Fig. 5-24) and the flexor tendon is then repaired. Repair of one or both digital arteries and both digital nerves is performed.

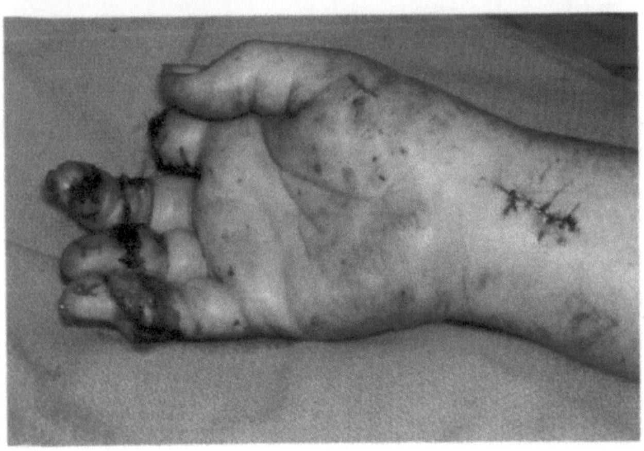
i

i. At the end of the procedure, there are three fingers with good neurovascular repair and intact proximal interphalangeal joints. The index finger is in the ring finger position, and the ring finger is in the small finger position (Fig. 5-21).

5.6.3 Ring Avulsion Injury (Fig. 5-33)

a. This 38-year-old fireman sustained a ring avulsion injury with devascularization of the finger and avulsion of the soft tissues to the distal phalangeal level.

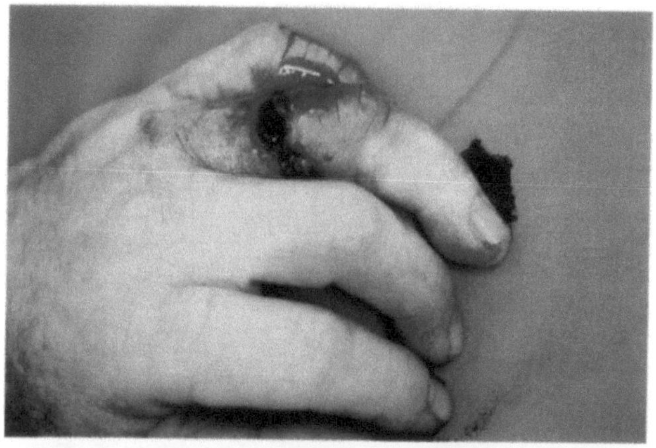

a

b. Both digital nerves are intact, but the digital arteries have been severely damaged and the digit has no vascularity. A vein graft has been harvested and reversed for use in the arterial reconstruction. The artery must be resected proximally and distally back to where it is normal. After transecting the artery, the intima should appear normal under high-power magnification. Often, the first normal segment of artery will be beyond the first uninjured branch.

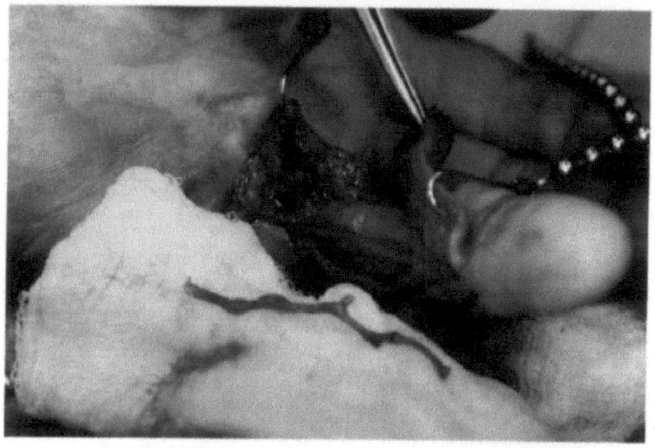

b

c. A vein graft is also used to repair the vein.

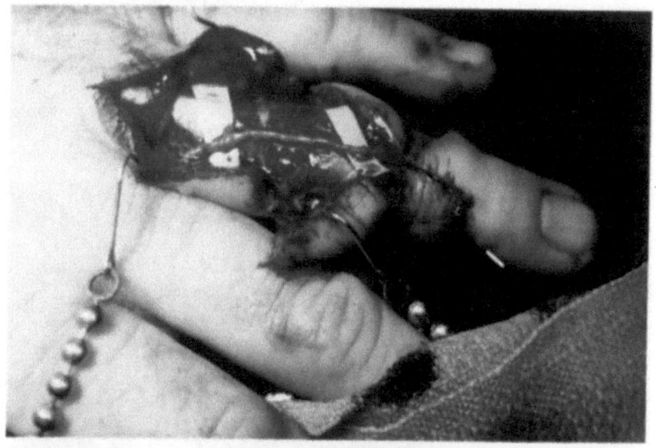

c

d and e. An excellent functional result with normal sensation can be achieved following this type of injury.

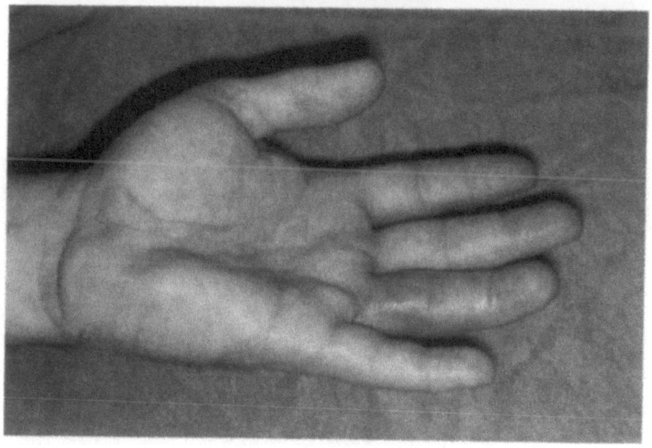

d

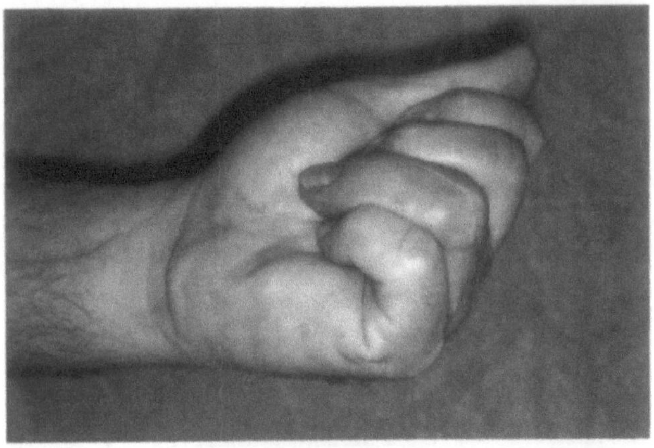

e

Fig. 5.33e

5.6.4 Vein Graft Harvesting (Fig. 5-34)

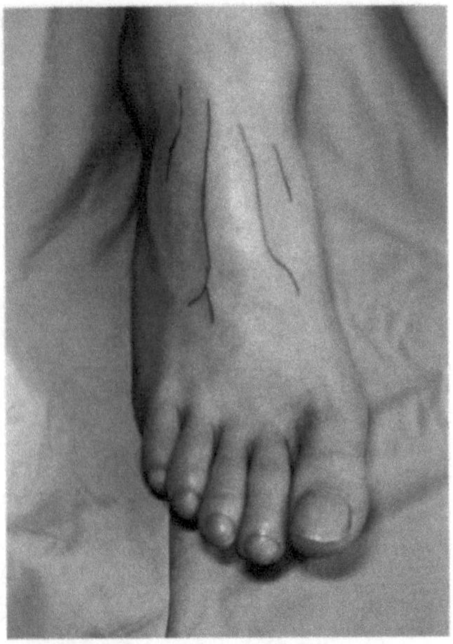

a

a. The thigh tourniquet is adjusted so that blood pressure is between systolic and diastolic; this makes the veins on the dorsal aspect of the foot and ankle stand out so that they can be marked. The smaller of the veins on the dorsum of the foot are generally of appropriate size for use in the fingers. The veins found at the ankle are used for wrist and more proximal repairs.

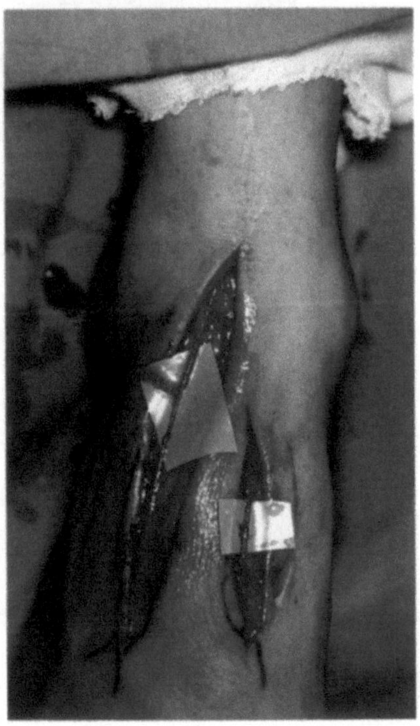

b

b. In dissecting the veins, all side branches are tied. The small branches are tied on the side closest to the parent vein with 9-0 nylon suture while the larger ones are tied with 6-0 silk. The opposite side can be coagulated with a bipolar coagulator. Heparinized saline (100 units/cc) is flushed through the vein graft prior to its use. One end of the vein graft is marked to make sure the vein will be appropriately reversed for arterial repairs; otherwise, venous valves will not allow blood flow. Great care in vein harvesting will decrease the problems of spasm and leakage at the recipient site.

5.7 Selected Bibliography

Biemer E (1981) Salvage operations for complications following replantation and free tissue transfer. Int Surg 66:37

The author found thrombosis following replantation to be largely on the venous side. He treated this with thrombectomy, heparin, dextran, and aspirin. Clinical presentation and causes are discussed. (In my experience, thrombosis occurs about as frequently in the arteries as it does in the veins. Prompt reoperation and placement of vein grafts provides the best chance of salvage.)

Chow JA, Bilos ZJ (1983) Forearm replantation. Long-term functional results. Ann Plast Surg 10:15

The surgical technique and results of forearm replantation are described. The importance of excellent nerve repair is emphasized and the authors' rehabilitation program is discussed.

Chow JA, Bilos ZJ, Chunprapaph B (1979) Thirty thumb replantations. Indications and results. Plast Reconstr Surg 64:626

Thumb function has been assessed to be 40% of hand function, so almost all thumb amputations should be replanted. The functional result is generally good. The demands for motion in the thumb are not as great as for the fingers, so most of the patients who had interphalangeal joint fusions had good thumb function. Bone was generally shortened 6–10 mm. (I feel that bone shortening should be minimized but may be indicated to allow nerve repair. For vessel damage, vein grafts are preferable to bone shortening. Shortening bone more than 10 mm should be done only rarely.)

Cooney WP III (1978) Revascularization and replantation after upper extremity trauma. Experience with interposition artery and vein grafts. Clin Orthop 137:227

The problem of failed replantation in cases of severe crush or avulsion injury is described. For improved survival, the use of patient selection criteria, interpositional artery or vein grafts for diffuse vessel damage, and anticoagulants are discussed. Some contraindications to replantation are also given.

Earley MJ (1986) The arterial supply of the thumb, first web and index finger and its surgical application. J Hand Surg 11B:163

This article details the vasculature of the thumb, index finger, and palm, including the anomalies. Variations of the princeps pollicis artery should be noted as well as the relative vessel size that can be expected (e.g., the radial digital artery of the thumb is consistently smaller than the ulnar digital artery).

Gordon L, Leitner DW, Buncke HJ, et al (1985) Partial nail plate removal after digital replantation as an alternative method of venous drainage. J Hand Surg 10A:360

The technique of venous outflow through the nail bed in combination with systemic anticoagulation is described. The authors consider this the method of choice for treating the problem of venous engorgement after digital replantation when venous anastomosis is not possible.

Gordon L, Monsanto EH (1987) Skeletal stabilization for digital replantation surgery. Use of intraosseous wiring. Clin Orthop 214:72

Different patterns of intraosseous wiring are described. These patterns allow mobility in the proximal and distal joints, which is important for postoperative therapy.

Graham BH, Gordon L, Alpert BS, et al (1985) Serial quantitative skin surface fluorescence. A new method for postoperative monitoring of vascular perfusion in revascularized digits. J Hand Surg 10A:226

This method of monitoring replanted and revascularized parts is described.

Harris GD, Finseth F, Buncke HJ (1980) The hazard of cigarette smoking following digital replantation. J Microsurg 1:403

The harmful effect of cigarette smoking following replantation surgery is well known, and patients should be cautioned about this danger before their procedure.

Ikuta Y (1978) Method of bone fixation in reattachment of amputations in the upper extremities. Clin Orthop 133:169

This article discusses the surgical procedures for replanting amputated limbs and digits. The details of bone fixation of the upper arm, elbow joint, forearm, wrist joint, hand, and digits are included.

Jones NF, Jupiter JB (1985) The use of Y-shaped interposition vein grafts in multiple digit replantations. J Hand Surg 10A:675

The use of Y-shaped vein grafts is described. The single proximal limb is anastomosed to the common digital vessels, and the two distal limbs are anastomosed to two digital arteries.

Jupiter JB (1986) Replantation. In Watson N, Smith RJ (eds): Methods and Concepts in Hand Surgery. London, Butterworths, p 270

The author describes the indications for and techniques of replantation that are used at the Massachusetts General Hospital. Some useful osteosynthesis techniques are also described.

Khuri SM (1986) Tension band arthrodesis in the hand. J Hand Surg 11A:41

The technique of tension band wiring for arthrodesis of small joints is described. A similar technique is used for fracture fixation.

Komatsu S, Tamai S (1968) Successful replantation of a completely cut-off thumb. Case report. Plast Reconstr Surg 42:374

This was the first report of a successful digital replant. The replanted thumb does not flex at the interphalangeal joint because the flexor tendon was not repaired. Repair of the digital nerve was postponed for fear of damaging the artery. The historic moment when circulation returned is recounted in this landmark article. (Even for today's most experienced replant surgeons, the moment when circulation returns is always accompanied by a sense of relief and accomplishment. Today, if possible, all structures are repaired at the initial replant procedure.)

Kutz JE, Hanel D, Scheker L, et al (1983) Upper extremity replantation. Orthop Clin North Am 14:873

The types of injuries encountered in replantation cases and indications for replantation are described. Cooling technique, the details and order of repair of various structures, and pitfalls (especially unrecognized blood loss) are discussed. Postoperative management is described, including some monitoring techniques.

Leung PC (1980) An analysis of complications in digital replantations. Hand 12:25

The etiology of and possible remedies for the complications of replantation are considered. Both of the early problems of vascular compromise – bleeding and infection – and the late problems of stiffness, deformity, and nonunion are discussed.

Malt RA, McKhan CF (1978) Replantation of severed arms. Clin Orthop 133:3

This is the classic and historic first case of limb replantation. The patient, a 12-year-old boy, arrived at the Massachusetts General Hospital 30 minutes after his right arm was severed below the elbow. An excellent long-term functional result was achieved, which is unusual for a replanted limb avulsed at this level, even for today. Young age and low ischemia time figure prominently in the decision to replant the entire upper limb.

May JW, Toth BA, Gardner M (1982) Digital replantation distal to the proximal interphalangeal joint. J Hand Surg 7:161

In this series of 24 replanted digits, the authors achieved a 96% survival rate and a mean active range of motion of the proximal interphalangeal joint of 95° with 11-mm two-point discrimination. Early return to school or work was possible. This group of patients who underwent replantation at this level was the first such series to be analyzed, and it is important to be familiar with this article when considering the indications for replantation.

Meyer VE (1985) Hand amputations proximal but close to the wrist joint. Prime candidates for reattachment (long-term functional results). J Hand Surg 10A:989

This retrospective analysis of 49 hand amputations demonstrates that a generally favorable outcome can be achieved with reattachment – 80% had excellent or good results.

Moneim MS, Chacon NE (1985) Salvage of replanted parts of the upper extremity. J Bone Joint Surg 67A:880

Fifteen replanted parts were reexplored to attempt salvage after vascular problems developed. Arterial occlusion was found in 11, while both arterial and venous occlusion occurred in four. Eight of ten vein grafts were successful. Thrombectomy was performed in six parts but was successful in only one.

Nakamura J, Kinoshita Y, Hama H, et al (1980) Successful replantation of four fingers by a single common digital artery anastomosis. J Microsurg 2:53

This article describes a case of four-finger replantation at the metacarpophalangeal joint level. All four digits survived, based on the third common palmar digital artery alone. Angiography showed transverse branches between the digital arteries on either side of the index, long, and ring fingers just proximal to the metacarpophalangeal joints. In replantations at this level (metacarpophalangeal), it may be possible to supply more than one digit through the repair of a single artery.

Nissenbaum M (1980) A surgical approach for replantation of complete digital amputations. J Hand Surg 5:58

An incision dorsal to the midaxial line allows dissection of the palmar and dorsal flaps in order to expose the digital arteries and veins. The details of exposure are described.

Nunley JA, Goldner RD, Urbaniak JR (1987) Skeletal fixation in digital replantation. Use of the "H" plate. Clin Orthop 214:66

Use of the AO H-plate is advocated for transverse fractures of the metacarpals and proximal phalanges.

Nunley JA, Koman LA, Urbaniak JR (1982) Major upper extremity replantation. Orthop Trans 6:512

Twelve complete and 27 incomplete amputations proximal to the wrist are reviewed.

Nunley JA, Spiegl PV, Goldner RD, et al (1987) Longitudinal epiphyseal growth after replantation and transplantation in children. J Hand Surg 12A:274

Epiphyseal growth continues after replantation and transplantation if the vascular supply is maintained. The average increase in length achieved during the follow-up period, which ranged from 27–81 months, was 92% of normal.

O'Brien BMcC, Macleod AM, Hayhurst JW, et al (1974) Major replantation surgery in the upper limb. Hand 6:217

Seven cases of replantation proximal to the wrist are described in detail. Three were later amputated, one for infection and two for extensive muscle and skin damage. Although the other four patients regained a functional extremity, the risks of such replantation must be kept in mind.

Phelps DB (1978) Should a torn-off little finger ever be replanted? Plast Reconstr Surg 61:592

Phelps comments on a previous article describing the replantation of a small finger that had been avulsively amputated at the metacarpophalangeal joint level. Function is unlikely to be good, but the technical possibility of replanting an avulsively amputated small finger can be extrapolated to the thumb or a multiple digit injury, in which case the indication would be different. Vein grafts should be used more or less routinely for such replantation.

Pho RWH, Chacha PB, Yeo KQ (1979) Rerouting vessels and nerves from other digits in replanting an avulsed and degloved thumb. Plast Reconstr Surg 64:330

The transfer of vessels from one digit to another is described as an alternative to vein grafting in replanting the avulsed thumb. Transfer of the dorsal digital nerves is also described.

Sekiguchi J, Ohmori K (1979) Youngest replantation with microsurgical anastomoses. Hand 11:64

Children tend to achieve excellent function following digital replantation. Replantation in children often depends on vessel size, which fortunately is often proportionally larger than expected if judging from the size of the child. Vascular spasm is often a problem, and the importance of adequate analgesia, antispasmodics, and a warm ambient temperature is emphasized. This article describes digital replantation in a 12-month-old patient.

Shafiroff BB, Palmer AK (1981) Simplified technique for replantation of the thumb. J Hand Surg 6:623

Anastomosing vein grafts to the digital vessels of an amputated thumb simplifies positioning of the hand for the vascular repairs.

Tamai S (1982) Twenty years' experience of limb replantation. Review of 293 upper extremity replants. J Hand Surg 7:549

The author discusses his extensive experience in replantation, and includes indications, levels of amputation, ischemia time, postoperative management, results, and many other factors that are important to the replant surgeon.

Tupper JW (1978) Techniques of bone fixation and clinical experience in replanted extremities. Clin Orthop 133:165

This article describes various methods of bone fixation as the first step in replantation. Vein grafting is preferred to bone shortening for direct vessel opposition. Clinical experiences with failed replants are discussed and recommendations to improve results are given.

Urbaniak JR, Evans JP, Bright DS (1981) Microvascular management of ring avulsion injuries. J Hand Surg 6:25

Ring avulsion injuries are classified and their management is described. The categories of injury are (1) *circulation adequate* – standard bone and soft-tissue treatment is adequate; (2) *circulation inadequate* – vascular reconstruction preserves viability (reasonable functional results were achieved); and (3) *complete degloving or amputation* – replantation is possible but the functional result is unpredictable. Good judgment is needed in deciding whether or not these kinds of amputations should be replanted. Results, sensation, and range of motion are reviewed.

Urbaniak JR, Hayes MG, Bright DS (1978) Management of bone in digital replantation. Free vascularized and composite bone grafts. Clin Orthop 133:184

The surgical technique of bone shortening; the management of joint injuries; and nerve, vessel, and tendon repair are described. A simple, longitudinal Kirschner wire is used for fixation. Today, more rigid fixation that does not involve the proximal or distal joints is preferred.

Urbaniak JR, Roth JH, Nunley JA, et al (1985) The results of replantation after amputation of a single finger. J Bone Joint Surg 67A:611

Fifty-nine patients who underwent single-finger replantation were reviewed; 86% of the digits survived. If the replantation was distal to the proximal interphalangeal joint, the average range of motion in that joint was 82°; if proximal to this joint, the average range of motion was 35°.

Vlaston C, Earle AS (1986) Avulsion injuries of the thumb. J Hand Surg 11A:51

Seven patients who had avulsion injuries of the thumb underwent replantation. Similarities among the injuries and the routine use of vein grafts are emphasized.

Weiland AJ, Villareal-Rios A, Kleinert HE, et al (1977) Replantation of digits and hands. Analysis of surgical techniques and results in 71 patients with 86 replantations. J Hand Surg 2:1

This article reviews 86 replants with regard to functional outcome. The patient population is described, and the location and type of injury are given. The surgical technique is detailed, and results over the 5-year period between 1970 and 1975 are reviewed. The discussion includes selection criteria and contraindications to replantation.

Yamano Y (1985) Replantation of the amputated distal part of the fingers. J Hand Surg 10A:211

The zones of replantation distal to the proximal interphalangeal joint, based on vascular anatomy, are described. Arteries in zone 1 (just proximal to the nail) were anastomosed, and venous egress was provided by "fishmouth drip vessels." Other authors have used leeches (Foucher G [1986] J Hand Surg 11A:456) or bleeding through the nail bed (Gordon et al. 1985) to accomplish venous egress. Experience with 87 digits is described.

Yoshimura M, Shimada T, Imura S, et al (1987) The venous skin graft method for repairing skin defects of the fingers. Plast Reconstr Surg 79:243

The technique and use of small flaps nourished by an underlying vein are described.

6 Regional Indications

6.1 Soft Tissue

The potential benefits of microvascular tissue transplantation are outlined in Sec. 2.1. Free tissue transplantation enables immediate elevation of the injured part, early mobilization in hand cases, and reconstruction in a single operation. As important as all of these factors is the advantage of being able to choose from a variety of different tissues. This allows the surgeon to tailor the surgical solution to the specific nature, site, and size of the clinical problem. A tissue that satisfies a number of requirements can be chosen. The various attributes to be found among the different tissues include variable size, vascularity, the ability to contour to the wound's dead space, sensation, limited mobility of the flap on the deeper tissues, and the ability to be combined with bone to form a composite transplant for the treatment of combined soft-tissue and bone defects. Once the decision to perform a microvascular transplant has been made, the choice of tissue must be carefully considered.

6.1.1 The Hand

6.1.1.1 Dorsum

If the tendons and paratenon are intact, split-thickness skin grafting generally suffices. If they are not intact, if bone is exposed or missing, or if later tendon reconstruction will be needed, a microvascular transplant may be the best solution. Thin, pliable skin with a mobile subcutaneous layer is needed to mimic the skin that naturally occurs in this region, and to allow subsequent tendon reconstruction. The *lateral arm flap* (Fig. 2-5) is ideal for this purpose. The *scapular flap* (Figs. 2-2 and 2-4) is more bulky but can be used for large defects that involve the forearm. The *dorsalis pedis flap* (Fig. 2-1) is of appropriate thickness, but the donor site is a problem and outweighs the primary advantage of this flap in providing sensation. Muscle or fascial flaps are not as pliable, and tendon reconstruction is more difficult under these flaps compared with cutaneous flaps. Two-stage tendon reconstruction is used routinely under muscle flaps.

If both the dorsum and palm need cover, separate slips of the *serratus anterior* can be applied to both sides of the hand (Fig. 1-5). Massive injuries may require a very large flap to drape over the hand, in which case the *latissimus dorsi* transplant can be used (Fig. 1-8). Occasionally, a composite transplant which consists of bone and soft tissue will be needed. The *composite dorsalis pedis transplant*, which includes the second metatarsal or metatarsophalangeal joint and tendons, can be used for a single metacarpal (Figs. 4-19 and 4-24). The *iliac crest osteocutaneous* transplant can be used for multiple metacarpal loss that occurs in conjunction with an extensive soft-tissue wound.

6.1.1.2 Palm

While cutaneous flaps are often too mobile to be ideal cover in the palm, the *serratus anterior muscle flap* is small and contours well (Figs. 1-4, 1-6, and 1-7). The split-thickness skin graft tends to be quite serviceable, and breakdown is unusual. Another option is the *lateral arm flap*, and for small defects, a narrow *dorsalis pedis flap* is useful (Fig. 2-1). Both the dorsalis pedis and lateral arm flaps provide sensation, which is an advantage when they are used in the palm. These flaps can be tailored to treat defects on adjacent fingers (Fig. 2-9). The *"retrograde" radial forearm flap*, also an option for the palm, is thin and can regain sensation (Fig. 2-7).

6.1.2 Upper Arm

The latissimus dorsi can be mobilized with or without a cutaneous component and be brought subcutaneously down the upper arm to cover most defects in the upper arm or elbow region. Dissection of the neurovascular pedicle and division of the muscle insertion allows more distant transfer of the muscle. If the latissimus dorsi and other local flaps are unavailable, microvascular transplantation may be necessary.

6.1.3 Forearm

Frequently, *groin or abdominal pedicle flaps* can be used in this region. If infection is present, a *microvascular muscle flap* may be preferable (Fig. 1-3). Major acute wounds may also be treated with a *microvascular cutaneous flap*, which allows elevation of the extremity and early hand therapy (Fig. 2-2). Because muscle flaps may break down if used across major flexion creases, a musculocutaneous transplant is often preferable, placing the cutaneous portion of the transplant across the flexion crease (Fig. 1-26).

6.1.4 Heel

Reconstruction of the heel remains an extremely difficult challenge. Subsequent breakdown, pain, and difficulties with ambulation are all evidence of the repeated pressure between the ground and the calcaneus. Following a devascularizing injury of the heel, it is difficult to ascertain how much tissue will become necrotic (Figs. 1-19 and 1-21). Because of the skin's thickness in this region, it takes 7–10 days before the amount of necrosis becomes evident.

Ideally, the tissue replacement should have limited *shear* on the deeper structures, some sensation, and be a good match in terms of size. Muscle tissue has little mobility early on, but it tends to become more mobile as it atrophies, and several debulking procedures are usually necessary. Still, muscle tissue or fascia is better than a purely cutaneous flap.

The *dorsalis pedis flap*, *lateral arm flap* (Figs. 2-3 and 2-6), *deltoid flap*, and *tensor fasciae latae transplant* (Fig. 1-21) all have the potential for *sensory return*. The choice among these flaps depends on the defect size (Fig. 1-1). The tensor fasciae latae flap must be oriented longitudinally along the sole. If placed transversely, it will be too bulky. If none of these flaps will be of appropriate size, the latissimus dorsi musculocutaneous transplant may be useful in some situations (Fig. 1-19).

6.1.5 Leg and Thigh

For a variety of clinical problems in the leg, microvascular transplants should be used when rotation flaps or other local procedures will be inadequate. One such problem is the major acute wound, which requires cover either immediately or within 1–2 weeks after surgery (Fig. 1-2). All necrotic or potentially infected tissue must be *meticulously debrided* before the wound is covered. In more chronic situations, metal plates or prostheses can be covered (Figs. 1-14 and 1-15) and osteomyelitis treated (Figs. 1-9 through 1-13, and 1-16).

Muscle tissue is preferred in the lower extremity, and in most situations, muscle covered with split-thickness skin graft provides the best contour. Muscle tissue is also effective in filling dead space (Figs. 1-14, 1-16, and 1-17), and the infection rate is extremely low. If bulk is needed because the defect is substantial, a musculocutaneous transplant may be advantageous.

6.1.6 Amputation Stumps

If possible, the knee or elbow joint should be salvaged to provide the best ultimate function and rehabilitation. Short below-elbow or below-knee amputation stumps with wounds require good soft-tissue cover if they are to be saved. *Musculocutaneous transplants* are generally best in such situations, providing good cover over the bone stump. The cutaneous island provides additional padding and durable cover. Debulking the flap is usually needed 6 to 9 months later to decrease the mobility of the transplant once the swelling has subsided and the transplant has atrophied somewhat. A tissue expander may be used to expand the cutaneous portion of the transplant or the surrounding skin to achieve cutaneous cover over the entire stump (Fig. 1-22).

6.2 Bone

The indications for vascularized bone transplantation and the choice of transplant are considered in Chapter 3.

When bone defects occur in conjunction with major soft-tissue defects, the staging of reconstruction is important. Simultaneous soft-tissue reconstruction and bone grafting (vascularized or nonvascularized) can be performed (Fig. 3-2) early after injury or in situations where infection has not been a problem. It is safer, especially in previously infected wounds, to first provide stable soft-tissue cover, usually by muscle transplantation (Figs. 3-3 through 3-5). Thereafter, once healing without evidence of infection has been achieved, various bone grafting options can be considered.

6.3 Composite Loss (Zhong-jia 1987)

In some situations, combinations of bone, soft tissue, and toe transplants can be used to reconstruct difficult problems. The vascular pedicle of one transplant is anastomosed to the second. In this way, a fibula transplant can be combined with overlying soft tissue, or a toe can be transferred along with a cutaneous transplant. However, such procedures require a large operating team and should be reserved for the surgeon experienced in microsurgery. In addition, if vascular problems develop and the transplant does not survive, the magnitude of the loss is greater, so the patient must fully understand this risk.

6.4 Selected Bibliography

Zhong-jia Y (1987) Combined transplantation of soft tissues. Plast Reconstr Surg 79:222

Double microvascular transplants which combine bone, soft-tissue, and toe transplants are described.

7
Recipient Site Preparation

In most circumstances, operating time can be minimized if two surgical teams work simultaneously. Two separate instrument setups are needed for transplantation to previously infected areas. Arteriograms are seldom necessary for the donor site, but they should usually be obtained for the region of the recipient site, especially if there has been previous trauma to the area. Arteriograms are not usually done in small children.

In both the leg and the forearm, it is imperative to know which vessels are supplying the foot and hand, respectively. A retrograde dorsalis pedis pulse can be diagnosed by applying pressure to occlude the posterior tibial artery while simultaneously palpating the dorsalis pedis artery. An Allen test in the hand is important. One may encounter a dominant radial artery or radial and ulnar arteries that supply separate regions (Figs. 2-1 and 1-26) (Sec. 2.9, Jones and O'Brien 1985).

The recipient vessels must be chosen and dissected with care if the need for long vein grafts is to be avoided. The most frequently used recipient vessels are listed in Table 7-1.

Table 7-1. Recipient vessels most frequently used in microvascular surgery.

Site	Recipient vessels
Hand	*Radial artery* on the dorsal aspect of the hand, just before it enters between the two heads of the first dorsal interosseous muscle (end-to-side or end-to-end) (Fig. 4-19) *Common digital vessels* (Fig. 4-11) *Palmar arch* (Fig. 2-1)
Forearm and elbow	*Radial artery* (Figs. 3-2 and 4-4) (*Ulnar artery* occasionally)
Upper arm	Branches of the *brachial artery* (microvascular soft-tissue transplants are unusual in this region)
Heel	*Posterior tibial artery* (Fig. 1-15)
Leg	*Anterior tibial artery* (found by following the small pedicles between the extensor hallucis longus and the extensor digitorum longus) (Figs. 1-9 and 1-12b) *Posterior tibial artery* (Fig. 1-10)
Posterior knee and distal thigh	In the presence of a good anterior tibial artery supplying the foot, the *posterior tibial artery* can be swung back and used in retrograde fashion (Fig. 1-16)
Posterior knee and distal thigh (*continued*)	*Branch of the popliteal artery* to the medial gastrocnemius *Other branches of the popliteal artery* around the knee *Femoral artery* in the region of the adductor hiatus
Anterior and lateral knee, and distal thigh	In the presence of a good posterior tibial artery supplying the foot, the anterior tibial artery can be dissected into the leg, divided, and swung back and used in retrograde fashion; it may be helpful to bring the artery deep to the tibialis anterior (Fig. 1-14)
Proximal thigh	*Lateral circumflex artery* (or the pedicle to the tensor fasciae latae) *Medial circumflex artery* (or the pedicle to the gracilis)
Hip region	*Inferior epigastric artery* (Fig. 1-17) *Lateral circumflex artery* (or the pedicle to the tensor fasciae latae) *Medial circumflex artery* (or the pedicle to the gracilis)
Spine	*Intercostal arteries* (Fig. 3-9)

If no other vessel is available, the same vessel can be used a second time for a second transplant. This strategy depends on the bed of the first transplant, which, if satisfactory, will provide adequate supply. I have used this approach on four occasions without problems, but careful judgment and caution must be exercised (Fig. 3-8). Clamping the pedicle and observing the vascularity in the transplant is wise, and other vessels should be used if available.

8 Monitoring

In few areas of surgery is failure as immediately apparent as in microvascular transplantation. Such failure represents an enormous loss to the patient. A tissue survival rate of over 95% is acceptable but cannot be achieved without a focused effort. Approximately 10–15% of transplants will need reoperation to salvage them after vascular problems arise, and these will make the difference between an acceptable and an unacceptable tissue survival rate.

Occasionally, a faulty arterial or venous repair must be redone, but this remedy is only feasible if the problem is detected very shortly after thrombosis. Far more frequently, a vein graft is required. This graft is either anastomosed to a different recipient artery or vein, or the same vessel is used more proximally, out of the zone of injury (Fig. 1-15). One of the most common causes of vascular failure results from the use of damaged vessels in this *zone of injury*. Vessels must be very carefully scrutinized under high magnification for any irregularities of the intimal lining; if these exist, the vessel must be used more proximally, even if it means having to use a vein graft.

Transplant salvage by *reoperation* is only effective if thrombosis is diagnosed *within hours* of its occurrence (Fig. 8-1). In most cases, an experienced observer can make the diagnosis of arterial or venous compromise through careful scrutiny of the transplant. However, this determination is difficult in some situations, such as if the patient is dark-skinned or very pale-skinned, or if the replanted part has been injured, macerated, or blistered. Also, an experienced observer may not always be available because of staffing or shift changes. These factors make a reliable monitor important.

The *ideal monitor* should be simple to use, continuous, quantitative, and noninvasive (Tables 8-1 and 8-2). In addition, direct monitoring of the capillary circulation in the tissue itself is preferable to monitoring the more proximal vessels. After all, it is *this* tissue that must survive for the transplant to be successful (Fig. 8-2f). Unfortunately, the ideal monitor for every transplant and every situation does not exist, but many different kinds of monitors are available. The following is my *approach* to monitoring transplants and replants.

If a skin surface is available, one of two kinds of monitors can be used. The *pulse oxymeter* (Fig. 8-2a) has all the necessary features outlined above, but it can only be used when the transmitter and receiver in the apparatus face each other. This requirement means that it can be used in toe transplants and replants of all types when it can be placed around the end of a finger (Fig. 8-2b). It cannot be used for a cutaneous transplant. The *dermal fluorimeter* (Fig. 8-2c) can be used on any skin surface, including digits or cutaneous transplants. An injection of fluorescein is administered

Table 8-1. Monitoring in microsurgery.

Type of transplant	monitor
Replant	Pulse oxymeter
Toe	Pulse oxymeter
Cutaneous	Fluorimeter
Muscle	Clinical observation; implanted temperature probe
Bone (buried)	Implanted temperature probe

Table 8-2. Comparison of the pulse oxymeter and dermal fluorimeter.

Pulse oxymeter	Dermal fluorimeter
Very simple	Simple
Reading is continuous	Read every 2 hours
Quantitative	Quantitative
Noninvasive	Requires an IV injection
Useful only on digits	Useful on all skin

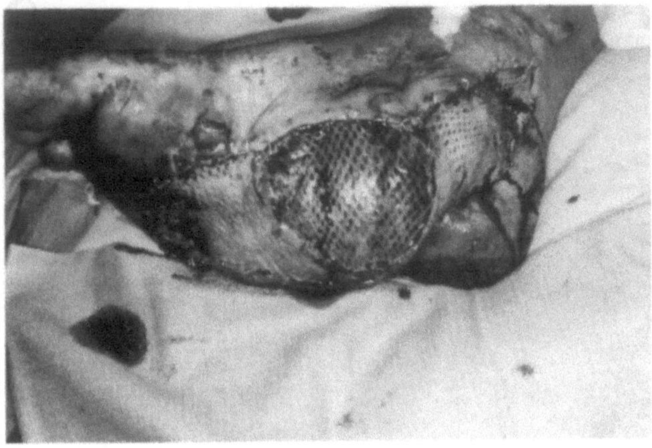
a

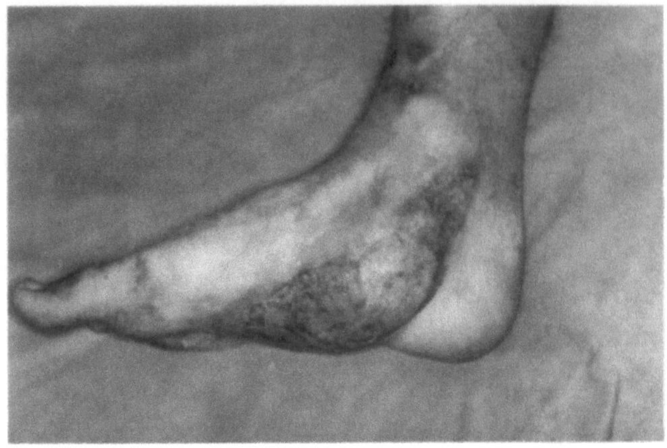
b

Fig. 8-1. a. A flap to the heel became congested about 2 hours after transplantation. A diagnosis of venous thrombosis was made, and a vein graft was used to reconstruct venous outflow within the hour. The arterial inflow remained brisk throughout. **b.** Salvage of this transplant was possible through reoperation, and a good result was ultimately achieved.

every 2 hours, which occasionally may produce mild nausea (Fig. 8-2d).

Neither of these monitors can be used on *muscle tissue*. *Venous congestion* in muscle is usually quite obvious because the blue discoloration and swelling are diagnostic. Quite frequently, the first sign of venous thrombosis will be *increased bleeding*, and the dressings become soaked. Such an event should always be taken as a very serious sign (Fig. 8-1).

Arterial thrombosis may be more difficult to diagnose. An empty, dry, and pale appearance of the muscle without adherence of the skin graft indicates this problem. A 25-gauge needle can be used to carefully prick the muscle tissue well away from the vessels and close to the distal end of the muscle. Even the tiniest drop of active, bright red bleeding can reassure the surgeon. Blue bleeding indicates a venous problem. If no bleeding can be demonstrated, reexploration is the safest procedure. When problems are suspected in a transplant, the dressing should be removed and the entire transplant exposed. Other techniques of monitoring muscle can be used but are not completely reliable. Implanted temperature probes are used most often (Fig. 8-2e).

Bone transplants without a cutaneous component can be followed by serial technetium scans to confirm vascularity. The results are not reliable or early enough to dictate surgical intervention. The implanted temperature probe is the only available method of reliably monitoring this kind of transplant (Fig. 8-2e). Some surgeons, however, prefer not to use an implanted device in a previously infected area, and these devices can also be cumbersome.

Even with the best monitors, a high success rate can only be achieved if vigilance is maintained by the surgeon, assistants, house staff, and nurses, and aggressive reexploration is initiated as soon as a problem is suspected.

---▷

Fig. 8-2. a. A *pulse oxymeter* was used to monitor this toe transplant. The pulse oxymeter measures hemoglobin saturation. It is simple to use, gives a continuous and quantitative readout, and is entirely noninvasive. Its only drawback is that it can only be used in digits because the transmitting and receiving probes in the monitor must face each other. It is useful for monitoring both replants and toe transplants. We are investigating probes that will function on flat surfaces such as skin and muscle. **b.** The pulse oxymeter will read between 96% and 100% if vascularity is adequate. With arterial compromise, the hemoglobin saturation will drop to 60% within a 5- to 10-minute period. If venous compromise occurs, the hemoglobin saturation will drop to approximately 85% within an hour of this complication. **c.** The *dermal fluorimeter* is relatively simple to use and the measurement cycle is repeated every 2 hours. The apparatus gives a quantitative readout and can be used on any transplant or replant that has skin. It requires an intravenous injection of fluorescein, which occasionally causes nausea. **d.** In using the fluorimeter to monitor a skin surface, a baseline reading is taken, after which a 1-cc intravenous injection of fluorescein (the amount used for an average-size adult) is administered. A second reading is taken 10 minutes later. With adequate arterial inflow, a marked rise in the fluorescein measurement of at least 30–50% will occur. A third reading is taken 1 hour after the injection; if adequate venous outflow is present, this reading will show a substantial drop from the 10-minute peak level. At 2 hours, the level will drop to a point near the original measurement. The cycle is then repeated. With *arterial compromise*, the initial rise following intravenous injection will not occur. With *venous compromise*, the drop after the 10-minute peak will be absent and the fluorescein readings will continue to rise. The fluorimeter is less reliable when used to monitor muscle tissue because the drop in fluorescein level may be much slower. **e.** Implanted temperature probes are placed on either side of the vascular anastomosis and sutured into position with a 9-0 or 10-0 nylon suture. The difference in temperature across the anastomosis is measured. With thrombosis of the anastomosis, the temperature distal to the anastomosis will drop. **f.** Monitoring may be directed at three levels of the circulation: (1) *Arteries and veins* – the arterial anastomosis

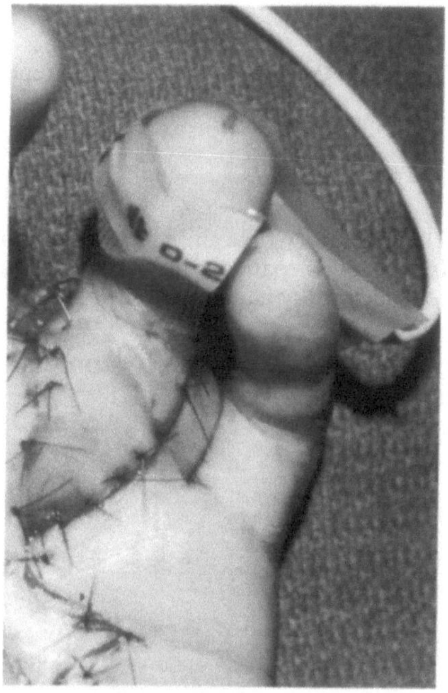
a

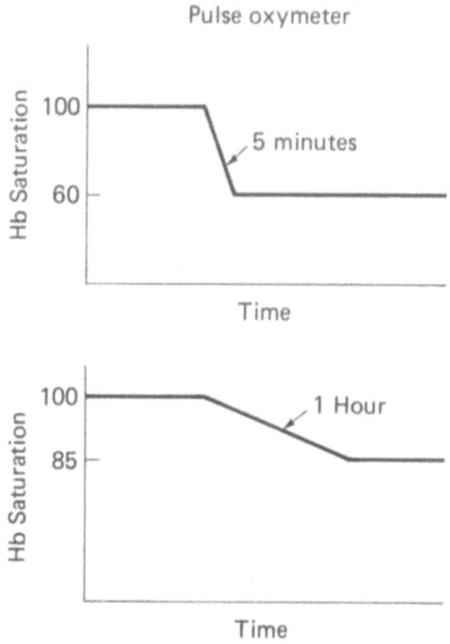

b

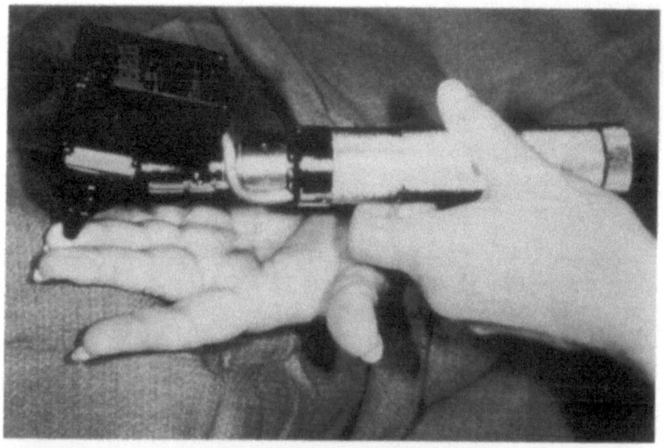

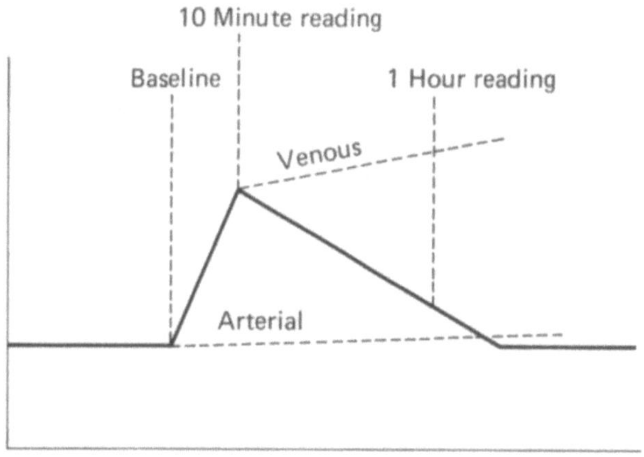

d

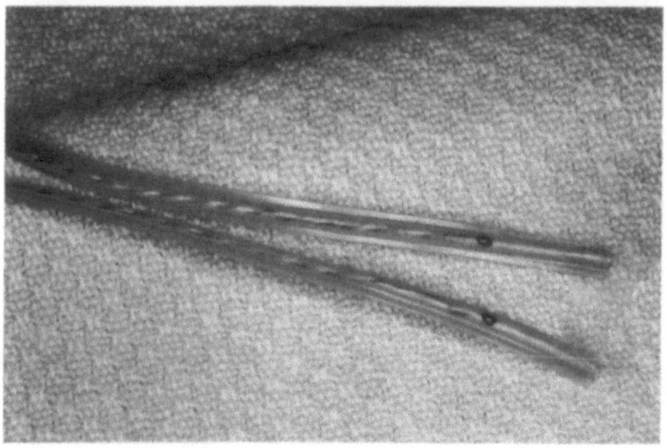
e

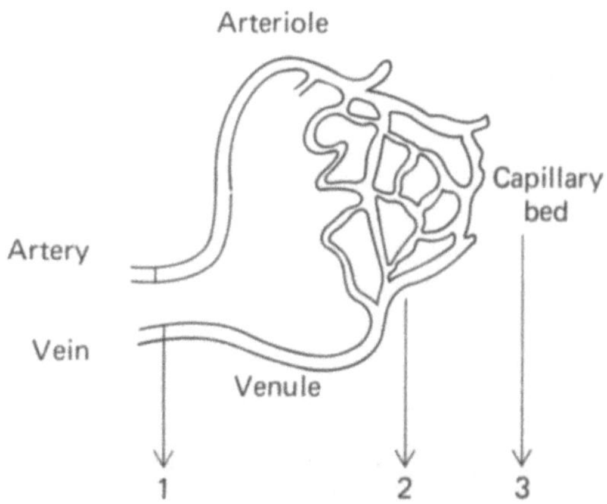

f

may be monitored directly with implanted temperature probes or Doppler monitors. (2) *Capillaries* – because this is the region where gas exchange occurs, the ideal monitor will measure the circulation at this level. Both the pulse oxymeter and dermal fluorimeter do exactly that. Even with patent anastomoses, circulation under certain conditions will not reach the capillary bed. This failure occurs with kinking of vessels, with other disturbances that cause pressure on the vessels distal to the anastomosis, or following lengthy ischemia of the transplant, where no recirculation and oxygen exchange occur distally. (3) *Surface* – indirect methods of measuring circulation include the surface temperature probe.

Selected Bibliography

Graham BH, Gordon L, Alpert BS, et al (1985) Serial quantitative skin surface fluorescence. A new method for postoperative monitoring of vascular perfusion in revascularized digits. J Hand Surg 10A:226

The use of the dermal fluorimeter in replantation is described.

May JW, Lukash FN, Gallico GG, et al (1983) Removable thermocouple probe microvascular patency monitor. An experimental and clinical study. Plastic Reconstr Surg 72:366

The laboratory data on and clinical application of this method are described. In two of 18 patients in whom the technique was used, venous thrombosis coincided with an abnormal reading.

Severinghaus JW (1986) Pulse Oxymetry. New York, Springer-Verlag

Index

Abdominal pedicle flaps, indications for, 174
Acetabular reconstruction, bone transplantation in, 79
Amputations
above-elbow, 149, 150
below-elbow, 145, 148
care of parts in, 151
in hand, replantation of. *See* Replantation
lower-extremity, 149, 150
multiple-level, 149
stump coverage in, 19, 21, 174
at wrist, 145, 147, 148
Arm flap, lateral, 51–52, 54, 56
anatomy of, 58
compared with scapular flap, 52
in hand wounds, 3
indications for, 173
surgical technique, 59–60
Arterial system of hand, assessment of, 24, 57, 65, 101, 177
Avulsive digital injuries, replantation in, 144–145, 146–147, 163
surgical technique of, 167–168

Bone transplantation, vascularized, 69–92
in acetabular or proximal femur reconstruction, 79
in avascular necrosis of hip, 79
choice of bone in, 79
in congenital disorders, 69, 70–71
fibula in, 74, 75, 79, 82–87
historical aspects of, 69
iliac crest in, 72, 78, 79, 88–91
indications for, 69–79, 174
monitoring of, 180
postoperative care in, 92
skin with. *See* Osteocutaneous transplants
in spine defects, 79, 80
in traumatic defects, 69–78
extensive, 69, 71–77
short, 69, 78
in tumor resection defects, 78–79
Brachial artery, 58
as recipient vessel, 177

Composite tissue transplants, 55, 115–116. *See also* Musculocutaneous transplants; Osteocutaneous transplants
indications for, 174
Congenital defects
bone transplantation in, 69, 70–71
toe-to-hand transfers in, 96–97, 107, 113
Contour defects, muscle transplants in, 11, 16
Cutaneous nerve
femoral, lateral, 42
of forearm, 58, 65
Cutaneous transplantation, 49–58
bone with. *See* Osteocutaneous transplants
choice of, 51–57
deltoid, 57
indications for, 174
dorsalis pedis, 50, 52, 55, 56, 57. *See also* Dorsalis pedis flap
for flexion creases, 49
groin flap, 49, 57
indications for, 174
in hand, for dorsum coverage, 5, 49, 53, 54
historical aspects of, 49
indications for, 49, 173–174
in large defects, 49, 51, 52
lateral arm flap, 51–52, 54, 56. *See also* Arm flap, lateral
monitoring of, 179
muscle with. *See* Musculocutaneous transplants
postoperative care in, 66
radial forearm flap, 50, 55, 57. *See also* Radial forearm flap
in replantations, 157–158
scapular flap, 51–52, 53, 56. *See also* Scapular flap
sensation restoration in, 49, 50, 54, 55
in toe transplantation, 129
split-thickness
covering muscle transplants, 3, 26, 74
foot closure with, 65
temporary, 5
temporoparietal fascial flap, 57
in toe-to-hand transfers, 101

Dead space filling, muscle transplants in, 11, 15
Debridement procedures, 5, 9, 153
Deltoid flap, 57
indications for, 174
Digital artery, 139
Digital vessels, common, as recipient vessels, 108, 177
Donor sites
in fibular transplant, 79, 81
in muscle transplants, 25, 26, 45
in toe-to-hand transfers, 98–100
in wrap-around procedure, 99, 126
Dorsalis pedis artery, 55, 117
Dorsalis pedis flap, 50, 52, 55, 56, 57
anatomy of, 63
in composite tissue transplant, 55, 116
foot closure in, 65
indications for, 173, 174
surgical technique, 63–64

Elbow
above-elbow amputations, 149, 150
below-elbow amputations, 145, 148
latissimus dorsi transplant in wounds of, 22, 24
Elderly patients, microvascular procedures in, 19, 52
Epigastric artery, inferior, 88
as recipient vessel, 16, 177

Fascia lata. *See* Tensor fasciae latae musculocutaneous transplants
Fascial flap, temporoparietal, 57
Femoral artery as recipient vessel, 177
Femoral cutaneous nerve, lateral, 42
Femoral reconstruction, proximal, bone transplantation in, 79
Fibula transplant, 74, 75, 79, 82–87
  anatomy of, 82–83
  compared with, iliac crest, 79
  donor site in, 79, 81
  surgical technique, 84–87
Fingers. *See* Hand
Flap. *See* Transplant
Flexion creases, coverage of
  cutaneous transplants in, 49
  musculocutaneous transplants in, 24, 26
Fluorimeter, dermal, 20, 159–160, 179–180
  compared with pulse oxymeter, 179
Foot
  amputations of, 149–150
  closure of
    grafts in, 65
    in toe-to-hand transfers, 124, 128
  toe-to-hand transfers. *See* Toe-to-hand transfers
Forearm
  amputations in, and replantation, 145, 148
  radial forearm flap. *See* Radial forearm flap
  reconstruction with soft tissue, 174
Free flap. *See* Transplant

Gracilis muscle transplantation, 1, 26–30
  anatomy in, 26–28
  donor site in, 25, 26
  as functional muscle, 23
  in osteomyelitis, 8, 9
  pedicle of, 26
  in plate coverage, 14
  size and shape of, 1
  surgical technique, 28–30
  vessel dimensions in, 24
Gracilis musculocutaneous transplant, in heel wounds, 19
Groin flaps, 49, 57
  indications for, 174

Hand
  amputated, banking in axilla, 5
  cutaneous transplants for dorsum of, 5, 49, 53, 54
  functional muscle transplants in, 22, 105
  lateral arm flap for, 3
  replantations in. *See* Replantation
  scapular flap for, 3
  separate radial and ulnar arterial supplies to, 24, 57, 65, 101, 177
  serratus anterior muscle transplant to, 3, 4, 5, 6
  soft tissue coverage of, 173
  toe transplantation to, 95–134. *See also* Toe-to-hand transfer
  transposition of digits in, 145, 152, 153, 164–165
Heel reconstruction, 174
  muscle transplants in, 12, 17, 18, 19, 20
Hip, avascular necrosis of, bone transplants in, 79

Iliac arteries, 88
Iliac crest transplants, 72, 78, 79, 88–91
  anatomy of, 88–89
  compared with fibula transplant, 79
Iliac vein, deep circumflex, 90
Ilium, 88
Infected wounds, muscle transplants in, 9, 10, 11, 12, 74, 76
Inguinal canal, 88
Inguinal ligament, 88
Intercostal arteries as recipient vessels, 80, 177

Latissimus dorsi muscle transplants, 1, 30, 36–39
  anatomy in, 30
  in contour defects, 16
  donor site in, 25, 26
  as functional muscle, 23
  indications for, 173
  in infected wounds, 12
  in lower-extremity trauma, 2
  serratus anterior with
    in dead space filling, 15
    in hand, 7
    surgical technique, 40–41
  size and shape of, 1
  surgical technique, 36–39
  in upper-extremity trauma, 2
  vessel dimensions in, 24
Latissimus dorsi musculocutaneous transplants
  in amputation stumps, 21
  in elbow wounds, 24
  in heel wounds, 17, 18
  in osteomyelitis, 10
  in radiation injury, 13
  surgical technique, 39–40
Leg and thigh reconstruction, soft tissue for, 174

Metatarsal artery, first dorsal, 117
Metatarsal ligament, transverse, 117
Monitoring procedures, 179–181
  dermal fluorimeter in, 20, 159–160, 179–180
  implanted temperature probes in, 180, 181
  pulse oxymeter in, 159, 179, 181
  signs of thrombosis in, 180
Muscle transplantation, 1–48
  in amputation stumps, 19, 21
  atrophy of, 26
  choice of, 24–26
  in complex wounds, 19
  in contour defects, 11, 16
  in dead space coverage, 11, 15
  donor site in, 25, 26, 45
  functional, 22–23
    in lower extremity, 23
    in upper extremity, 22, 105
  gracilis muscle in, 26–30. *See also* Gracilis muscle transplantation
  in heel wounds, 12, 17, 18, 19, 20
  in high-risk patients, 19, 22
  historical aspects of, 1
  indications for, 1–24, 173–174
  in infected wounds, 9, 10, 11, 12, 74, 76
  latissimus dorsi in, 1, 30, 36–39. *See also* Latissimus dorsi muscle transplants
  monitoring of, 180
  in osteomyelitis, 8, 9, 10
  pedicles of, 24
  postoperative care in, 46
  in prosthesis or plate coverage, 11, 14
  in radiation injury, 9, 13
  serratus anterior muscle in, 1, 30–36. *See also* Serratus anterior muscle transplant
  size and shape of, 1, 25–26
  split-thickness skin graft with, 3, 26, 74
  in traumatic wounds, 2, 3–9
    lower extremity, 2, 3, 75
    timing of, 5
    upper extremity, 2, 3
  vessel dimensions in, 24
Musculocutaneous transplants, 24, 26
  for flexion creases, 24, 26
  in heel wounds, 19
  indications for, 174
  latissimus dorsi, 39–40. *See also* Latissimus dorsi musculocutaneous transplants
  tensor fasciae latae, 1, 42–45. *See also* Tensor fasciae latae musculocutaneous transplants

Nerve repair in replantations, 156–157
Nutrient artery of fibula, 82

Obesity, muscle transplants in, 19
Obturator nerve, 26
Osteocutaneous transplants, 72, 79
  dorsalis pedis, 173
  iliac crest, 173
Osteomyelitis, muscle transplants in, 8, 9, 10

Osteosynthesis
in replantations, 153–154, 155
in toe-to-hand transfers, 101
Oxymeter, pulse, 159, 181
compared with dermal fluorimeter, 179

Palmar arch as recipient vessel, 50, 177
Pectoralis major transplant as functional muscle, 23
Peroneal artery, 82
Peroneal nerves, 117
Plantar artery, deep, 117
Plantar ligament, 117
Plantar nerve, medial, 117
Plate coverage, muscle transplants in, 11, 14
Pollicization. *See* Toe-to-hand transfer, in thumb reconstruction
Popliteal artery as recipient vessel, 177
Pulse oxymeter, 159, 181
compared with dermal fluorimeter, 179

Radial artery
lack of communication with ulnar artery, 24, 57, 65, 101, 177
as recipient vessel, 72, 102, 115, 177
Radial collateral arteries, 58
Radial forearm flap, 50, 55, 57
anatomy of, 65
indications for, 173
surgical technique, 65–66
Radiation injury, muscle transplants in, 9, 13
Recipient site preparation, 177–178
in toe-to-hand transfer, 97–98, 124, 177–178
Rehabilitation after replantations, 160–161
Reoperations
reuse of blood vessels in, 78, 178
vein grafts in, 14, 179, 180
Replantations, 139–168
anesthesia in, 151
antibiotics in, 151
anticoagulation in, 152
arterial repair in, 154, 156
in avulsive injuries, 144–145, 146–147, 163
surgical technique in, 167–168
care of amputated parts in, 151
contraindications to, 149–150
debridement in, 153
dressings in, 158
emergency department care in, 150–151
fasciotomy in, 158, 159
at forearm, 145, 148
indications for, 139–149
ischemia time in, 145, 151
late reconstruction in, 161–162
monitoring of, 159–160, 179
dermal fluorimeter in, 159–160
pulse oxymeter in, 159, 181
multiple-finger, 141, 142
surgical technique in, 164–166
nerve repairs in, 156–157
osteosynthesis in, 153–154, 155
planning of, 152–153
postoperative care in, 158–161
reexploration of, 160
rehabilitation in, 160–161
Scribner shunts in, 145, 148, 151, 152
single-finger, 139–141
between proximal and distal joints, 140–141
distal phalanx, 139–140
proximal, 141, 150
skin grafts in, 157–158
surgical technique in, 151–158, 163–168
tagging of structures in, 142, 152, 153
tendon repair in, 140, 154
thumb, 141, 142–144
in crush or avulsion injuries, 144
surgical technique in, 163–164
transmetacarpal, 145
and transposition of digits, 145, 152, 153, 164–165
vein grafts in, 144, 153, 163, 167
harvesting of, 168
venous drainage in, 140
nail bed removal for, 156, 159
venous repairs in, 157
at wrist, 145, 147–148

Scapular arteries, 60
Scapular flap, 51–52, 53, 56
anatomy of, 60–61
compared with lateral arm flap, 52
in hand wounds, 3
indications for, 173
surgical technique, 61–63
Scribner shunts in replantations, 145, 148, 151, 152
Second transplants, reuse of vessels in, 78, 178
Sensation restoration
in cutaneous transplants, 49, 50, 54, 55
in toe transplantation, 96, 129
Serratus anterior muscle transplant, 1, 30–36
anatomy of, 30
donor site in, 25, 26
as functional muscle, 23, 105
in hand, 3, 4, 5, 6
indications for, 173
in infected wounds, 11
latissimus dorsi with
in dead space filling, 15
in hand, 7
surgical technique, 40–41
size and shape of, 1
surgical technique, 34–36
vessel dimensions in, 24
Sickle cell disease, muscle transplants in, 16, 19
Skin grafts. *See* Cutaneous transplantation
Spine defects, bone transplants in, 79, 80
Subscapular artery, 60

Tagging of structures, in replantations, 142, 152, 153
Temperature probes, implanted, 180, 181
Temporoparietal fascial flap, 57
Tendon repair
in replantation, 140, 154
silastic rods in, for hand, 5
Tensor fasciae latae musculocutaneous transplants, 1, 42–45
anatomy of, 42
donor site in, 25, 26
in heel wounds, 20
indications for, 174
surgical technique, 44–45
vessel dimensions in, 24
Thoracic nerve, long, 30
Thoracodorsal artery, 30
Thoracodorsal nerve, 30
Thrombosis
arterial, 180
venous, 180
Thumb
reconstruction of. *See* Toe-to-hand transfer, in thumb reconstruction
replantation of, 141, 142–144
surgical technique, 163–164
Tibial arteries, 117
as recipient vessels, 8, 9, 11, 13, 14, 15, 177
Toe-to-hand transfer, 95–134
in adactyly, 98
anatomy in, 117–119
arterial system of hand and foot in, 101
choice of toes in, 97–99
clay model of, 101, 105, 113
and comparison of metacarpophalangeal and metatarsophalangeal joints, 95, 96
in congenital defects, 96–97, 107, 113
donor site in, 98–100
in wrap-around procedure, 99, 126
finger reconstruction in, 98, 108–109, 110, 111, 113
thumb with, 98, 112, 114
foot closure in, 124, 128
great toe as the donor in, 98–99, 100
in thumb reconstruction, 97
transplantation technique, 120–124
wrap-around procedure for, 96, 97, 104, 124–126
historical aspects of, 95–96
indications for, 96–97
interphalangeal joint in, 96, 133
metatarsophalangeal joint in, 96, 115–116, 131–132
monitoring of, 179
osteosynthesis in, 101
parts of toes in, with sensate skin, 96, 129–130

postoperative care in, 134
preoperative planning in, 101
recipient site considerations in, 97–98, 124, 177–178
second toe as the donor in, 99, 100
in thumb reconstruction, 97
transplantation technique, 126–128
skin flaps in, 101
surgical technique, 120–133
in thumb reconstruction, 97–98, 103, 104, 105–107
fingers with, 98, 112, 114
great toe in, 97
hand preparation in, 124
second toe in, 97
wrap-around technique in, 96, 97, 104, 124–126
in trauma, 96
in tumor resection defect, 96
venous system of hand and foot in, 101
web spaces in, 96, 101
wrap-around technique in, 96, 97, 104, 124–126
donor site in, 99, 126
Transplant. *See* Arm flap, lateral; Bone transplantation, vascularized–fibula in, iliac crest in; Composite tissue transplants; Cutaneous transplantation–deltoid, dorsalis pedis, groin flap, lateral arm flap, radial forearm flap, scapular flap, temporoparietal fascial flap; Gracilis muscle transplantation; Latissimus dorsi muscle transplants; Latissimus dorsi musculocutaneous transplants; Musculocutaneous transplants; Pectoralis major transplant as functional muscle; Serratus anterior muscle transplant; Tensor fasciae latae musculocutaneous transplants; Toe-to-hand transfer; Wrap-around procedure in toe-to-hand transfer
Transposition of digits, 145, 152, 153, 164–165
Trauma
bone transplants in, 69–78
muscle transplants in, 2, 3–9
toe-to-hand transfer in, 96
Tumor resection defects
bone transplants in, 78–79
toe-to-hand transfer in, 96
Ulnar artery, lack of communication with radial artery, 24, 57, 65, 101, 177

Vein grafts
in reoperations, 14, 179, 180
in replantation of digits, 144, 153, 163, 167
harvesting of, 168
Venous drainage in replantations, 140
nail bed removal for, 156, 159
Venous repairs in replantations, 157
Venous system of hand and foot, assessment of, 101

Web spaces in toe-to-hand transfers, 96, 101
Wrap-around procedure in toe-to-hand transfer, 96, 97, 104, 124–126
donor site in, 99, 126
Wrist amputations, and replantation, 145, 147–148

MIX
Papier aus verantwortungsvollen Quellen
Paper from responsible sources
FSC® C105338

If you have any concerns about our products,
you can contact us on
ProductSafety@springernature.com

In case Publisher is established outside the EU,
the EU authorized representative is:
Springer Nature Customer Service Center GmbH
Europaplatz 3, 69115 Heidelberg, Germany

Printed by Libri Plureos GmbH
in Hamburg, Germany